ETHICAL DIMENSIONS
in the Health Professions

ETHICAL DIMENSIONS
in the Health Professions

Seventh Edition

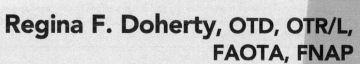

Regina F. Doherty, OTD, OTR/L, FAOTA, FNAP
Professor and Director
Department of Occupational Therapy
School of Health and Rehabilitation Sciences
MGH Institute of Health Professions
Boston, Massachusetts

Foreword by

Ruth B. Purtilo, PhD, FAPTA
Professor Emerita
Creighton University, Omaha, Nebraska and
MGH Institute of Health Professions,
Boston, Massachusetts

ELSEVIER

Elsevier
3251 Riverport Lane
St. Louis, Missouri 63043

ETHICAL DIMENSIONS IN THE HEALTH PROFESSIONS,   ISBN: 978-0-323-67364-8
SEVENTH EDITION

Library of Congress Cataloging Number : 2020944565

Senior Content Strategist: Lauren Willis
Director, Content Development: Ellen Wurm-Cutter
Senior Content Development Specialist: Kathleen Nahm
Publishing Services Manager: Shereen Jameel
Project Managers: Radhika Sivalingam/Umarani Natarajan
Senior Book Designer: Bridget Hotette

Printed in the United States of America

Last digit is the print number: 9 8 7 6 5 4 3 2 1

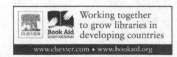

Working together
to grow libraries in
developing countries

www.elsevier.com • www.bookaid.org

With gratitude to
the patients, families, professional colleagues, and students
whose experiences have taught me
volumes about the value and meaning of care.

Foreword

Since you are pausing here at the Foreword before pursuing the next leg of your journey into this textbook, I am happy to be among the first to welcome you to your initial or deeper study of professional ethics. This is the seventh edition of *Ethical Dimensions* and I, as the author of the first and subsequent editions up until this current one, have been afforded the privilege of being at the head of the receiving line! You are joining 40 years of readers who have since gone on to professional careers in all areas of the health professions across a wide variety of settings. I take delight in introducing you to this current edition in which my revered colleague Regina Doherty has assumed sole and primary authorship. Understandably, since the release of the first edition in 1981, the content has evolved steadily to ensure it remains a living document for you and your generation. It is similar to any living entity, including ourselves, that must not lose hold of the core foundations that ground our identity and guide our growth while adapting to current situations to stay truly alive to ourselves and fit for the purposes that help us stay relevant to others. Looking back, each edition reflected an increased understanding of professional ethics as an integral aspect of professional identity. The contents of each also has benefited from a growing number of ethics colleagues whose ideas, research, and insights have enriched our overall understanding of key developments. This edition follows that pattern, bringing in several significant examples of the exciting environment awaiting you in your professional career and affirming again how essential ethical reasoning and discernment is for staying abreast of emerging as well as long-standing challenges and opportunities.

You may wonder what you should bring along on this journey. Bring who you are as a person—your personality, major influences on whom you have become, your hopes, dreams and fears. Bring your curiosity and the motivations that have brought you to your decision to become a health professional. Bring your beliefs about how to lead a good life, how you should treat others, and what you expect from them in return. In your study of ethical dimensions in the health professions, the two terms *profession* and *ethics* are the signposts guiding you along the path of preparing for a fulfilling career: A profession signifies a societal group whose members have taken on an age-old, role-related societal identity in addition to a personal one. Professionals are seen and judged as persons, but they also voluntarily have promised society to competently use specialized skills for the benefit of its individuals and groups. Professionals promise to abide by specific standards and guidelines that help individuals and societies stay on the path of protecting and promoting cherished human values. Ethics denotes the essence of what this societal identity requires of professionals in terms of their attitudes, moral character traits, duties, conduct, and constraints in the service of honoring these values.

Professional ethics has been shaped by philosophers such as Aristotle and Hippocrates; prophets and leaders of the world's greatest religions; naturalists; novelists; feminist and racial activists; forward-thinking leaders in the health professions; and behavioral, biological, and social scientists, to name a few. This is the rich environment in which we authors go about our project of providing a written map for you, updating it with each subsequent edition.

In the expanding market of teaching materials in ethics and related areas, the publishers of *Ethical Dimensions* have continued to publish new editions of this book. They rely on data of consistently substantial numbers of copies sold, years of repeat adoptions by instructors, and an ever-widening breadth of programs finding it useful, as well as its high ranking by formal review bodies designed to evaluate the quality of such teaching materials. As authors naturally we welcome this kind of positive feedback for our efforts and the opportunity to continue. Yet, Christine Cassel (coauthor of the first edition), Regina Doherty (coauthor of editions 5 and 6), and I have remained primarily motivated by other criteria. One criterion is our observation that a significant number of readers who first encountered *Ethical Dimensions* have chosen to keep it around throughout their professional career. For instance, it makes my day when I meet professionals at meetings and elsewhere who produce their dog-eared volume or, in more recent years, show me that when they upgraded their computer, they brought this book along. I will not be surprised if Regina Doherty or I find you doing the same.

As any author is likely to do, Dr. Doherty and I have reflected on why this book has such staying power. When we pose this question to users, two major lines of reasoning come up time and again. I'll share each in turn because they get to the more elemental issues that motivate us to present you with this new edition.

The first is that the material proves to be a *reliable lifelong reference*. This is not a big surprise to us. The basic utility of *Ethical Dimensions* is that it is a vehicle to provide evidence of why ethics really matters. No aspect of professional formation rests on a deeper, more enduring foundation than professional ethics, and you will find that this point is aptly elucidated in Regina Doherty's first chapters. From the authors' combined personal experiences as clinicians, educators, administrators, and researchers in the health professions we can confidently declare that professional ethics does not embody airy fairy unattainable ideals. We nudge learners like you toward understanding that ethics content and skill acquisition are basic orienting points on a compass designed to guide health professionals through everyday decisions. This compass is set to unfailingly point professionals in the direction of basic human values, anchoring humans in the effort to survive and thrive. Its sweet spot is experienced as integrity between personal and professional dimensions of one's existence in which self-interest and the interests of others intersect. Learners who go on to assume leadership positions across the spectrum of professional roles remind us that professional ethics remains relevant by providing toeholds for solid moral footing while individual, institutional, and societal situations evolve. This is crucial because the professions themselves are among the keepers of the keys of some basic values needed for individuals, societies, and our planet to survive and thrive.

Initially I was more surprised by a second area of our readers' judgment, namely that this book remains on their short list of keepers as a trustworthy *source of reassurance.* Of course! On reflection I am reminded of the prescient physician-author Atul Gawande's study of how to decrease errors in complex problem-solving situations that carry high stakes. He took three high-stakes situations: the operating room, pilots on overseas flights, and the kitchens of 5-star restaurants. The one constant that brought about a significant decrease in errors was a checklist. The health professional's role inherently is a high-risk situation with basic human well-being placed in our hands. And we authors have yet to meet a health professional who is so self-assured that they can sail through their career without facing professional encounters that are deeply disquieting. All of us seek reassurance at such moments. The discomfort may take the relatively benign form of a vague shadow of doubt that threatens to spoil an otherwise perfect afternoon. Other times it swoops in to shake one to the core as it settles, vulture-like, on the branches of one's day. The discomfort may arise from uncertainty regarding the best practice in a course of treatment and evaluation or their analogies in other professional roles. This warning sign warrants attention. Disquieting professional ethics encounters may take similar shapes. At the same time, ethics challenges tend to sink to the base of the trunk—the very foundations—of professional identity, posing a threat to the health professions' deep roots of meaning and values. A high-alert signal sounds that the health professional's action may compromise the very well-being of the involved parties, most importantly, the patient and family who hold the rightful place at the center of care. When this alert sounds, moral courage and resilience are required.

One advantage of the professional era you are entering is that interprofessional care teams increasingly are the norm for addressing complex treatment, policy, and administrative decisions in the health professions.

Throughout this book the forms these institutional and societal resources take are brought to your attention. It is marvelously reassuring to learn that you are not alone, and, in fact, some may be sharing–or successfully have found a resolution–to your quandary. Together you can create a checklist that is more likely to be inclusive of what is at stake than you can achieve alone. The discovery that yours is not a unique, unresolvable situation gives rise to hope–the hope that tragic error will be avoided. The light will break through with all interested parties moving forward together.

But there is a distinct kind of disturbance involving ethical challenges. Ethicists have several terms for it, summed up in the phrase *moral distress*. Sometimes a clear singular path forward does not emerge because of the sheer complexity of authentic human encounters involving cherished values. The good news is that there also are resources for this type of situation. I remember a colleague saying that integrity is a human condition with claws–claws that cling for dear life to our basic resolves, its function to help us be who we promised to be, and do what we ought to do. It does not stretch my imagination too much to think of the current edition of this book as a "member" of the healthcare team adding its large body of data and support to the human members. It provides its own type of reassurance that personal and professional integrity can be protected.

In conclusion, I thank our readers who claimed that *Ethical Dimensions* is a lifelong reference tool and a trusted source of reassurance throughout one's career. Each response has helped me to reflect on it and joyfully arrive at the same conclusion. It *is* a type of checklist. It includes the steadfast grounding of basic concepts continuously chiseled and refined from the earliest days of the professions, down to earth methods that allow complex situations to be viewed and analyzed as separate but related aspects of the whole, and criteria for what constitutes a "good outcome." It shares illustrations highlighting the stunningly beautiful diversity of the human condition and how we humans cling to a shared basic hope to survive and thrive. The authors' desires to engage *with* reader-learners and not just lecture *to* them prompted such features as questions for thought and discussion, text inserts encouraging reflection, and exercises for individual and group learning. If this relatively slender volume provides reassurance each step of the way that being a health professional is a high calling demanding much but offering a lifeline of deep satisfaction and fulfillment, we would have succeeded in meeting our own highest hopes for you! Happy trekking!

Ruth B. Purtilo, PhD, FAPTA
Professor Emerita
Creighton University, Omaha, Nebraska and
MGH Institute of Health Professions, Boston, Massachusetts

What's New in This Edition

The seventh edition of *Ethical Dimensions in the Health Professions* reflects the growing body of evidence that knowledge and skills in ethics supports compassionate care delivery and professional well-being. This text gives readers the basic tools to efficiently recognize ethical issues, build understanding, and competently work toward the resolution of complex problems. Readers of previous editions will notice signature features carried through and updated in this edition, among them a caring response as the overarching goal of professional practice, major prototypes of ethical problems, the six-step process of ethical decision making, narrative accounts to illustrate relevant ethics themes in everyday practice, built-in reflection exercises, summary statements, and questions for thought and discussion in each chapter. Federal statutes and regulations that have ethical bearing in practice have been added and updated. Content has been expanded to highlight contemporary topics in healthcare ethics, with updated references and research integrated throughout.

In Section I, the reader is introduced to fundamentals of morality and ethical study as they apply to the health professions. An emphasis is placed on professional integrity and the increasing role of interprofessional collaborative practice in the delivery of compassionate, patient-centered care. The importance of attending to the sociocultural determinants of health is reinforced, along with updated literature on how cultural humility and inclusive practices can more fully engage patients and families, meeting the moral commitment to improve health outcomes for all. Section II begins with a focus on how expertise and responsibility evolve throughout one's professional career. It includes an expansion of content related to interprofessionalism and increased attention on clinician well-being in the health professions. Strategies to support moral resilience, prevent burnout, and promote self-care are introduced, with emphasis on cultivating self-awareness, mindful practice, moral courage, and a culture of workplace wellness. Section III reflects updated national standards and challenges in confidentiality, electronic health communications, data protections and privacy, social media, informed consent, and clinical research.

Section IV gives new attention to the current understanding of disability and participation in society, a focus seldom incorporated into general healthcare ethics texts. The importance and complexity of quality-of-life ethical decisions that honor patient's values across the life span are highlighted. Given the evolving emphasis on data-driven decision making, the quadruple aim, and quality measurement in healthcare, expanded literature on the scientific effects of compassion on patient outcomes, patient safety, clinician well-being, and organizational performance is also provided. In Section V, the reader is presented with ethical decision making set within the societal reality that some level of limitation, ranging from moderate to severe, almost always exists in healthcare goods and services. Major social, economic, and cultural conditions in which justice deliberations in healthcare arise are described, as is the professional's expanded moral agency and duties in justice situations. Timely topics such as health disparities and scarcity caused by healthcare supply chain shortages, climate change, and natural or human-made disasters are discussed. These final chapters also highlight opportunities for participation in ethical issues in which the roles of the health professional and the citizen meld locally and globally.

The seventh edition stands on the shoulders of the previous six, grounded securely in theory and those enduring concerns that have supported the need for professional ethics and ethical professionals since the beginning of healthcare. It also builds on the abiding conviction that health professionals can and should assume a strategic position from which to help shape ethical practice in today's healthcare environment so that it embraces and protects cherished societal values. I hope that *Ethical Dimensions in the Health Professions* will provide you with the tools needed to be an ethically competent and resilient health professional. My hope is that you will engage with patients, families, and interprofessional colleagues in conversations and reflections in the "moral spaces" along your journey in professional ethics. This journey is, I believe, a key to finding self-fulfillment in professional life.

Regina F. Doherty

Acknowledgments

Edition Seven

I owe a debt of gratitude to the health professions students and colleagues I have had the opportunity to teach and learn from at my respective places of past and current employment, including the MGH Institute of Health Professions, Tufts University, and the Massachusetts General Hospital. My interprofessional collaborations on ethics committees and national commissions throughout my career have expanded my understanding of how ethical issues impact the lives of patients, families, health professionals, care delivery systems, and societies. I have benefited greatly from the generosity, guidance, and caring support of mentors throughout my professional journey. The previous editions of this book were coauthored by my dear mentor, colleague and friend, Ruth Purtilo. I thank Dr. Purtilo for her wise counsel, support, insights, and outstanding ideas, which have advanced the field of professional ethics and have greatly impacted my scholarly trajectory. Forty years ago, Ruth and Dr. Christine Cassel, launched *Ethical Dimensions in the Health Professions* into the bestselling ethics text it is today. Through vision and commitment, these inspiring women leaders advanced the development of ethics knowledge and skills in countless health professionals, and as a result, ensured that *care* was always central to the healthcare provided to patients and families across the globe.

Last, a heartfelt thanks to my family. To my parents, Vincenzo and Yvonne, who taught me the importance of virtues and empowered me to pursue my goals; to my husband, Dan, whose deep support and respect for my professional endeavors nourishes my work and life; and to my daughter, Olivia Grace, whose inquisitive spirit and open heart is a source of motivation, boundless joy, and optimism for the future.

Regina F. Doherty

Notes to Instructors on Using This Edition

The core purpose of this book is to provide tools for addressing common ethical issues in the health professions. The tone of this book is practical throughout, designed for people on the front lines of healthcare decision making. The aim is that both instructors and students will find it user friendly. I encourage you to use the content in this text to create experiences that help your students learn to think, reason critically, communicate, and actualize their roles as moral agents, health professionals, and citizens.

General Framework

As you will note from the table of contents, the chapters in this text invite the reader to participate in reflection and analysis on various ethical dimensions in the health professions. The text is divided into five sections, with the first section introducing readers to the foundations of ethics and subsequent sections guiding them through the application of ethical reasoning in professional roles, patient relationships, chronic and end-of-life care, and social contexts of healthcare. Whether focusing on confidentiality in the use of social media, the complexities of research for individuals with disabilities, or the role of the health professional in policy decisions, emphasis throughout the text is placed on health professionals as moral agents whose competency in ethical analysis and reflection supports best practice and the delivery of quality care.

The six-step ethical decision-making process is a signature feature of this text. It has been used by health professionals across a wide variety of practice settings to reflect on, analyze, and move toward resolution of ethical problems. It is woven throughout each chapter and applied to each clinical narrative. A summary of the six-step process is outlined in the table that follows.

The Six-Step Process of Ethical Decision Making

The Six Steps	Building Blocks
Step 1: Get the story straight – Gather relevant information	Attend to the details of a situation. Gather as much relevant information as possible to get the facts straight. Learn to distinguish the clinical, legal, and ethical content in the narrative describing the situation.
Step 2: Identify the type of ethical problem	Prototypes of ethical problems (e.g., moral distress, ethical dilemma) help to organize the details of a narrative into the appropriate category (or categories) for ethical analysis. Moral agency and shared agency support the health professional and the interprofessional care team when ethical tensions arise.
Step 3: Use ethical theories or approaches to analyze the problem	The skills of ethical reasoning are put into play. Foundational theories, approaches, and methods of ethics (i.e., moral virtues, rights, duties, and principles) serve as guidelines and conceptual frameworks. They are tools for recognizing, analyzing, and working to resolve ethical problems.
Step 4: Explore the practical alternatives	Determine the realistic, ethically supported options for carrying through with appropriate action. Openness and creativity are essential.
Step 5: Complete the action	In this step, action is required. Resolve and moral courage are needed.
Step 6: Evaluate the process and outcome	Reflect on the ethical decision, action, and outcomes to generalize information and insight (for both the individual health professional and the interprofessional care team) into what can be learned for future situations. Reflection is an essential step. It supports the development of moral resilience and a culture of clinician well-being.

Each chapter contains:
- A *Narrative* to illustrate key themes in the chapter.
- Educational *Objectives* for the chapter.
- *New Terms* introduced in the chapter.
- A list of *Key Concepts* used in the chapter and where each first appeared in the book.
- *Reflection* exercises throughout the text allowing readers to pause for their own response during their study when a key concept or point has been made.
- Numerous *Summary Statements* within each chapter and at the end of each chapter to help guide the reader along.

- *Questions for Thought and Discussion* at the end of each chapter for group discussion or individual reflection. These include additional cases along with other exercises that can be used by instructors and readers to reinforce the main points of the chapter.
- *References* for those interested in learning more about a particular topic.

Objectives

Through studying this book and discussing the Questions for Thought and Discussion section, readers will be able to:

1. Increase their knowledge and understanding of the ethical dimensions of professional practice.
2. Appreciate how effective interprofessional care teams collaborate to achieve a shared common good, supporting optimum health outcomes.
3. Identify how the goal of a caring response factors into a wide range of ethical issues in professional practice.
4. Recognize the nature and scope of moral agency as an individual health professional and shared agency as a member of the interprofessional care team.
5. Effectively apply ethical reasoning with the help of a straightforward problem-solving method designed for ethical situations.
6. Become competent in applying widely used ethics theories, approaches, and concepts to address ethical challenges across a wide variety of settings in professional practice.
7. Recognize current and long-standing themes in professional ethics, and cite examples of concrete ethical situations in clinical practice and health policy.
8. Appraise the quadruple aim and integrate strategies that support moral resilience, self-compassion, and clinician well-being in the health professions.
9. Recognize the ethical issues that present in the societal context of healthcare and the health professional's role in analyzing and resolving ethical problems to justly serve patients, families, and communities locally and globally.
10. Select resources that are useful for more in-depth study of professional ethics.

Contents

S E C T I O N   **IV**
Ethical Dimensions of Chronic and End-of-Life Care, *291*

Guide to Ethical Narratives in Text

Introduction to Ethical Dimensions in the Health Professions

1

Morality and Ethics: What They Are and Why They Matter

Objectives

The reader should be able to:
- Define morality and ethics and distinguish between the two.
- Define integrity and understand its relationship to fundamental moral beliefs and values in the health professions.
- Describe the relationship of personal, group, and societal moralities that health professionals must integrate into their role and everyday practice.
- Delineate values of an interprofessional care team that are consistent with professional morality.
- Describe the functions of a health professions code of ethics.
- List three ways in which ethics is useful in everyday professional practice.
- Compare the basic functions of law and ethics in professional practice.
- Identify some laws and policies that protect the personal moral convictions of health professionals while upholding the ethical gold standard of respecting human dignity.

New terms and ideas you will encounter in this chapter

plateaus	societal morality	ethics committees
morality	group morality	constitutional law
moral development	moral community	statutory law
moral judgment	professional morality	administrative law
values	interprofessional care	licensing laws
moral values	team	common law
moral duty	code of ethics	state interests
moral character or virtue	Hippocratic Oath	moral repugnance
personal morality	ethics	
moral integrity	ethicists	

Introduction

Your journey into the world of healthcare ethics begins with a story. In this story and throughout this textbook you will meet patients, health professionals, families, and others who face challenges posed by their situations and the healthcare environment. Their stories illustrate the types of ethical issues you yourself may face as a caregiver, a member of an interprofessional healthcare team, a patient, or a family member. This book emphasizes basic ethical themes woven through the stories, which allows you to examine them for their unique or interesting characteristics and to assess the role each plays in the overall scheme of professional practice.

The following story introduces you to the Harvey family and the healthcare system into which they are catapulted after the tragic events of a beautiful late spring day.

❤ The Story of the Harvey Family and the Interprofessional Care Team

Drew Harvey was undoubtedly one of the most popular students at Mountmore College. In his senior year, he was captain of the college basketball team, which had had its best season ever, going to regional competition, and he had his own band that played every Saturday night at the local pub, *The Mole Hole*. He had played more than studied during his first 2 years of college, never having had to "crack the books" in high school. But after his sophomore year, he worked as an assistant to a physical therapist who treated the members of the locally based professional football team during their summer training. When he returned in his junior year, he announced that he was going to become a physical therapist. He buckled down and gained an almost straight "A" record, without having to give up basketball or the band.

Then a violent incident occurred the weekend before commencement that rocked the entire university community. Drew's band was playing at a local pub at an event reserved for graduating students and their friends. At the end of the first set, just as Drew was acknowledging the band members to the applause and howls of the audience, he suddenly staggered; blood splattered across his forehead as he fell forward off the platform. After a moment of stunned silence, someone screamed, "He's been shot!" Pandemonium broke out. Everyone frantically dialed 911 on their cellular phones. Drew mumbled, a confused and frightened look on his face, "What's going on?" and then lost consciousness. He was rushed to the emergency department of a hospital where a bullet was determined to have lodged in his skull, penetrating it above his left temple. The emergency room team flew into action. Confused students and police swarmed everywhere.

After 10 days in the intensive care unit (ICU), Drew regained consciousness. The shunt that had been placed in his skull to relieve the swelling of his brain was working well. He was beginning to focus his gaze, and he was attempting to communicate. Drew spent a total of 20 days in the ICU, after which he was transferred to the neurology floor. At a family meeting, the hospitalist told Drew's mom, Alice, that Drew's condition was stabilized and the goal would be to get him home soon. "Home!" Alice gasped. "How can we possibly manage at home? He can barely talk; he can't walk and can't go to the bathroom alone!" The social worker explained that Drew's student insurance did not cover inpatient rehabilitation but that the Harveys would be referred to Mountain Home Health, a home healthcare agency for continued nursing and rehabilitative services. Over the next week, the interprofessional care team noted Drew's improvement, and he was discharged home with the support of his family and home care services 1 month following his injury.

At home, Drew's right arm and hand regained motor function to the point that he could almost dress himself. He could not walk or shower independently because of spasticity in his right leg. His vocabulary was limited, but he increasingly caught himself when he used a wrong word. Because of his progress, the case manager authorized another 4 weeks of home occupational therapy, physical therapy, and speech therapy services.

Mr. and Mrs. Harvey were understandably anxious but very supportive throughout the entire recovery, encouraging their son toward as much independence as possible and offering support when needed. Drew's older brother made some adjustments in the Harveys' home to accommodate Drew's limited mobility and made himself available to help his parents so that they could go out at least once a week without worrying about leaving Drew at home alone.

The home care team working with Drew had grown attached to him and his family. They rejoiced with every sign of progress and struggled with him through the frustration and sadness that accompany such a traumatic experience. But the health professionals are now faced with a difficult situation. Drew is 4 weeks into his care plan and a treatment review is due. Understandably, when no measurable progress can be shown, authorization for treatments (and therefore the reimbursements for them) will be discontinued.

Drew's speech and progress in performing activities of daily living in the home setting have reached a plateau. However, the team as a whole has not reached an agreement regarding whether more improvement may be on the way. Maybe he will be able to avoid lifelong use of a wheelchair and become more independent in his daily tasks if his physical and occupational therapy treatments are not discontinued at this critical juncture. Maybe his language and cognitive skills will continue to improve after a brief plateau. But his university's health plan insurers use success ("outcome") measures that make it unlikely he will continue to be reimbursed for therapy costs in the home setting. The health professionals know that continued payments for treatment depend on their report of his continuous progress. They have also come to realize that Drew's student insurance covers 60 days of home healthcare but only a total of 15 outpatient therapy visits, which makes his transition to the next level of service even more challenging. Drew's mom, Alice, has emailed the home care agency to ask for a team meeting. In her email she writes, "I have heard some talk of potential changes in Drew's care plan. I want to make sure we talk about this together since our goal is for Drew to return to school and live independently."

Professionals who work with patients like Drew know that his care team faces a critical and delicate situation. The rate of "progress" in care recovery is not always constant. It may be marked by periods of rapid improvement interspersed with other periods of almost no perceptible change (*plateaus*). Moreover, different team members may see varying degrees of improvement because each continues to see the patient through the lens of progress in his or her area of expertise. Yet many insurance plans or other methods of payment for services make little or no allowance for these plateau periods, and treatment is generally discontinued when gains cannot be shown at a consistent rate. In this case, a patient must have a symptom that becomes acute again before treatment can be reinstituted. In summary, although progress eventually does end, the failure to allow for a plateau period often results in the patient's premature discontinuation from treatment altogether. This is precisely the problem that faces the home care team who is treating Drew Harvey.

 Reflection

Suppose you are a member of the interprofessional care team working with the Harvey family. What should you do?

- Should the team "bend the truth a little," reporting that Drew continues to make daily progress in *all* areas so that he is less likely to lose an opportunity for possible further functioning in others?
- Should you cut and run from the team as a whole and insist that they tell the truth that he has reached a plateau in the area of therapy you are providing, knowing that Drew will be discontinued from all interventions?
- What other alternatives to an "either/or" solution to this problem should you and your teammates pursue?
- An even broader scope may be encompassed. Should you get involved in trying to change the insurance company policies that put the team in this difficult situation in the first place? How could you and your team advocate for the Harveys?

Jot down what you think are the most important challenges that face these health professionals involved with Drew Harvey's situation, regardless of whether they are suggested in the text:

_____

_____

_____

_____

Responses to these challenges are not found in the textbooks that deal with the technical skills of your chosen field. You are beginning to use your understanding of morality and how ethics figure into your professional life if you are concerned with one or more of the following questions:

- What is right or wrong conduct for you in this situation and why?
- What are your duties to everyone involved and what are your (and everyone else's) rights?
- What issues arise because you, individually, *and* the team are accountable for the decisions made?
- What are the character traits you want to preserve?
- What constitutes fairness for all patients in similar situations?

To simplify, what is involved in showing Drew and his family that you care? These considerations may even make you think about what type of society you want to help build in your professional career. In all of these areas of your professional life, you are dealing with morality and moral values.

 Summary

Facing difficult human questions about right and wrong conduct, duties, rights, character traits, and fair treatment is the focus of professional ethics.

Morality and Moral Values

When *morality* is mentioned, you may think of what you were told to do or not to do as a child. You are right. That is a part of morality. But morality is a much richer set of ideas than that. From the earliest societies onward, people have established guidelines designed to preserve the very fabric of their society. The guidelines become a natural language and behavior that describe the way things ought to be and what types of things we should value. Most members of society accept these guidelines, allowing the assumptions on which morality is based to prescribe decisions about many aspects of daily life.

Morality is not simply an intellectual exercise. Individuals and groups act out of strong convictions about what is right or wrong and good or bad. We shape our lives and reputations around our beliefs. A part of human development called *moral development* has been studied to show that adults instill these assumptions into children at a deep emotional level so that acting on the guidelines becomes not only habitual but also provides confidence that the right decision was taken. Viewed collectively, these guidelines constitute a society's morality.

Morality is relational. It is concerned with relationships between people and how, ultimately, they can best live in peace and harmony. The goal of morality is to protect a high quality of life for an individual, group, or the community as a whole. Ethicists Beauchamp, Walters, and colleagues summarize it this way: "Certain things ought or ought not to be done because of their deep social importance in the ways they affect the interests of other people."[1]

Morality is also context dependent. A *moral judgment* is needed when the particulars of a specific situation arise. When the members of the home care team were faced with being advocates for Drew, they were forced into thinking of him in very specific terms as a unique human in relationship to his family, to social groups such as his university classmates, and to society.

Morality includes values, duty, and character. No matter what the specific circumstances are, you always need to consider three distinct areas of morality.

* *Values* are the language that has evolved to identify intrinsic things a person, group, or society holds dear. Not all values are *moral values* of course. For instance, some things are cherished for the beauty, novelty, or efficiency they bring to our lives. Things that uphold our ideas of what is needed for morality to survive and thrive are viewed as moral values. Many moral values describe qualities that support individuals in their desire to live full lives and that allow them to pursue their own basic interests and provide help for others to do so. Others reflect qualities of groups within society that highlight our need for cooperation. We ascribe moral value to character traits of persons, groups, and societies, too, making moral judgments of their praiseworthy or blameworthy traits. A compassionate person is judged as praiseworthy, and a cruel group, such as a gang, is judged as blameworthy; a just society is judged as praiseworthy, and one that holds its citizens in a grip of terror is judged as blameworthy.
* *Moral duty* is a language that has evolved to describe actions. Not all duty is moral duty, just as not all we value is of moral value. Moral duty describes certain actions required of an individual, group, or society if each is to play a part in preventing harm and building a human foundation that can thrive.
* *Moral character or virtue* is a language used to describe traits and dispositions or attitudes that set the groundwork for us to trust each other and to

provide for human flourishing in times of stress. Common examples are compassion, courage, honesty, faithfulness, respectfulness, and humility. These traits, taken together and exercised regularly, make up what we mean when we say a person is "of high moral character." As a child, you acquired parts of your morality from family and friends, reading, television, films, the Internet, religious teachings, and experiences in school and extracurricular activities.

Reflection

Consider some sources that have informed your understanding of your own moral values, duties, and praiseworthy character traits.

Who or what have been four important influences on your understanding of moral guidelines that are worth trying to live by?

_____

_____

_____

_____

Name three people you admire for living exemplary moral lives. They may be people who you know personally, lived historically, or you learned about only by reputation. What makes them admirable?

_____

_____

_____

Think of groups (e.g., sports teams, church or civic groups, workplace teams) you have observed or in which you participated. Name two rules each group abides by that reflect basic moral necessities for them to achieve their goals.

_____

_____

Personal, Societal, and Group Morality

As a member of the health professions, you must reckon with at least three subgroups of morality: your personal morality, societal morality, and the group morality of the health professions, including the additional considerations that arise in team-delivered care. Fortunately, large areas of overlap are found.

Personal Morality

Personal morality is a collage of values, duties regarding conduct, and character traits each person adopts as relevant for his or her life. It is "who you are" as a unique moral being among others. Becoming intimately familiar with your own moral identity will serve you well. In other words, take care to "know thyself" as counseled by the ancient sage Plutarch in 650 BC. Doing so enhances the self-understanding needed to take on the responsibilities and tasks of your professional role. Your personal morality is also the foundation stone from which you can try to understand and respect the personal morality of patients, colleagues, and others with whom you come into professional contact. To illustrate, the interprofessional team treating Drew Harvey will not be successful if all members are not aware of their own moral values and beliefs as the individuals and team encounter the moral values and beliefs of the Harvey family. Without this deep self-awareness, it is impossible to discern why you respond to another with the feelings, emotions, and judgments that arise in the course of your communications and decisions.

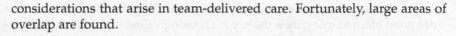 *Reflection*

List five key components of your own personal morality (e.g., lying is wrong; I should be kind to myself and others; everyone deserves respect).

_____

_____

_____

_____

_____

Try to think of a situation in your role as a health professional when one or more of these guidelines may be needed. If you cannot come up with one at the moment, keep this page earmarked and come back to it when you are faced with a real-life challenge or are reflecting on other stories in later chapters of this text.

Personal Morality and Moral Integrity

One of the most essential resources in your professional life is your own *moral integrity.* You experience a sense of integrity when you act in accordance with the values that make up your personal morality. Everyone has an idea of a good life, and integrity is the key to choosing values and actions that support the ideals of that life. The term *integrity* comes from the Latin *integritas*, which means unimpaired condition, sound, whole, undivided. It is easy to understand how living by the guidance of your personal morality helps you maintain a clear sense of "who you really are" when challenges arise. The reward is that you can maintain a sense of unified purpose, direction, and action in different kinds of situations. Cynda Rushton summarizes it well:

> *Integrity is not merely doing what is morally or ethically justified but doing so with the properly nuanced knowledge, intention, and attitude. Skillfully enacting one's values and commitments requires ongoing discernment, practice and opportunities for course corrections along the ways. Integrity is not only a moral ideal—it requires commitment and discipline to live the values and principles one espouses rather than to merely profess them.[2]*

Put simply, moral integrity is the integration of character and conscience. Sustaining moral integrity requires an ongoing commitment to reflection and refinement, especially when it is challenged. Table 1.1 provides some helpful "I" statements for you to reflect on as you consider aligning personal integrity with your role as a health professional.

Societal Morality

Large components of personal morality are drawn from a morality that is shared with others in society. *Societal morality* contains values and ideas of duty or character that spring from deep cultural beliefs about humans and their relationship with God (or the gods in some cultures), with each other, and with the natural world. Societal morality becomes codified in laws, customs, and policies. In the United States, the founding fathers and mothers who risked crossing oceans and leaving behind almost every security tried to capture the common denominator of their societal morality in the

Table 1.1   Integrity Begins With "I"

- I know what I stand for.
- I walk the talk—I live my values in each moment.
- I am open and listen wholeheartedly.
- I ask the hard questions.
- I embrace difficult, or potentially unknowledgeable, questions.
- I listen to the call of conscience.
- I am courageous in response to moral adversity.
- I inquire and am curious to discover what will serve.
- I speak out for what I stand for.
- I act even when doing so is difficult or consequences unpleasant.
- I am responsible and accountable.

From Rushton CH, editor: Moral resilience: transforming moral suffering in healthcare, New York, 2018, Oxford University Press.

statement "all are created equal" and therefore everyone should have an equal chance at "life, liberty, and the pursuit of happiness."

Almost always, some tensions exist between personal and societal morality. These tensions are played out in societal debates, with individuals and groups taking sides to try to influence laws and policies. Two current healthcare-related debates deal with the morality of abortion and assisted suicide. Others focus on the appropriate limits of the use of the natural environment for human purposes; the moral rights of embryos, undocumented immigrants, prisoners, or others; and the use of taxes for the purpose of providing basic human services to individuals living in poverty. Can you name some others? A free society always generates lively debate, and your personal values serve as one source of engaging meaningfully.

Group Morality: The Health Professions and Interprofessional Care Teams

Every member of society, except perhaps the most isolated recluse, joins or is swept into one or more subgroups of society by virtue of being a member of a religious group, a workplace culture, a club, a service organization, an ethnic cluster, or other deep group affiliation. The moral guidelines adopted by a subgroup constitute its *group morality*. A good way to capture the essence of group morality is to think of it as a *moral community* within the larger society. One such community is the health professions.[3] Thinkers from various fields of study have noted that professionalism involves specific moral and other assumptions, a subset of group morality that the authors of this text suggest can be summarized as *professional morality*. Professional morality embraces moral values, duty, and character traits that do not apply equally or at all to others in society, although it goes beyond a strictly personal morality to a public statement. For instance, citizens in general are not morally required to offer help to another in need of medical attention. Health professionals are. Citizens are not morally required to keep in confidence information they hear about another. Health professionals are. Citizens are not morally required to be nonjudgmental about another's character. Health professionals are. Your fiduciary duty as a health professional is discussed in other parts of this book, notably in Chapters 2, 9, and 11.

As you saw in Drew Harvey's process of recovery, a segment of the professional moral community is the *interprofessional care team*. Almost every care plan involves a team of professionals working together. Team rules embody, but at times may conflict with, one or more general moral guidelines that make up one's personal or individual professional morality. Remember that effective teams are grounded in a shared purpose to support the common good in healthcare,[4] which is not about what is best for a singular practitioner; rather, it is about what is best for the patient. Core to the interprofessional care team's functioning are the value on common goals and assumptions of cooperation such as loyalty to and honesty with each other. Professionals must communicate, collaborate, and negotiate across professional boundaries to ensure the delivery of quality care.[5] Understanding the strengths and challenges of this form of healthcare delivery and the group morality aspects of it is so important that an entire chapter is devoted to the interprofessional care team (see Chapter 7).

Summary

You are a member of a group in a special type of relationship with others in society because of your professional role. The moral guidelines taken together make up a group morality called *professional morality* that can be thought of as a moral community. One aspect of this moral community is the presence of interprofessional care teams. Ideally, the values and moral expectations that arise from the professions and interprofessional care teams are aligned with your personal and society's values, but full agreement is not guaranteed in all cases.

One significant resource that describes the details of professional group morality as it applies specifically to your chosen field is the *code of ethics* of your profession.

Professional Codes of Ethics

Your profession's code of ethics emerged from an historical understanding that professionals are in a position to have a powerful positive or harmful influence on others. The code guides practice and promotes integrity. It is a visible acknowledgment that, as a group, professionals are granted societal privileges; however, with these privileges comes the responsibility to conduct themselves in ways that are acceptable not only to other members of the group but also to the larger society. The ancient oaths, such as the familiar *Hippocratic Oath* (Box 1.1), were statements that swore their group intent to the gods to practice in specific ways that reflected a commitment to human well-being. Although codes do not require the actual swearing in of the ancient oaths, the oaths often are recited during ceremonies, marking the student's progress toward becoming a professional.

Most codes are produced by the profession's national association and reflect the collective wisdom about how members should conduct themselves as professionals, which gives the items in the code an authoritative collective voice for that profession. A shortcoming of the current approach to codes of ethics is that almost all focus primarily or solely on the moral guidelines of a single profession, leaving as secondary or absent the fact that care is almost always delivered by interprofessional care teams.

Be that as it may, why is knowledge of your code important?

Box 1.1   Hippocratic Oath

I swear by Apollo the Physician, by Aesculapius, Hygeia, and Panacea, and all the gods and goddesses, making them my witnesses, that I will fulfill according to my ability and judgment this oath and this covenant:

To hold him who has taught me this art as equal to my parents and to live my life in partnership with him, and if he is in need of money to give him a share of mine, and to regard his offspring as equal to my brothers in male lineage and to teach them this art—if they desire to learn it—without fee and covenant; to give a share of precepts and oral instruction and all the other learning to my sons and to the sons of him who has instructed me and to pupils who have signed the covenant and have taken an oath according to the medical law, but to no one else.

I will apply dietetic measure for the benefit of the sick according to my ability and judgment; I will keep them from harm and injustice.

I will neither give a deadly drug to anybody if asked for it, nor will I make a suggestion to this effect. Similarly I will not give to a woman an abortive remedy. In purity and holiness I will guard my life and my art.

I will not use the knife, not even on sufferers from stone, but will withdraw in favor of such men as are engaged in this work.

Whatever houses I may visit, I will come for the benefit of the sick, remaining free of all intentional injustice, of all mischief and in particular of sexual relations with both female and male persons, be they free or slaves.

What I may see or hear in the course of the treatment or even outside of the treatment in regard to the life of men, which on no account one must spread abroad, I will keep to myself holding such things shameful to be spoken about.

If I fulfill this oath and do not violate it, may it be granted to me to enjoy life and art, being honored with fame among all men for all time to come; if I transgress it and swear falsely, may the opposite of all this be my lot.

Edelstein L: The Hippocratic Oath: Text, Translation and Interpretation. "The Hippocratic Oath: Classical Version." Reprinted with permission of The Johns Hopkins University Press.

- Your code is your profession's most succinct statement of its professional (group) morality. It is literally a codified shorthand of your larger moral role in society as a member of a special moral community.
- Your code is a protector of your own best interests as a professional committed to a patient's well-being. Patients, families, policymakers, or others may ask you to do things that you judge are not in accordance with your professional moral judgment. The code likely provides support for your position if your deliberations fall within the common denominator of the moral guidelines detailed in your code.

- Your code also provides a measuring rod for you to engage in continual self-improvement in practice. In a complex situation, you can refer to it to ask "How do I measure up against the moral standards and specific directives outlined in my code?" and "How am I doing?"

 Reflection

Find the code of ethics of your profession.

Note: You can usually find your code on the website of your professional association. For example, a nurse in the United States can refer to the American Nurses Association website, a physical therapist to the American Physical Therapy Association website, and so on.

When you have found your code, compare the core concepts of the ancient Hippocratic Oath and of your code.

_____

_____

List the major items in your code that you believe could apply equally well to any other health profession.

_____

_____

Which items, if any, seem to be specific only to the members of your chosen profession?

_____

_____

Which items in your profession's code of ethics apply to the specific situation of the interprofessional care team treating Drew Harvey?

_____

_____

Would your code help the team members in the decision they have to make? If so, how could they use it?

_____

_____

Institutional Policies

The group morality of the health professions should be embedded in the policies, customs, and practices of healthcare institutions. The world would be perfect if members of the professions could rely completely on these policies; fortunately, they are reliable guides for most decisions you will have to make. The idea of a professional embodies a moral conviction that each and every patient will get the type and amount of care that is needed. The identified patient is the sole focus of an interprofessional healthcare team's interventions.[6] But what about other patients with similar clinical conditions? Policies function to try to create a just environment for all like-situated patients; this in turn may mean that, because of scarce resources, limits are set, which result in practices that do not seem to place the individual patient's well-being at the front and center of operations. The first instinct for many professionals is to see institutional policy as so far removed from the real purpose of healthcare that they believe the interests of patients have been unnecessarily compromised for other goals of the institution, such as efficiency, financial solvency, or competing priorities not related to patient care. Exemption from having to abide by an institutional policy that a person or group believes is morally questionable may not be assured. The predicament in which the health professionals find themselves regarding Drew Harvey's care presents a traditional professional morality challenge because we can safely assume that most of them find it personally wrong to falsify details about his immediate rate of improved function. At the same time, their duty of due care for him means that some of them probably blame institutional policies governing home healthcare as being unfair policies.

These situations are by no means limited to the health professions. People of strong moral grounding through the ages have had to come to grips with institutional policies that grate against their personal or group moral values and duty. An historical example comes from another professional group, the clergy.

The Christian Reformation in 1500s Europe took place when the morality of some religious leaders came into conflict with the policies and patterns of moral conduct in their religious institution. The famous statement, "Here I stand. I can do no other," exemplifies the moral breaking point persons or groups sometimes reach. The phrase is attributed to reformist priest Martin Luther, as he nailed 95 objections to the official church policy regarding the practice of indulgences to the door of All Saints Church in Wittenberg, Germany.

 Reflection

There are many historical and contemporary examples of moral breaking points between policies and what individuals or groups deem to be morally necessary. Take a moment and jot down a few with which you are familiar.

_____

_____

The good news is that, overall, the policies of healthcare and other institutions almost always help prevent you from having to participate in processes, procedures, or other activities that run counter to your personal and professional moral integrity. Before accepting a position in an institution, it is always a good idea to become well informed of the job expectations outlined in its policies.

Summary

Moral values, duty, and expectations of character occur at the level of personal life, within one's society, and with various groups. For professionals, professional group morality is recorded in oaths, codes, and other practice guidelines that govern this moral community. Interprofessional care teams and institutional policies may add additional moral considerations that foster conduct consistent with high moral standards of personal and professional morality.

From the Moral to the Ethical

You have learned that morality provides a basis for moving successfully through many daily actions: I will stop at this stop sign; our team will not cheat on this play. However, occasionally the naturalness comes to a gradual or screeching halt. Should I trust my feelings about what I am seeing in the treatment of this patient? Does our past experience on the team count here? The author has heard several metaphors that characterize this situation. "I thought I saw the solution clearly, but the edges went blurry and gray." "I call it my 'oops!' moment!" "Suddenly I felt like I was up a creek without a paddle."

These "Stop—Look—Listen!" reactions are a means of protecting ourselves against straying from the morality that we have learned to rely on habitually as we go about our daily lives. The reactions signal that something does not "fit right" in the situation. Take them as healthy alerts that something potentially harmful is threatening your moral integrity and practices.

Ethics is the discipline that waits in the wings as a health-restoring resource when moral policies and practices fail to do the job alone.[7] Ethics takes moral assumptions that are operative at the personal, group, or societal level and provides a language, method, and tools for evaluating them to create a better path for yourself and others.

Ethics: Study and Reflection on Morality

Ethics is a systematic study of and reflection on morality: "Systematic study of" because it is a discipline that uses special methods and approaches to examine moral situations and "reflection on" because it consciously calls assumptions about our morality into question. The goal is to highlight what does and does not fit in a particular situation. Ethics is a process that sees "what is" and asks "what really ought to be?"

Without this level of questioning and reflection, individuals, groups, and whole societies have no way to create more viable habits or customs as situations change. Originally, approaches to moral analysis were developed as areas of philosophy and theology. Today, the social sciences and other disciplines have added to the number and types of approaches. You will have an opportunity to learn more about them in Chapter 4.

The study of ethics takes the following question as its unchangeable gold standard.

> The gold standard: What do human dignity and respect demand of us?

Starting from this standard, the following questions arise in respect to specific situations:

- Do our present moral values, conduct, and character traits pass the test of further examination when measured against the gold standard?
- When conflicts arise, which moral guidelines are helpful in this situation and why?
- When a new situation presents uncertainty, what new thinking is needed and why?
- Overall, what aspects of present moralities most reliably guide individuals, groups, and societies on a new path consistent with honoring the gold standard?

You were introduced to codes of ethics previously in this chapter. How do they fit into the larger picture of ethics as we are now describing it? Fundamentally, they are a combination of moral, practical, and, in some areas, legal starting points for ethical deliberation. Take the case of the decision that faces the team members treating Drew Harvey in his home setting. Your code or even the combined codes of all of your team members does not do the full work of ethics for you and your teammates. In additional to the guidelines in the code, you must add your own critical thinking and attention to morally complex problems with the help of ethical theory and methods.

The websites and professional literature of many health professions associations now offer ethics case examples or opinion pieces that apply to your profession. Fortunately, many now also feature situations that place you as a member of an interprofessional care team. Such adjuncts to ethical codes are superb learning opportunities for you.

Ethicists and Ethics Committees

Ethicists have as their primary career activity the work and teaching of ethics. Medical ethicists or healthcare ethicists specialize in healthcare issues. At the level of clinical practice, they consult with care teams and families to help them recognize and analyze problems that arise, which helps clarify the moral values, duties, and other aspects of morality in a specific situation. Their role on the interprofessional care team is so important, that since 1992, institutions accredited by The Joint Commission have been required to have a process in place that allows staff members, patients, and families to address ethical issues.[8] The goal of ethics consultation is to help resolve difficult moral problems if possible. Ethicists support individuals and teams, who are at times driven by time or other external pressures, to reach thoughtful conclusions in complex moral situations (Fig. 1.1). Ethicists also work as consultants in the design of ethical policies and institutional practices.

In many institutions today, *ethics committees* serve the same purpose as an individual ethics consultant and usually include ethicists, other professionals, and laypeople. In this regard, they function as another type of care team. Ethics consultants and ethics committees focus on addressing uncertainty or conflict regarding value-laden concerns in the healthcare context.[9] But ethics is not the work of ethic consultants or ethics committees only. Ethics is the work of everybody.

ⓢ Summary

Ethics is the study of and reflection on everyday morality. It functions as a fundamental resource and takes specific forms when someone assumes a special role such as an individual health professional or member of an interprofessional care team. Ethics codes are a starting point for insights and guidance, but the complexity of healthcare today requires professionals to go beyond them to become skilled in analyzing complex moral issues in everyday practice. Ethicists specialize in bringing ethics understanding to the clinical and institutional care setting.

The Moral and Ethical Thing to Do

You commonly hear someone say, "That is the moral and ethical thing to do." The terms *moral* and *ethical* are used interchangeably. We suggest you use them more purposefully, however, because after what you have just

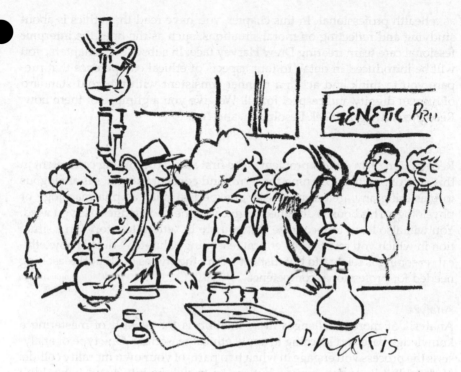

"I FIND IT HARDER AND HARDER TO GET ANY WORK DONE WITH ALL THE ETHICISTS HANGING AROUND."

Fig. 1.1. Copyright ScienceCartoonsPlus.com.

learned, that phrase should have more meaning for you. The "moral thing to do" means that the traditions, customs, laws, and other markers that an individual, group, and society call on for habitual moral guidance allow you to proceed with confidence in your course of action. The "ethical thing to do" means that the course of action that would be taken in the everyday moral walk of life has been reflected on and your moral judgment has dictated that it still seems the right thing to do (or refrain from doing). Fortunately, most situations allow you to act both morally and ethically.

Use of Ethics in Practical Situations That Involve Morality

The scholarly discipline of ethics has always been interesting from the point of view that its subject matter has immediate relevance for everyday life. Aristotle and others in the classical Greek era called ethics "practical philosophy." This interest has led to the development of ethicists and ethics committees discussed previously. We now turn to your own ethical formation as a health professional. In this chapter, you have read that ethics is about studying and reflecting on moral situations, such as the ones the interprofessional care team treating Drew Harvey face. In subsequent chapters, you will be introduced in detail to four aspects of ethical competence that prepare you to think and act in a manner consistent with the gold standard of human dignity and respect for all. We give you a glimpse of them now: Recognize, Analyze, Seek Resolution, and Act.

Recognize

Recognition of an ethical problem is the first step to becoming competent in this area of practice. Learning the terms and concepts of ethics is analogous to mastering any area of professional expertise, such as pharmacology or physiology. This book is designed to give you the knowledge base you need. You will also learn to recognize that you are in "ethics territory" in a situation in which you must apply ethical reasoning. Chapter 4 details how ethical reasoning is related to but distinct from other types of clinical reasoning needed for professional competence.

Analyze

Analysis of moral challenges in a situation is the reward of mastering a knowledge base and learning to apply ethical reasoning. One type of analysis is the process you engage in when two parts of your own morality collide: "I shouldn't lie to my spouse, but the truth will be bitter and I shouldn't hurt them either." Analysis also requires you to pay attention to the deeply human aspects of the specific situation you are facing.

 Reflection
The famous medieval physician Galen fled Rome during the plague. He analyzed his personal morality and decided he had to flee on behalf of his wife and children, whose lives he knew were threatened by the plague. We are told that for the rest of his life he had nightmares about failing in his professional morality because he had abandoned his patients to certain deaths. In other words, his knowledge and analysis of his personal and professional values, sense of priorities among his duties, and his character collided head on. Do you think his analysis served him well in resolving his dilemma? Did he do the right thing? Why or why not?

_____

_____

_____

_____

Answers to these questions require that your own analysis about his situation include a consideration of the facts available to you and your reasoning about right and wrong, the conflicting priorities he faced, the psychological dynamics he had to navigate, his professional obligations, and the practical consequences of his alternatives. Analysis uncovers relevant details to help inform possible directions toward resolution and purposive action. Although Galen's situation was extreme, the process of analysis you used to engage his conflict is the same process you probably used to think about which direction Drew Harvey's care team ought to take.

Seek Resolution

The point of ethical reasoning is to work toward resolution of a complex moral situation. Obviously, this is what Drew Harvey's healthcare team needs to do. One approach to finding resolution is to try to build consensus among the various concerned parties (e.g., team members, the patient, his family, the institution). Some ethics approaches focus on how to resolve issues when no consensus is reached or when consensus does not seem to fully address the moral conflicts embedded in the situation.[10] In many healthcare institutions, the ethics consultant or ethics committee can be called on to add insight and counsel in the most challenging instances.

Act

Purposive action stems from analysis and thoughtful work toward resolution. The health professionals involved with Drew Harvey's potential discharge from their care are looking for direction to act purposefully and preserve the moral integrity of the entire community.

> **Summary**
>
> Acknowledgment of the value of recognition and analysis of moral problems that ultimately serve as a guide for purposeful action have led to a resurgence of interest in ethics in many areas of everyday life. Healthcare ethics is one such area of applied ethics.

Legal Protections for Your Ethical Decisions

Legal protections come in the form of case law *(constitutional law)* as a result of court decisions from the lowest courts to the supreme or high courts of the land that set legal precedence for future similar situations; legislation *(statutory law* or statutes) passed through Congress or parliament; and legally binding regulations *(administrative law)* promoted through a state's or national government's regulatory bodies, such as the U.S. Department of Health and Human Services.

How Does Law Factor Into Professional Morality?

National and state or provincial laws embody and codify moral values and types of duty that should govern individual and institutional conduct related to the health professions and provide legal interpretations of key professional issues. For example, laws outline the conditions under which health professionals have the license or privilege to practice in a state, province, or territory. Laws provide clarification about informed consent, confidentiality, and conditions related to a health professional's competence, among many other issues. Each of these is based on moral values relevant to the health professional–patient relationship, on an understanding of professional duty, and on societal expectations of the type of moral character professionals cultivate and exhibit. Many health professions programs today wisely include a course on healthcare law governing their profession; if you do not have one in your program of study, web and other resources also are available for you to learn about the legal dimensions of your practice.

As a general rule, laws and moral standards of a society seem to support each other. But you should not expect the same guidance from laws or policies that you receive from ethical codes and vice versa. Each has its special function. For a succinct summary of major distinctions between law and ethics, the subsequent chart from the work of Jennifer Horner is helpful.

Morality[a]	
Law	*Ethics*
Defined by government	Defined by individual and community
Based on concepts of justice and equality	Based on how we define a good, worthwhile, or meaningful life
Formal rules for resolution of complex problems	Informal guidelines for resolution of complex problems
Uniformity	Some uniformity; respectful of diversity
Minimum standard of behavior ("at least")	Ideal or aspirational ("better" or "best")
Coercive (penalties for misconduct)	Noncoercive ("dictates of conscience")
Rules of law enforced by regulatory authorities and courts	Standards and exhortations by custom, professional standards, discussion, and persuasion
"Must"	"Should"

[a]Widely held societal values (universal, ultimate, impartial, other-regarding).
From Horner J: Morality, ethics and law: introductory concepts. Semin Speech Language 24(4):269–273, 2003.

Protections

As you think about living within the dictates of your conscience and professional morality in seriously contended moral issues, keep in mind the following general resources available to professionals through laws and policies.

Licensing Laws

Professionals become certified, registered, or licensed to practice nationally and within a particular state or jurisdiction after the completion of all formal professional preparation requirements. Written into the *licensing laws* that govern professional practice are both responsibilities and protections or rights. Among the rights is your right to practice within the dictates of your practice guidelines and own convictions. This right is weighed against the reasonable expectations of patients or families who come to you for professional help.

State Interests

Common law (i.e., law that comes into practice over time through the lived life of a community) dictates that there are *state interests*, that is, a responsibility to intervene on behalf of persons under four extreme circumstances: (1) to save their life, (2) to prevent their suicide, (3) to protect them from harm as an innocent third party, and (4) to protect them as a bearer of the "integrity of the professions." This final cause for legal intervention obviously applies to professionals only. It has evolved because of circumstances in which health and other professionals have been faced with requests by patients or clients or have been dictated to by policies to act in ways that are believed by a court to be contrary to the true moral and legal social role of a professional. This protection must be appealed to on a case-by-case basis.

Moral Repugnance

Moral repugnance came into the health professions literature with the U.S. Supreme Court decision *Roe v. Wade*, which made abortion a legal right. A conscience clause allows individuals who believe that participation in abortion procedures is morally wrong to be exempt from having to do so. An important aspect of this provision is that the procedure itself is key to whether this exemption is upheld. It is not a protection against, for example, your refusal to treat patients whose lifestyles are morally unacceptable to you. Therefore it is a limited but important protection. Many have argued that a request to assist in the lethal procedures that cause death in capital punishment fall under the protection of this notion. The same is true for medically administered euthanasia, which is legally permissible in select states and countries. This conscience clause operates as a conscientious objection analogous to conscientious objection in situations of war.

Limits of Protection

In summary, society and many institutions that deliver high-quality healthcare are aware of the need for your personal protection so that in your professional role you can perform acts that the layperson cannot, and you are provided a recourse in those hopefully rare circumstances in which you feel morally compromised by something you are expected to do in that role. Some legal cases involve the entire interprofessional care team, but more often, laws are still designed with an individual legal agent in mind. In either situation, the final burden of proof rests on why you or the team refuses on moral grounds to participate in an action or take a position contrary to the norm. You may be able to find support in one of the previously mentioned legal mechanisms that have been developed. The best recourse is to know your own moral values and reasons for your decisions and have good justifications to support them. In team situations, there is strength in engaging the range of moral values and understanding of what morality requires of each individual. Fortunately, most health professionals seldom experience the deep, troubling tension of being in a situation they believe compromises their personal and professional moral convictions.

 Summary

Protections that provide legal conditions that permit you to practice and allow you to follow the dictates of your own conscience are provided through federal and state or other more local legal mechanisms. However, the final burden of proof for your refusal or request for exemption from usual and customary procedures falls on you. Some legal protections now are designed to take into account the moral responsibility of a healthcare team for decisions that involve two or more members of the team.

Summary

This chapter is but one step in your lifelong journey in professional ethics. You have chosen a career path that requires complex moral judgments regarding patient care, health policy, and other aspects of professional life. Many of these judgments are made within the context of an interprofessional care team. This chapter has introduced you to some basic ways of thinking about the sources of morality on which you can draw, the general relevance of ethics to your everyday professional life, and some legal protections you can expect. As you study the subsequent chapters, you will be better able to appreciate the contribution of these considerations.

Questions for Thought and Discussion

1. Search your local or other national news source for a story about healthcare that involves moral values or duties.
   a. What is the basic point of the piece? What is the reporter saying?
   b. What does the writer or reporter suggest are the main moral issues raised in this situation? Do you agree? Why or why not?

2. You learned in this chapter about personal, group, and societal moralities. Identify a value in your own personal morality and describe that value's relationship with the morality of a group or society in which you currently live. Use the following box to compare the moralities.

Personal value	Group value	Societal value

References

1. Beauchamp TL, Walters L, Kahn JP, et al: *Contemporary issues in bioethics*, Belmont, CA, 2007, Wadsworth Publishing.
2. Rushton CH, editor: *Moral resilience: transforming moral suffering in healthcare*, New York, 2018, Oxford University Press.
3. Austin W: The ethics of everyday practice: healthcare environments as moral communities, *Adv Nursing Sci* 30(1):81–88, 2007.
4. Interprofessional Education Collaborative. *Core competencies for interprofessional collaborative practice: 2016 update*. Washington, DC, 2016. Available at www.ipecollaborative.org/resources.html.
5. Doherty RF, Peterson EW: Responsible participation in a profession: fostering professionalism and leading for moral action. In Braveman B, editor: *An evidence-based approach to leading & managing occupational therapy services*, 2nd ed, Philadelphia, 2015, FA Davis.
6. Haddad A, Purtilo R, Doherty R: *Health professional and patient interaction*, 9th ed, St. Louis, 2019, Elsevier.
7. Berlinger N: Perspective: helping people out, *Hastings Cent Rep* 39(1):53, 2009.
8. The Joint Commission: *Comprehensive Accreditation Manual for Hospitals*, 2019, Joint Commission Resources.
9. Arnold RM, et al: *Core competencies for healthcare ethics consultation*, 2nd ed, Chicago, 2011, American Society for Bioethics and Humanities.
10. Moreno J: *Deciding together: bioethics and moral consensus*, New York, 1995, Oxford University Press.

2

The Ethical Goal of Professional Practice: A Caring Response

Objectives

The reader should be able to:
- Describe the basic idea of a caring response and its function in healthcare.
- List some types of claims on professionals and the reasoning supporting that patient interests generally must take priority.
- Describe patient-centered care.
- Compare caring expressed in friendships or family life and caring expressed in a professional relationship.
- Identify the two components of professional responsibility and why both are essential for a caring response.
- Understand how cultural humility and cultural competence ensure a caring response.
- Identify sociocultural determinants of health and appreciate their impact on health outcomes.
- Discuss how the ethical concept of justice figures into the intent to meet the goal of a professional caring response.
- Discuss some burdens and benefits of being a caregiver as they arise in the health professional–patient relationship.

New terms and ideas you will encounter in this chapter

a caring response
care
care plan
claim
patient-centered care
relationship-based care
technical competence

professional
   responsibility
due care
accountability
responsiveness
right
human rights

social determinants of
   health
cultural competence
cultural humility
health inequity
justice

Topics in this chapter introduced in earlier chapter	
Topic	*Introduced in chapter*
Ethics gold standard	1
Interprofessional care team	1
Professional morality as a group morality	1
Moral community	1
Code of ethics	1

Introduction

The goal of professional ethics is to arrive at *a caring response* in situations you encounter throughout the course of carrying out your professional role and its functions. In Chapter 1, we introduced the ethics gold standard of upholding every person's dignity in your professional relationships. We now introduce *care* as the fundamental means by which you can recognize whether or not you are practicing according to that standard.

Some ethics texts do not spend much time focused specifically on the notion of care, however, students and professionals alike often measure their professional effectiveness and satisfaction by whether they can conclude that they did a good job of caring for patients. Still, when asked, they do not find it easy to grasp fully what care is. This is not too surprising because, as one wise colleague put it succinctly:

> You can't bottle care. It is not a formula. Just as in a loving relationship there is no one formula, so it is with care. Whatever is expressed as care has to be authenticated by going deeper into the spirit through which it is offered. Care connects you not only with the other but also reflects back who you are as a human being. In this regard it is not like the contributions you make through applying your technical expertise. At the same time this is what makes care the special gift of a health professional and patient relationship because it sets you squarely in a human to human encounter where not only your patients' well being but your own is at stake. You must work together to find the shape that a caring response will take in each case.[1]

The effect and science of care has been well established throughout the years. A recent review traces a long history of care as the central feature that divides the mere science of medicine from its essential quality. The investigators showed that recent physiological and neuroimaging studies indicated positive findings in patients who believed that their professionals really cared. They based their conclusion on the professionals' attitudes and conduct, not just their technical expertise.[2]

Although the deep motivations for expressing care are personal, some expressions of professional caregiving are so similar that almost everyone can recognize them. As noted in Chapter 1, this goal seldom is fully reached alone: The whole team is needed to collaborate in efforts to show the patient that "We've got your back!" "We are on your side!" "Your dignity is safe with us!" As noted in the previous quote, the specific shape this care takes in a specific patient's *care plan* depends on what each member of the inter-professional care team collaborating with the patient and the patient's loved ones comes up with that helps preserve the patient's dignity. At the same time, this chapter shares some themes and expressions of care that will help you learn how others have come to recognize and use this key component of a successful professional career.

 Summary

A caring response is the ethical goal of every health professional–patient relationship. It is the key to honoring a patient's dignity. Care requires a human-to-human exchange that needs participation by all involved. The goal is realized most often through the interactions and collaborative contributions of the interprofessional care team.

After these introductory chapters, you will have many opportunities to consider different types of situations in which you must determine what a caring response involves; every situation will be an adventure into the unknown territory of another unique person's values, preferences, and life experiences. To get started, consider the following story that highlights some challenges that Pat Jackson, a physician assistant, and the interprofessional care team encounter as they try to live by their intention to promote a caring response.

 The Story of Pat Jackson, the Interprofessional Care Team, and Mr. Sanchez

---

Pat Jackson was excited to be invited into a rural group practice in her home state. During her hiring interview, she found the team of physicians, nurses, technologists, therapists, and others compatible with her own commitment to high-quality healthcare. She told the team how she had welcomed the opportunity to attend school in a large city but now was eager to return as a physician assistant to the type of rural setting she had so enjoyed as a child. The group was impressed with her enthusiasm and the several academic and humanitarian awards she had received during her training.

So it was a terrible moment for her when, with the honeymoon period barely over, she misdiagnosed Mr. Sanchez's symptoms of asthma as a temporary allergic response attributable to the very high pollen count that month. (You will return to this part of the story later in the chapter, but for the moment, read on.) Mr. Sanchez came to the clinic with a characteristic stuffy nose and watery eyes she had seen several times earlier in the week. Although his wheezing concerned her, she was eager to leave work that Friday evening in time to keep her commitment to serve at a community church supper down the road from where she lived. Her initial response to being paged by the departing receptionist had been annoyance at having to see yet one more patient. "Stop thinking this way," she chided herself.

Assuredly, this patient did look more miserable than others she had seen that week, but in an interprofessional care team meeting on Wednesday, the discussion included how much the presenting symptoms of pollen allergy can vary among migrant workers who come to harvest the fields during this season. Many workers developed allergies they had not encountered previously. When she asked him whether he had ever had such symptoms before, Mr. Sanchez wheezed, "No, señora." She noted that he may or may not have completely understood her question. Still, his "No, señora" seemed emphatic enough that she did not think she needed to run after her colleague who was just getting into his car but could pose the question to Mr. Sanchez in his native language. Noting her hesitance, Mr. Sanchez said, "Gracias, thank you, okay me." "Thank me for what?" she thought. He did not look okay. But overall, she was relieved that he was another pollen sufferer she could quickly send on his way with a prescription to relieve his respiratory stuffiness and wheezing.[3]

Many issues can be raised in this story, but your opportunity here is to focus on your opinion about Pat's professional mandate to provide a caring response to Mr. Sanchez's problem.

Reflection

When Mr. Sanchez came to the clinic, did Pat reflect attitudes and conduct that are consistent with your assumptions of how a caring professional should respond?

Yes____ No____ Somewhat____

If you answered yes or somewhat, which aspects of her approach are consistent with your assumptions?

_____

_____

Most readers also sympathize with Pat's situation. Do you? If so, what is the basis of your sympathy about her responses when he arrived? Are they sufficiently understandable that any shortcomings in her approach are relatively inconsequential?

_____

_____

Jot down some thoughts about what role other members of the interprofessional care team play in ensuring a caring response to Mr. Sanchez.

_____

_____

As in many ethical challenges, Pat's situation contains details that can cause you to see more than one side of the story, which is when ethical analysis becomes a resource. We discuss this at more length in Chapter 5. At the moment, our attention is on whether or how she was expressing care.

The Patient as the Focus of a Caring Response

A caring response involves a claim on you as a professional to give priority to optimizing positive results and minimizing damage to the patient. What is meant by a claim? A *claim* is a request made verbally or nonverbally based on the expectations people have of your professional role. It says, "Give me your expert attention." You know that your professional role involves many types of relationships, with patients or clients and other times with families, professional teammates, research participants, policymakers, and the public; the list is not complete if you fail to include your relationship with yourself. For instance, an unfair conclusion is that Pat's desire to serve the larger community at the church supper and to build personal relationships there was unreasonable. Each and every one of the parties you will encounter comes with claims on your time, services, expertise, or other type of attention. From time to time, you will find yourself torn between more than one of them, just as Pat did. She understood that her patient Mr. Sanchez had a strong claim on her to be treated with dignity and have her full attention. But still, her desire to be caring of herself by participating in a social event on this Friday night in her newly adopted town understandably was pressing in on her while she was trying to treat him, and no one would fault her for the wish to meet new people there.

L *Reflection*
Stop here and think about your day so far. What competing claims on your time, attention, or other resources have you already faced?

_____

_____

Competing claims are part and parcel of everyday life. But the ethical dimension of Pat's professional role helps her to set priorities in relation to

Mr. Sanchez with the awareness that when other claims tempt her to override this priority, there must be very compelling reasons to do so.

Patient-Centered Care

Patient-centered care is a term adopted in the health professions literature to emphasize the imperative that professionals keep their focus on the values and well-being of their patients. To be truly patient centered, you as the health professional, must engage with the patient, family, and other members of the interprofessional care team to plan a course of action that matters most to the patient.[4] The U.S. Center for Medicare and Medicaid Services defines person and family engagement as working with patients and families in

> *defining, designing, participating in and assessing the care practices and systems that serve them to assure they are respectful of and responsive to individual patient preferences, needs, and values. This collaborative engagement allows patient values to guide all clinical decisions and drives genuine transformation in attitudes, behavior, and practice.[5]*

The central theme is that a patient's values, concerns, and informed preferences have more moral weight in your everyday clinical decision making than anything else calling for your attention. Patient-centered care acts as the orienting point on the professional's moral compass when deciding what direction to take at a crossroads of decision making between two or more priorities.

You can easily see that patient-centered care means that the care is tailored to fit each patient *as a unique person,* not simply as a diagnosis or collection of symptoms. This focus on the whole patient frequently is challenged in an era of clinical specialization. A particular disease, symptom, body part, or biological system can capture the attention of an individual professional, or the patient can be divided up according to the expertise of different members of the interprofessional care team. The dehumanizing effect that this fragmentation has on the health professional and the patient is illustrated in Fig. 2.1. Two guidelines toward avoiding this mistake are close attention to details about the patient as a person and use of individualized appropriate communication tools for each patient situation.

The Patient as a Person: Attention to Details

As obvious as this guideline sounds, today's stimulus-rich environment offers distractions at every turn. Pat was distracted by her desire to get out of the clinic that Friday night when Mr. Sanchez needed her full attention. Something as mundane as a cell phone buzzing at your waist can divert you from what a patient is trying to express through verbal or nonverbal means. And the care team itself can engage in conversation triggered by something the patient says or does that cuts into your line of thought and

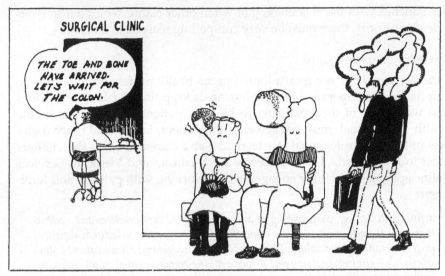

Fig. 2.1. A dehumanized view of patients. *(From Purtilo R: Kapital II: Att upprätta en relation. In Vård, vårdare, vårdad [translation: Care, care giver, receiver of care], Stockholm, 1978, Esselte Studium, p. 139.)*

attention.[6] In an era in which our attention span is shorter and shorter as a result of the constant sources of input, being self-aware, mindful, and present are important tools for actively listening to the patient's story. Shifting the conversation from "what's the matter?" to "what matters to you?" cues you to listen better and engage patients and families as genuine partners in care decisions to improve health, quality, and value.[7]

Seek Appropriate Communication Tools
Patient-centered approaches also highlight that the form of communication with the patient either can profoundly enhance your ability to arrive at a caring response or throw the focus of care off-kilter. For instance, Pat Jackson may or may not have communicated basic information to Mr. Sanchez, but a high probability exists that he would have felt more cared for as a person if she had included her interprofessional care team colleague who knew how to communicate with him in his native Spanish. With an interpreter's support, Mr. Sanchez may have opened up with more detailed information that would have provided a better clinical picture overall. And in today's technology-intensive world, new avenues of effective communication are arising. For instance, creative adaptations of video game concepts are being developed within healthcare that a few years ago would have not been imagined as a tool for patient communication and education.[8] Effective communication is so important that we devote an entire chapter to it (see Chapter 10).

Most of the discussion so far has been about direct care. However, about a decade or so ago, a group of U.S. health professionals took the challenge of a professional caring response to the level of healthcare institutional practices and policies. The Minneapolis-based consulting company, Creative Health Care Management, Inc., introduced the concept of *relationship-based care*, which emphasizes that intentional presence by healthcare providers is a catalyst that transforms care at the systems level of institutions and policies and on the interpersonal level.[9] Note the inferences to paying attention and selecting appropriate forms of communication in one of their values statements:

> *Caring is a **conscious, intentional decision** to interact with others with compassion, mutual respect **and open and honest communication**. Caring activity promotes meaningful connections between human beings and is built on the knowing that we're all in this together. Such connection facilitates healing and prevents isolation.*

◎ Summary

In your practice, you will be torn by competing claims for your attention. Your primary professional priority is the patient. Patient-centered care and relationship-based care are concepts that help remind you of this priority and enhance the probability that your response can and will be tailored to suit each individual.

Three Characteristics of a Caring Response

So far, you have learned that a professional caring response is not a set formula (i.e., it cannot be bottled) and that, at the same time, some general guidelines that point in that direction are paying attention to each person as a unique individual and working toward effective communication. Attention is now turned to how a professional caring response can further be understood with a comparison of conduct appropriate in the health professional–patient relationship and that for other significant relationships.

Navigation Between Friendly and Professional Conduct

A professional caring response includes aspects of conduct that are identical to the ones you show toward a friend or relative. So, let us begin with your own experience.

 Reflection
If you have been to a physician, therapist, or other health professional for an ailment recently, what are some aspects of your exchange that

were similar to those you might have with a friend or family member and that you would characterize as signs of their care for you?

_____

_____

If you listed some things you each did that were sensitive to making each other comfortable, showed mutual regard for the other, or were light and in appropriate good humor, they are apt examples of everyday caring relationships. These are the human sensitivities, affection, and politeness that also bolster a patient's belief that you care about him or her.[10] This friendly caring calls on your creativity to meet another person in ways consistent with that person's personality and unique needs. It may include taking the extra few minutes to attend to a bedridden patient's personal hygiene needs (e.g., putting her water glass and toothbrush within reach), decreasing physical discomfort (e.g., offering a support pillow or straight-back chair), or complimenting a patient. Acknowledging a patient's birthday or anniversary can bring a smile. And the professional caring that is in common with other human relationships also goes deeper, of course, so that basic trust and appreciation develop between you. Given just the little we know about Pat Jackson and Mr. Sanchez, this is a good moment to reflect on some things she could have done to show basic human caring toward him.

Summary

A caring response includes common everyday expressions of kindness and thoughtfulness that create trust and lay foundations of a professional relationship.

At the same time, a health professional's relationships with patients are different too, with moral and legal dimensions not fully applicable to other relationships. Therefore a caring response must mean something more than common everyday expressions of affection, nurturance, or protectiveness associated with care.

Reflection
Examine the picture of these friends in Fig. 2.2. What do you see that may not seem appropriate for a health professional–patient relationship?

_____

_____

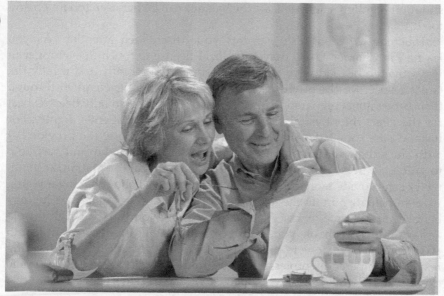

Fig. 2.2. Friend relationship is pictured (vs. a health professional–patient relationship). *(From iStock: iStock.com/peepo.)*

Their physical proximity is one cautionary message. A governing characteristic of your professional caring response is that you must not cross psychological, physical, and sexual boundaries that could make the patient responsible or responsive to you in ways that go outside of (or create opposition to) the healing core of the relationship.[11] For instance, if you have just been faced with a big disappointment, pouring your heart out to a patient like you would to a friend not only may take attention from the patient's issues but also may create a feeling that you are the one who came to be cared for instead of the patient. An apt question to ask yourself is "Does my conduct help keep the patient and me focused on the health-related matters that I am competent to address through extensive training in my field?" This point of difference is what distinguishes you and members of the patient's interprofessional care team from other caring people in the patient's life. Communication also figures in regarding the type of information you solicit from the patient. And so a second question to ask yourself is, "What do I and the team need to know about the patient to provide the best care possible?" You will likely come to know other things too, but your intent should be guided by this "need to know." Pat did not cross the line of personal sharing—she could have explained to Mr. Sanchez that she was running late for another appointment. Instead, her conduct suggests to the reader that she may have erred on the side of not taking the initiative to solicit enough "need to know" information about his history and symptoms. Their situation highlights how delicate the balance can be between too much and too little.

Touching a patient also warrants your disciplined attention. As you learned in Chapter 1, you may have legal license to touch this stranger in ways that go beyond what a nonprofessional can morally and legally do. Great respect for the privileges health professionals have earned through their professional preparation must be enveloped in an equally deep respect for the effect the physical contact may have on the patient's dignity. For instance, the knowledge that Mr. Sanchez is a farm laborer can provide Pat with clues about the environment in which he lives each day and may help to guide her in how to approach him. His age, sexual orientation, and ethnicity can provide more clues as to how he may feel about having a young woman palpate him on the face, neck, or trunk and ask questions he may believe are a private matter. As a reader making your way through the examples in this textbook, you will be able to further flesh out what health professionals have done in different situations to provide a friendly caring response tempered by professional role boundaries and to identify ways to exercise the discipline of staying focused on the patient's needs.

Care Expressed Through Technical Competence

A professional caring response depends on competently and conscientiously carrying out your professional duties. The bottom line is that, without *technical competence* or expertise, the goal of a caring response cannot be achieved. The patient's trust goes beyond the hope that you will offer a kind or even generous personal response to the clinical issue that has brought this person to you. Your technical expertise places you in a unique position to aid persons in maintaining or regaining health (or relief of suffering or a peaceful death) in ways that they cannot achieve without you. Fortunately, professionals today can rely more than ever before on evidence-based practices that help ensure optimal clinical outcomes.

Many clinical approaches make use of the tools of modern medical technology. The concern that technology will take the place of more traditional types of hands-on treatments often is discussed in the literature.[12] Because both professionals and patients are at risk of putting too much trust in what technology can do, misuse can lead to untoward or harmful effects and you will benefit by taking advantage of the caveats as well as the opportunities that modern technological discoveries in your field offer.[13] However, that being said, technology is an important extension of more traditional understandings of how to apply one's technical expertise and should be welcomed. Moreover, the interprofessional care team enhances the likelihood of success; their combined technical expertise distinguishes what one professional acting alone can achieve from the combined competence of all. The well-coordinated efforts of the team give patients the best chance of feeling that their dignity as a whole person is upheld. In short, competent application of your technical skills is in itself an essential component of a caring response.

Summary
A professional caring response includes the conscientious expression of technical competence. In most cases, the optimal result is reached through the coordinated efforts of the interprofessional care team because the many faceted aspects of the patient's situation can be more fully assessed. Modern technology is an asset when used wisely as a tool of technical competence.

Care as Professional Responsibility

The idea of a caring response is also partially captured in the common phrase *professional responsibility*. In legal language, professional responsibility can be summarized with the term *due care*. Due care specifies what is reasonably expected of you in your role as a provider of professional service to a particular purpose.[14] You can see how technical expertise applies to this idea. Before we go into more detail, take a minute to draw on your common sense idea of responsibility.

Reflection

Previously in this chapter, you had an opportunity to identify some competing claims on you as you move through this day. Take it a bit further now and try to describe your understanding of your responsibilities to yourself or others involved in each of those claims.

_____

_____

_____

_____

Accountability and Responsiveness

From an ethical point of view, one of the most helpful interpretations of professional responsibility is that described by theologian Richard Niebuhr in his now classic book *The Responsible Self*.[15]

Professional responsibility = Accountability + Responsiveness

Accountability. The most common understanding of professional responsibility associated with the health professions grows out of the western philosophical traditions that emphasize the individual's functions in upholding the moral life. *Accountability,* holding one to account for one's actions, assumes that one is not only capable of acting in a certain way and has the appropriate knowledge to do so but is also free to go ahead unimpeded. Once those conditions are met, your decisions rest entirely with you.

Accountability also implies that an ethical standard exists against which one's actions can be measured. Recall that the ethical gold standard of healthcare is to uphold the patient's dignity. In one form or another, all accountability is related to upholding the dignity of ourselves and those with whom we are in a relationship. If you go back to examine your own profession's code of ethics through the lens of accountability, you will note that it is very duty oriented and describes the basic characteristics and conduct expected of anyone in your field. In that regard, we could all benefit from the sign that former U.S. President Harry Truman kept on his desk, "The Buck Stops Here," which means "I am the one who has to finally answer to what happens in those relationships where I am entrusted to uphold human dignity. In these situations, I deserve to be held to account."

Your own list of claims likely evoked different kinds of accountabilities you know that you and others are counting on to keep your relationships from self-destructing. Whether with a friend or spouse, with a patient, or sitting at the desk of a president, a caring response requires accountability. As you can quickly discern, accountability can also lead to abuse of the power invested in one by virtue of one's societal role. Part of a caring response in the health professions is not to take advantage of that position. It is within this framework that Niebuhr proposes the necessary complement of responsiveness.

Responsiveness. An important contribution by Niebuhr often overlooked in ethical discussions of responsibility is that it is relational. Accountability, taken alone, is unidirectional and does not require a detailed understanding of what one is being accountable *to,* and *why. Responsiveness* requires willingness to engage with the other to try to gain a deep understanding of the person or group to whom one is accountable and a willingness to adapt conduct to honor them. With this, we are back in the territory of paying attention to and communicating effectively with the other, those essential general ingredients of a professional caring response. The importance of adding responsiveness to the concept of responsibility is emphasized in this excerpt by ethicist Thomas Ogletree, who also highlights how creative a process effective caring is:

> *Responsive judgments are guided by the notion of what is fitting. The fitting action may be largely self-evident once we have grasped what is morally at stake in a situation. Yet it may emerge only gradually, through the thoughtful balancing of multiple variables in their negative and positive features. Moral imagination and discernment are as important to this balancing process as are conceptual precision and logical rigor. The reasoning involved, moreover, is often more akin to weaving a tapestry than to forging a chain.*[16]

Reflection

Given these insights, jot down some aspects of Mr. Sanchez's situation to which Pat Jackson and her colleagues must be responsive in choosing a course of action that meets the general requirements of accountability.

_____

_____

_____

In Chapter 4, you will be introduced to some approaches to ethics that show how over time the field itself is increasingly acknowledging the contributions of the patient's story in the professional's deliberation about morally right conduct that aligns with providing a caring response

Professional Responsibility and Rights

As you know, the idea of rights plays prominently in ethical and legal discourse regarding our responsibility toward each other, animals, and the environment. What is a right? Basically a *right* is a concept that identifies stringent claims or demands of one person or group on another. If I present you with something that is my right, you must honor this quality or need in me. The weight of your demand creates a duty for me to respond to it. For instance, in a founding document of the United States, the Declaration of Independence, we find the phrase that Americans are "endowed" with the rights of life, liberty, and the pursuit of happiness. If I have a right to life, you have a duty to help protect it and you certainly must not rob me of it. Therefore rights and duties are inextricably linked, although as you will learn in Chapter 4, not all duty-driven ethical theories or approaches rely (historically speaking) on the relatively recent concept of rights.

When rights are interpreted as applying to everyone alike, they are said to be *human rights*. The core idea of human rights is that they are an important means of expressing a common hope for humanity that flows beneath differences of culture, civilization, and ways of life, like the magma that flows beneath the earth's varied surface. We are born to nourish our life individually and as a society, and we have invented the language of human rights to try to help us understand what we must do to make this nourishment available to everyone when we are different in so many external ways.

Some rights are associated with healthcare and the health professional–patient relationship in the United States and other countries. Healthcare itself is viewed as a right in many parts of the world.

Reflection
If you think back to the relationship between Mr. Sanchez and Pat
Jackson, what do you believe are the rights of each?
The patient, Mr. Sanchez's, rights:

_____

_____

_____

_____

The health professional, Pat Jackson's, rights:

_____

_____

_____

_____

Compare what you wrote with the following commonly cited rights of
patients and health professionals.

The patient has a right to:
• Respect from the health professionals and healthcare system
• A clean and welcoming environment
• High-quality care
• Confidentiality of sensitive information
• Shared decision making about course of treatment
• Truthful information about one's condition to enhance self-determination
  about what to do in regard to treatment options

Health professionals have a right to:
• Respect from the patient
• Relevant information necessary for treatment to be effective
• Freedom to freely exercise clinical best judgment (i.e., professional
  autonomy)
• Fair payment for professional services

Critics of rights approaches point out that an emphasis on rights in healthcare has the following shortcomings:
• Rights are highly individualistic and emphasize the demands of one
  individual or group on another, thereby often obscuring their common
  interests or other interests that also are relevant to the situation.
• When rights conflict, very little within rights approaches exists to help to
  resolve the problem.

- Rights often are too general for the responder to determine which duties adequately meet the demand for a response. An example is the right to healthcare. My demand for health-related services based on my right to healthcare can be interpreted by you as anything from a right to a band-aid to all the services and goods you can provide.

Health professionals must pay attention to rights language found in ethics codes, policy statements, or institutional documents; in licensing laws; and in use by colleagues or patients. In each case, the language is designed to urgently summon a caring response to a request that is embedded in the demand. Your professional responsibility is to discern the particulars of such a response. You will discover that no one formula for implementing a professional caring response based on human rights fits all patients any more than it fits all nations, cultures, or civilizations. However, use of rights as a general guide takes the professional a long way toward understanding what is involved.

⊚ Summary

A professional caring response includes a specific understanding of responsibility toward others that includes accountability and responsiveness. A deep understanding of responsibility has evolved through the language of rights. Rights are stringent claims on someone else or society for a caring response to a person's or group's needs. Human rights usually are viewed as universal needs such as food, shelter, healthcare, and the protection of life itself. Rights claims may come from both health professionals and patients and help to shape professional responsibility and summon a truly caring response.

Sociocultural Determinants of a Caring Response

So far in this chapter, you have been reading about ways the goal of a professional caring response can be met. Several important such determinants are the challenges and opportunities that result from the rich diversity of patients, families, and other care providers. We will discuss them briefly here to support you in the delivery of evidence-based, client-centered, and compassionate care.

Cultural Differences

One key consideration is the rich, racial, ethnic, and cultural diversity of humans. Professionals and patients not only come in all sizes and shapes but also bring to their relationships their personal and group identities associated with their race, ethnicity, age, gender, sexual identity, sexual orientation, religion, geography, socioeconomical standing, nationality, and education. Together, these traits compose a person's or group's culture and help determine their understanding of health and how it should be addressed. *Cultural competence* is "an ongoing process in which the health-care professional continually strives to achieve the ability and availability to work effectively within the cultural context of the patient."[17] It includes not only ethnicity and race, but the intersection of ethnicity, race, gender, age, class, education, religion, sexual orientation, and physical ability, along with the unequal distribution of power and the existence of social inequi-ties.[18] Cultural competence is supported by an inclusive environment that upholds dignity and respect for all. To demonstrate cultural competence, all health professionals must engage in self-reflection and personal critique to nurture *cultural humility*. Cultural humility promotes cultural awareness, interpersonal sensitivity, reflection on power imbalances, learning from dif-ferences, and openness in clinical encounters.[19] It allows health profession-als to avoid unfair conscious or unconscious judgments or oppressive biases about other people's traditions, values, and beliefs. When we demonstrate cultural humility, we are more likely to understand and respect a patient's decision or action. Health professionals who engage in the lifelong process of cultural awareness engage more fully with their patients and meet their moral commitment to serve all patients, regardless of their cultural values, beliefs, or practices.

Reflection
What assumptions can you make about the cultural differences between Pat Jackson and Mr. Sanchez from the small amount of information you have about each of these parties?

_____

_____

Cultural differences among members of the interprofessional care team may also raise challenges and opportunities for effective teamwork.

Reflection
Look around the room of your classroom or clinic. What observations can you make about the cultural differences between you and your colleagues from the information you have about each of them?

_____

_____

Observations are an integral part of good clinical assessment. Reflec-tion on observations provides an opportunity to acknowledge key differ-ences and work through assumptions so that they need not be a barrier to achieving a caring response for the patient. Sometimes the smallest things can make the biggest impact.

Limited Resources and Justice Considerations

Several external factors can influence the good intent of a caring response being realized, and together, they can be recognized as *social determinants of health.* The World Health Organization defines social determinants of health as "the conditions in which people are born, grow, live, work and age. These circumstances are shaped by the distribution of money, power and resources at global, national and local levels."[20] Social determinants of health are mostly responsible for *health inequities*—the unfair and avoidable differences in health status seen within and between individuals, populations, and/or countries. Addressing social determinants of health is an essential step in improving health outcomes and reducing health disparities. Social determinants of health include factors such as race, socioeconomical status, education, neighborhood and physical environment, employment, and social support networks, as well as access to healthcare.[21] The ethical idea of *justice,* addressed in later chapters of this book and the focus of the final section, requires you to take into account how a particular important good or service can be distributed fairly among persons with similar needs. The rub comes when a limited supply of the valued good such as money, beds, or equipment, or even clinics, prevents professionals from providing enough of the valued good to a patient to satisfy what an optimal care plan requires. It also arises when there is a limited supply of health professionals or the time each can devote to a patient. If you think back to the rights discussion in this chapter, you can understand the moral bind this puts the professional in because rights suggest that your duty is to give each and every patient what he or she needs, and the full extent of meeting that expectation cannot always be met.

Limitation reminds us that ours is not a perfect world. Theories of distributive justice are available to help professionals think through the options. Policies and practices that focus on fairness are attempts to help come to the professional's rescue and are included for your more thorough consideration in later chapters

Limited Resources and Unjust Practices

At the same time, seemingly unjust policies and practices that arbitrarily tie the professional's hands sometimes occur.[22] A concern in the United States shared by many professionals (and prospective patients) is access to healthcare, in particular how it is made available, and how to ensure it is free of bias and discriminatory practices. Policies that give disproportionate advantage to those who are economically much better off are judged as one injustice in the U.S. system.

To better understand the relationship between Pat Jackson and Mr. Sanchez from the larger perspectives of sociocultural and justice considerations, consider the follow-up to what happened after he left the clinic.

 The Story of Pat Jackson, the Interprofessional Care Team, and Mr. Sanchez (continued)

During the interprofessional care team meeting the week after her interaction with Mr. Sanchez, Pat had the haunting feeling that she may have misdiagnosed Mr. Sanchez's problem. In the ensuing discussion, she was made more acutely aware that asthma can be a serious life-threatening health problem for the migrant field workers because it is exacerbated by allergic responses to pollen. Being so new to the environment and this population of patients, she previously had not been fully cognizant of this fact.

Pat also had not been employed at the clinic long enough to know that many migrant workers come with no healthcare coverage, but this, too, came up at the meeting. The administration of the health system in which the clinic is situated has not been supportive of the clinic giving the migrant workers the same welcome as "paying customers" and follow-up often falls short of ensuring effective long-term clinical management of the problem. Although this policy has not been put in writing, at the team meeting, several members expressed increasing distress at the quiet pressure they have felt to do only the minimal and move this population of patients out.

This increased Pat's own concern about her lack of diligence. "I should have documented his wheezing more fully," she thought. "If everyone who saw migrant workers would document their own distress about the suffering of these patients, our reports over time could have an impact on the hospital administrators who are the primary policymakers." This knowledge gave her sufficient motivation to make an appointment with the attending physician on the team to discuss her own distress further. He reminded her that owning up to one's shortcomings or mistakes as she had done is part of how good teamwork can continue to maintain its standard of excellence and that she had done the right thing by bringing it up at the meeting. He showed sympathy for how this could have happened because she was so new to this environment but also reminded her that due diligence is always required.[23]

The very next Friday, Mr. Sanchez was brought in by his supervisor, this time in acute respiratory distress. The receptionist helped him onto a stretcher and into a clinic booth, where a nurse placed an oxygen mask over his face and took his vital signs. The attending physician stood ready to perform resuscitation if necessary, frowning while he scanned the patient's clinical record. "Serious asthma attack," he said to the nurse. "Glad you were right here!" Pat hovered near the curtain of the treatment booth, her heart pounding. Now she knew beyond a doubt that she had misdiagnosed his problem during his initial visit. She was ambivalent about joining the nurse and doctor but felt a wave of gratitude to these teammates for being there.

New thoughts went through her mind. What if she was shunned by patients in this population because the word got out that she was not competent to treat them? Worse yet, what if stress and fear prevented the migrant workers from seeking medical care?[24] And what about her clinic's pride in providing quality care to Mr. Sanchez's previously underserved Latin community, even in spite of the administration's current resistance? Where would that community find clinical care if not with them?

Later that evening, Pat emailed her entire team to say that she wanted to be an agent in supporting the team's efforts to work with the administration toward a more just solution for the migrant population and other rural community members who could not access treatment. She wrote that her own commitment as a caregiver must include efforts to change policy or practices that seemed unfair (or at least required closer scrutiny) and offered to work with administration to find a more workable solution. She assured the others that she understood the institution's need to survive fiscally but that this should never warrant discrimination against a given population to balance the books. She invited others to join her because together they would probably increase the likelihood of coming up with strategies that would encourage the administration to invite discourse and, hopefully, make some changes.

In this follow-up to the first part of the story, we can see more clearly how attentiveness to patient diversity, justice considerations, and the professional's participation at the policy level are part and parcel of how a professional caring response is realized. The creative energies that lead to job satisfaction over the long haul can emerge to support these extended efforts at improving care.

Summary

A professional caring response must be understood within the limits of constraints imposed by bias, lack of cultural competence, limited resources, and unjust practices. Professionals are morally obligated to gain cultural proficiency and actively address the root sources of challenges to care imposed by limited resources and unjust practices or policies.

Burdens and Benefits of a Caring Response

At the core of all your caring, you have to be in touch with caring for yourself. That in turn means looking at all the ways caring in your professional role affects you. A caring response is such a fundamental goal in the health professions that sometimes the real burden and benefits of engaging in the professional relationship are overlooked. Hopefully this last section of this chapter helps rectify the oversight.

The Burden of Care

Although care is usually cast in a positive light for good reason, it is easy to ignore the reality that searching for a caring response and acting according to what it requires of you is a burden at times.

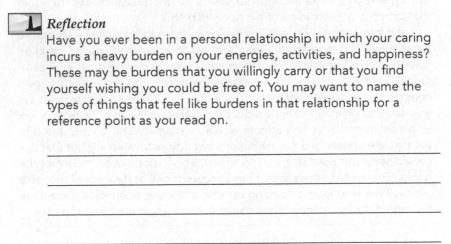

Reflection

Have you ever been in a personal relationship in which your caring incurs a heavy burden on your energies, activities, and happiness? These may be burdens that you willingly carry or that you find yourself wishing you could be free of. You may want to name the types of things that feel like burdens in that relationship for a reference point as you read on.

_____

_____

_____

_____

The burden of caring is not limited to personal relationships. When students in a graduate course in the health professions were asked to be brutally honest with themselves about negative feelings they had at times about caregiving, some expressed feelings that made them question if they were unfit for their professional role.

The answer is, not necessarily. It goes beyond the purpose of this text to unpack all the underlying conditions that might lead a professional to make such statements regarding the feelings about caring that arise from time to time. In Chapter 6, in which the focus is explicitly on caring for yourself, you will have an opportunity to explore how to overcome barriers to your own caring for others or find support that helps you not govern your responses to patients. For the time being, you have an opportunity to use this insight to prepare yourself for situations in which you do not automatically warm up to finding the caring response for a particular patient. We find it reassuring, for instance, that the burden Pat carried about her relationship with Mr. Sanchez was offset in part by her insight into the bigger picture of how she could express care at the larger institutional level. Although this cannot substitute for keeping the patient at the center of one's caring, it does help to keep the bandwidth of expressions of care before the reader.

Benefits for the Caregiver

Fortunately, overall, the amount of negative burden a caring response incurs usually is small compared with the benefits. Developmental psychology tells us that one of the most important ways in which adults gain a recognized place in society is through their contributions to that society's well-being. Professional caregiving benefits you by putting you in a position to participate in activities that society respects. For most health professionals, caregiving is also a basis for self-fulfillment and job satisfaction. Many can relate to the line in the prayer of Saint Francis of Assisi, "It is in giving that we receive." What do professionals receive? You often hear those who have been in the field for a long time recount how much their work has given them, including remarkable insights into their own humanness, in both its vulnerability and strengths; how they have been inspired by patients' "will to live" or gumption to continue on in spite of seemingly great challenges; and how the kindness and gratitude of patients and families help keep the professional going. What the research shows and most clinicians experience is that relationships with patients are the most meaningful and rewarding aspect of work as a health professional.[25]

How then does this understanding and awareness help to shape a truly caring response to a patient's situation? Your part in engendering mutual respect for what each offers the other as humans must burn at the core of the relationship. We can catch a glimpse of this when Pat Jackson began to take a second look at who Mr. Sanchez was when he came back a second time. It became an occasion for her to learn something important about herself and the kind of professional she wanted to be. It was an occasion for her to feel gratitude toward her team members who now were showing such care toward him. She had to move toward acknowledging that the primary thing an individual professional or interprofessional care team can offer is to tap into a patient's or group's desire of healthfulness and try to support it.

Summary
Although caring involves burdens for most professionals, they find that the benefits outweigh the burdens. A professional's acknowledgment of caring as a basic competence and resource tips the balance toward the likelihood that all, including themselves, benefit in the professional encounter.

Summary

This discussion of the ethical goal of a professional caring response supports thoughtful exploration into ways that care warrants special attention as health professionals strive to refine their unique contributions to individuals and societies. Looking ahead to the next chapters, you will be introduced to ethical challenges that present themselves in different forms or prototypes: moral distress and ethical dilemmas. Both call for you, the professional, to be guided by the goal of a caring response. You are now ready to take what you have learned about a caring response into the specifics of recognizing an ethical issue and submitting the situation to ethical analysis in your search for an ethically acceptable resolution and informed action. Indeed, for the rest of the text, the reader will be brought back time and again to the central role of care.

Questions for Thought and Discussion

1. As a health professional, you will be expected to provide a caring response to all kinds of people. Which populations of patients do you think will be the most difficult to truly *care* for and why? Give some specific examples of behaviors or other characteristics that you think would make caring about and for such patients especially challenging.
2. Describe a medical or dental visit in which something happened to make you feel that the professional's attention was not centered on you. What happened? What could the professionals and others in that environment have done to make you feel more like they were motivated by the goal of a caring response to you?
3. The emergency departments of major hospitals are a whirlwind of activity, with many life or death situations for patients who literally have just come through the door. When asked to reflect on care in the emergency room, a young nurse recently said to one of the authors, "There's no time for hand-holding here. We are too busy; it's life-or-death interventions 24-7."
   a. What are some examples of how the emergency room interprofessional care team can demonstrate a caring response to patients?
   b. Now do the same exercise in an operating room setting.
   c. And finally, do the exercise as an interprofessional care team member working in a locked residence for patients with advanced Alzheimer's disease.

References

1. Personal correspondence with Simon W. Davison, director, *LOK, LLC*, Oxford, England, August 1, 2014.
2. Harris JC: Toward a restorative medicine: the science of care, *JAMA* 301(16): 1710–1712, 2009.
3. Nelson W, editor: *Handbook for rural health care ethics: a practical guide for professionals*, Lebanon, NH, 2009, University Press of New England. Available at http://geiselmed. dartmouth. edu/cfm/resources/ethics/.

4. Interprofessional Education Collaborative: *Core competencies for interprofessional collaborative practice: 2016 update.* Washington, DC, 2016. Available at www. ipecollaborative.org/resources.html.

5. Center for Medicare and Medicaid Service: Person and family engagement strategy: sharing with our partners, 2019. Available at https://www.cms.gov/ Medicare/Quality-Initiatives-Patient-Assessment-Instruments/QualityInitia- tivesGenInfo/Downloads/Person-and-Family-Engagement-Strategy-Summary. pdf.

6. Charon R: *Narrative medicine: honouring stories of illness,* New York, 2006, Oxford University Press.

7. Institute for Healthcare Improvement (2017). *Person- and family-centered care overview.* Available at http://www.ihi.org/Topics/PFCC/Pages/Overview.aspx.

8. Loria K: *Game on: PT in MOTION,* August 2014, Alexandria, VA, 2014, American Physical Therapy Association, pp 16–21.

9. Koloroutis M, editor: *Relationship-based care: a model for transforming practice,* Minneapolis, 2004, Creative Health Care Management.

10. Kahn MW: Etiquette-based medicine, *N Engl J Med* 358(19):1988–1989, 2008.

11. Haddad A, Doherty R, Purtilo R: Professional boundaries guided by re- spect. *Health professional and patient interaction,* ed 9, St. Louis, 2019, Elsevier, pp 28–40.

12. Gutmann A: The ethics of synthetic biology: guiding principles for emerging technologies, *Hastings Cent Rep* 41(4):17–22, 2011.

13. Doherty RF: The impact of advances in medical technology on rehabilitative care. In Purtilo RB, Jensen GM, Brasic Royeen C, editors: *Educating for moral ac- tion: a sourcebook in health and rehabilitation ethics,* Philadelphia, 2005, FA Davis, pp 99–106.

14. Garner BA: *Black's law dictionary,* ed 10, Eagan, MN, 2014, Thomson West Publishing.

15. Niebuhr HR: *The responsible self: an essay in Christian moral philosophy,* New York, 1963, Harper and Row.

16. Ogletree T: Responsibility. In Post SG, editor: *Encyclopedia of bioethics,* ed 3, New York, 2004, Macmillan Reference USA Thomson Gale, pp 2379–2384 (quote, 2383).

17. Campinha-Bacote J: Patient-centered care in the midst of a cultural conflict: the role of cultural competence, *Online J Issues Nurs* 16(2).1, 2011.

18. Chiarenza A: Developments in the concept of 'cultural competence. In Ingleby D, Chiarenza A, Devillé W, Kotsioni I, editors: *Inequalities in health care for mi- grants and ethnic minorities (66-81),* Antwerp, 2012, Garant.

19. Campinha-Bacote J. Cultural competemility: a paradigm shift in the cultural competence versus cultural humility debate–Part I. *Online J Issues Nurs,* Jan 1;24(1), 2019.

20. World Health Organization. *The social determinants of health.* Available at https://www.who.int/social_determinants/sdh_definition/en/.

21. Artiga S, Hinton E: Beyond health care: the role of social determinants in promoting health and health equity, *Health* 20:10, 2018.
22. Grace P: Professional responsibility, human rights and injustice. In Grace P, editor: *Nursing ethics and professional responsibility*, Sudbury, MA, 2009, Jones and Bartlett Publishers, pp. 107–131.
23. Purtilo RB: What interprofessional teamwork taught me about an ethics of care, *Phys Ther Rev* 17(3):197–201, 2012.
24. Kuczewski Mark: Clinical ethicists awakened: addressing two generations of clinical ethics issues involving undocumented patients, *Am J Bioeth* 19(4): 51–57, 2019. doi: 10.1080/15265161.2019.1572812.
25. Chou CM, Kellum K, Shea JA: Attitudes and habits of highly humanistic physicians, *Acad Med* 89(9):1252–1258, 2014.

● 3

Prototypes of Ethical Problems

Objectives

The reader should be able to:
- Recognize an ethical question and distinguish it from a strictly clinical or legal one.
- Identify three component parts of any ethical problem.
- Describe what an agent is and, more importantly, what it is to be a moral agent.
- Name two prototypical ethical problems.
- Distinguish between two varieties of moral distress.
- Compare the fundamental difference between moral distress and an ethical dilemma.
- Describe the role of emotions in moral distress and ethical dilemmas.
- Discuss the role of locus of authority considerations in ethical problem solving.
- Identify four criteria to assist in deciding who should assume authority for an ethical decision to achieve a caring response.
- Describe how shared agency functions in ethical problem solving.
- Describe a type of ethical dilemma that challenges a professional's desire (and duty) to treat everyone fairly and equitably.

New terms and ideas you will encounter in this chapter

legal question	clinical question	shared agency
disability benefits	agent	moral distress
ethical question	moral agent	moral residue
prototype	locus of authority	ethical dilemma

Topics in this chapter introduced in earlier chapters	
Topic	Introduced in chapter
Ethical problem	1
Integrity	1
Interprofessional care team	1
Professional responsibility	2
A caring response	2
Accountability	2
Sociocultural determinants of health	2
Justice	2

Introduction

You have come a long way already and are prepared to take the next steps toward becoming skilled in the art of ethical decision making. The first part of this chapter guides you through an inquiry regarding how to know when you are faced with an ethical question instead of (or in addition to) a clinical or legal question. A further question is raised: How do you know whether the situation that raised the question is a problem that requires your involvement? This chapter helps you prepare to answer that question, too. You will learn the basic components of an ethical problem and be introduced to two prototypes of ethical problems. We start with the story of Bill Boyd and Kate Lindy.

 The Story of Bill Boyd and Kate Lindy

Bill Boyd is a 25-year-old soldier who lives in a large city. Bill served in the U.S. Army for more than 6 years and was deployed to both Iraq and Afghanistan for multiple military missions in the past 4 years. During his final deployment, Bill suffered a blast injury resulting in significant shoulder and neck trauma, a mild traumatic brain injury (TBI), and posttraumatic stress. He was treated in an inpatient military hospital and transitioned back to his hometown, where he moved into his childhood home with his mother.

Kate Lindy is the outpatient psychologist who has been treating Bill for pain and posttraumatic stress. Bill is in a structured civilian reentry program. This competitive program is administered by a government subcontractor; its goal is to help injured veterans find meaningful careers or employment on return from the front lines. Bill reports that he is struggling with the transition to civilian life. He originally was prompt in keeping his appointments but recently has missed almost all of his sessions. Twice Bill has arrived for his appointment more than 30 minutes late and smelling of alcohol. Kate informed Bill that she could not treat him in this condition and that if he continued to arrive in this state, she would need to discontinue therapy. Bill responded to Kate and said, "You have no idea what all of this is like. And don't even go there on the alcohol; like you have never had a drink on a bad day."

Kate is concerned about Bill. She calls his home and gets no answer. She then calls the case manager listed on his intake form. Kate tells the case manager about Bill's regularly missed appointments (three in the last 4 weeks). She also tells the case manager that Bill has been charged for the missed visits because he has not called to cancel, which is the billing policy of the institution where Kate is employed.

The manager responds that Bill does not qualify for transitional career/ employment services unless he is compliant with all outpatient care. She adds that in her experience patients like Bill have a hard time adjusting to the fact that they are no longer eligible for active duty.

The case manager says she will talk to Bill about the unacceptability of his failing to let the therapist know when he decides not to keep his appointment. In fact, if Bill keeps that up, the case manager continues, he will be kicked out of the civilian reentry program because the government cannot be expected to pay for his lack of responsibility. Kate responds that maybe Bill was unclear about the policy. The manager replies, "It doesn't matter. He's an army man; he knows better than that."

A week goes by. At the scheduled time for Bill's appointment, he again does not appear. Kate has been uneasy about the conversation with the manager, and when the time comes for her to fill out the billing slip for another missed appointment, she feels positively terrible.

Reflection

Do you share Kate's feelings that something is not right? If yes, what do you think the problem is? Jot down a few thoughts here and refer back to them as the chapter progresses.

_____

_____

_____

_____

Recognizing an Ethical Question

Health professionals face all types of questions in clinical practice. Some are ethical questions, others are not. Many times what may appear to be an ethical question is in fact something else, such as a miscommunication or a question about a clinical fact or a legal issue. Often complex clinical situations include clinical, legal, and ethical questions; part of your challenge is to distinguish them and sort them out for their relevance to the patient and the delivery of care.

The following exercise is designed to walk you through one example of an issue that includes clinical, legal, and ethical dimensions, with a description of why the last is an ethical question.

Is this an ethical question? Answer Yes or No:

Can a person status post traumatic brain injury (TBI) drive?

If you answered "no," you are correct. This is a *clinical question* because clinical tests and procedures can help answer it. Patients who pass various cognitive assessments and an on-road driving evaluation have the clinical ability to drive, and those who fail do not. Refer back to the story at the beginning of this chapter. In the narrative about Bill Boyd, Kate Lindy, and the case manager, what additional clinical information can help you better evaluate the situation?

Now consider the following question:

Must patients status post TBI comply with medical advice if they want to continue to drive?

Is this a clinical, legal, or ethical question? If you said "a *legal question*," you are on the right track. A tip-off is the word "must." As you learned in Chapter 1, the laws of the state and other laws are designed to monitor public well-being and enforce practices that protect the public good. Almost all states include procedures to help ensure road safety. Relevant information about people who are dangerous behind the wheel is found in part through clinical examinations. Clinical and legal systems are interdependent in that and other situations, so the decision to ignore clinical recommendations is not always up to an individual patient.

Now, go to the specific legal implications of Bill Boyd's situation. When the physician referred Bill for therapy, she assessed that the patient's discomfort was from a combat-related injury. The time may come when Bill wants to apply for *disability benefits* for his condition. Veterans disability benefits are legally enforced governmental programs in the United States to help protect members of the military from financial duress when injured during service duty. So a related legal question relevant to this situation is: Do patients have the right to benefits provided by the government if for any reason they miss prescribed treatment and the professional reports this?

Benefit eligibility usually requires that a patient comply with prescribed treatments; the fact that Bill missed multiple treatments may compromise his case. The case manager may choose to fight Bill's claim for disability benefits now that Kate has contacted the manager with this information.

Finally, consider this question, which is an *ethical question*. As you read it, think about why it is an ethical question.

● *Should people with TBIs who refuse to take a recommended on-road driving assessment be allowed to continue driving? If so, under what circumstances?*

The word "should" is the tip-off here. It points to something in society all have agreed to support, and each individual has a responsibility to help do so. Kate's reflection on whether she should have talked with Bill's case manager and her ambivalence about having to charge for treatments that she did not administer are examples of ethical questions about the wrongdoing or rightness of her actions that she was pondering.

⊚ Summary

Ethical questions can be distinguished from strictly clinical or legal questions, although all of these questions often arise in health professional and patient situations. An ethical question places the focus on one's role as a moral agent and those aspects of the situation that involve moral values, duties, and quality-of-life concerns in an effort to arrive at a caring response.

For your continued learning, several prototypes of ethical problems, into which many different everyday ethical questions will fit, are now introduced.

Prototypes of Ethical Problems: Common Features

What is a *prototype*? Prototypes are a society's attempt to name a basic category of something. Prototypes can be objects, concepts, ideas, or situations.[1] Prototypes of ethical problems are recognizable as a group by three features they have in common. Each of the prototypes in this chapter appears different from the others; in fact, each has a different role to play when ethical questions have arisen. That said, the first step into this venture is to become familiar with the same basic structural features found in all the prototypes of ethical problems:

A: A moral agent (or agents)
C: A course of action
O: An outcome
Each feature is discussed in turn.

The Moral Agent: A

Which of the following best describes your idea of a health professional as an agent?

A. A person with more than one basic loyalty; a deeply divided loyalty (e.g., a double agent).
B. A person who has the moral or legal capacity to make decisions and be held responsible for them (e.g., a signee on a contract).
C. A person who plans schedules or events (e.g., a booking agent).

If you answered "B," you are most clearly focused on the meaning of agency in the health profession roles you will assume. In ethics or law, an *agent* is anyone responsible for the course of action chosen and the outcome of that action in a specific situation. Obviously, being an agent requires that a person is able to understand the situation and be free to act voluntarily. Acting as an agent also implies intention: The person wants something specific to happen as a result of that action. A *moral agent* is a person who "acts for himself or herself, or in the place of another by the authority of that person, and does so by conforming to a standard of right behavior."[2]

Reflection

This book emphasizes your role as a moral agent in the health profession setting because, as a professional, you must answer for your own actions and attitudes. If you have observed a situation in which someone in your chosen field has had to act courageously, then you have observed a moral agent at work. Briefly describe what you observed and why you feel the responsibility fell to that person to be on the front line of the decision.

_____

_____

_____

_____

A moral agent intends the morally right course of action. The idea of responsibility that you learned about in Chapter 2 is in fact the description of what an agent does; when faced with an ethical challenge in the health professions, the actor assumes the role of a moral agent. Professional responsibility is exercised through moral agency, and professional accountability and responsiveness to the patient through ethical action. Kate and the case manager are both agents whose actions influence the outcome of Kate's efforts and affect Bill's health. As a health professional, Kate clearly is in the role of a moral agent.

Agents and Emotion

Moral agency is grounded in a relational context. The moral agent must have not only cognitive ability but also emotional capacity to demonstrate an attitude of respect for the other.[3] Both reason and emotion operate as part of your internal processor in which you can go and search to find the appropriate tools to exercise your professional responsibility. Much is said about ethical reasoning and problem solving in this book. Through the years, considerable debate about the significance of emotion in an agent's activity has taken place. Strict rationalists view emotion as too subjective and unpredictable to serve as a reliable guide. However, a burgeoning body of current professional and lay literature lends new knowledge about the role of emotion in decision making more generally to support the essential role of emotion in ethical decision making. Such well-regarded bodies as the Harvard Decision Science Laboratory conduct research on the mechanisms through which emotion and social factors influence judgment and decision making. From their work and the work of others, we find convincing arguments for assigning emotion at least two functions in ethics.

First, emotion is an "alert" system that warns you that you may be veering off the road of a caring response. When you encounter a morally perplexing situation, you, who will be accountable, feel discomfort, anxiety, anger, or some other disturbing emotion. Nancy Sherman, a contemporary philosopher who is working on the place of emotion in morality, proposes that emotions are "modes of sensitivity that record what is morally salient and... communicate those concerns to self and others."[4] Sometimes, an emotional response stirs a person out of lethargy and moves him or her into thinking and action on someone else's behalf.[5,6] In other words, your emotions help grab your attention and motivate you to "do something." We saw this in the process Kate was going through as she faced the reality of Bill's missed appointments.

Second, according to current research, emotion kicks in again at the point of decision making to complete the human picture of what is happening.[7] Even if you have been logical in your assessment of the ethical problem, emotion puts the last strokes on the canvas and brings the decision into focus as one example of how humans actually conduct their lives all around. In the end, emotion, attention, self-awareness, knowledge, and behavior interact with each other for real-time decision making.[8,9] Effective moral agents work to integrate emotional responsiveness with critical thinking, so, rather than disregarding emotion, they develop the right emotion suited to the situation.

⟳ Summary

An agent has responsibility for an action. A moral agent has a responsibility to act in a way that protects moral values and other aspects of morality. An ethical problem requires attention to both reasoning and emotion in the process of decision making. Emotion alerts, focuses attention, motivates, and increases one's knowledge about complex situations.

The Course of Action: C

The course of action includes the agent's analysis, the judgment process of discerning the best likely resolution to the problem, and the decision to act in accordance with that judgment. Because ethics problems are complex, they are often unpredictable and have competing imperatives. The next two chapters explain how this process works within the context of ethical problem solving with ethical theories and approaches, so more detail about that is not necessary now. Kate Lindy used the information she had to analyze the situation. One attempt at resolution was to call the case manager looking for Bill. Kate's emotional response afterward reflected a concern for her patient's well-being, even though she was irritated when she made the call; her discomfort suggests she was unsure she had exercised the correct moral judgment in what she said to the case manager. As we know, Kate also felt a sense of responsibility to bill for the scheduled treatments Bill did not receive, although she did not like this policy in her workplace. This back-and-forth reflection about what she was feeling and doing kept the course of action alive to the possibilities of what should happen.

The Outcome: O

The outcome is the result of having taken a particular course of action. Of course, the goal is that a caring response is achieved as a result of the whole process. More information is needed about what actually happened as a result of Kate's conversation and what she thought about it to know whether she considered it a good outcome for her patient Bill Boyd.

Some ethical approaches that you will learn to use in the next chapter place much more weight on the outcome; others place moral priority on the course of action. In everyday descriptions of ethics, this tension is sometimes referred to as the "ends" one achieves and the "means" used. The important point is that real-life professional situations require your full participation in all three features of an ethical problem. The decision of which of the features takes precedence in a particular ethical problem depends in part on the approach or theory you adopt.

> ### ⓢ Summary
>
> The two prototypes of ethical problems share three features in common: a moral agent (or agents), a course of action, and an outcome.

Considerations in Moral Agency

Locus of Authority

The role of the moral agent is not always easy. At times, one may have the emotional and cognitive capacity to act as a moral agent; however, constraints in the practice environment limit one's authority to respond. A *locus of authority* conflict arises from an ethical question of who should have the authority to make an important ethical decision. In other words, who is the rightful moral agent (A) to carry out the course of action (C) and be held responsible for the outcome (O)? Locus of authority problems most often arise when ambiguities exist about who is in charge (Fig. 3.1). Schematically, the situation looks like this:

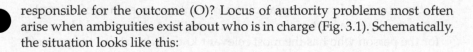

A_1 ————————————— O_1 vs. A_2 ————————————— O_2
　　　　　C_1　　　　　　　　　　　　　　　　　C_2

Fig. 3.1. Locus of authority problem. A, Moral agent (or agents); C, Course of action; O, Outcome.

Note that two people assume themselves to be appropriate moral agents (A_1 and A_2) and proceed along parallel (or even conflicting) courses of action (C_1 and C_2). As each analyzes the situation, they may come to different conclusions about how to achieve the best outcome (O_1 vs. O_2) for a patient.

This consideration of agency highlights that it does matter who has decision-making authority and say-so. In these situations, structural and team empowerment, which is discussed subsequently in this book, are vital to the nourishment of a moral culture.

Reflection
In the story of Kate Lindy and Bill Boyd, who do you think should make the decisions about whether to charge for missed treatments?
　The health professional who is providing the service?
　The supervisor of the unit?
　The institutional administrator?
　The government or some other, larger societal regulating body?
　The patient?
Give a brief explanation of your thinking to support your position.

_____

_____

_____

_____

Sometimes, no ambiguity or conflict exists, but reflection on the issue reveals that the wrong person has the authority. In that case, the situation creates moral distress. The challenge of determining the appropriate locus of authority is the topic of thoughtful reflection by ethicists and other individuals. In the context of the health professions, there are at least four ways of thinking about authority in healthcare decisions.
1. Professional expertise. You are in a professional role along with other people in different professional roles. This is the essence of interprofessional teamwork that characterizes so much of quality healthcare today. The role differences mean that you bring different spheres of expertise

to the situation. In some areas of the patient's care, each professional is an authority on a part of the whole picture. That alone should be a vote for the person who has the most relevant knowledge about the patient's condition and other factors that influence the situation.

2. Traditional arrangements. Traditionally, in the healthcare system, the physician has been the authoritative voice in healthcare decisions. The physician is considered to be *in* authority because of his or her office or position rather than (or in addition to) *an* authority because of special expertise. From this perspective, the medical director of the unit is the one to make a decision about what to do, although he or she may choose to invite advice and counsel from other individuals.

3. Institutional arrangements and mechanisms. Sometimes the decision about the authoritative voice comes from special institutional arrangements. For example, some tasks may be delegated to committees. In these instances, the committees or designated individuals assume specific task-related roles. This is really a variation of the first two roles, with the designated individuals in authority because of their expertise and the positions they hold. For example, the authority for making a decision regarding billing for missed treatments may be referred to a committee designed to deal with humane treatment of patients in unusual situations rather than billing solely as a financial issue.

4. The authority of experience. A voice of authority may emerge because of the insight that comes from experience. Situations always exist in which we seek the advice of people who have been in similarly perplexing situations and defer to their judgment. Kate Lindy may wish to seek advice for the next step from a supervisor, senior member of the professional staff, or other person judged to have the benefit of experience. This is seldom institutionalized as a formal mechanism for dealing with locus of authority challenges and is a variation of the professional expertise approach, which assumes that expertise often is refined with experience in a wide range of situations.

None of these sources should be taken for granted as the appropriate authority for all situations. The ethical gold standard remains what will result in a caring response for the patient.

Shared Agency

Given that care is increasingly provided by interprofessional teams, another consideration in moral agency is *shared agency*. As you recall from Chapter 1, the interprofessional care team is a group of care providers (including licensed health professionals, assistive staff, and ancillary support staff) who work together to deliver quality, evidence-based, and client-centered care. These teams share day-to-day concerns as they arise and work together to navigate practice while upholding professional responsibilities, values, and duties. When faced with the moral dimensions of professional practice, sharing concerns among the team members can create an atmosphere that nurtures ethical reflection. One question that often arises is: Who is the moral agent? Because the goal is to achieve a caring response, the care team may give consideration to shared agency. Shared agency is not to be taken lightly because it requires high levels of engagement from all team members. It entails a commitment to group discussion, collaborative decision making, and mutual trust. In the disposition to act on the intentions of the team over the individual, shared agency takes into account the previous discussion that at different times various members of the team may emerge as the appropriate authority when the actual decision making is imminent. A prerequisite for shared agency is that each team member is heard (including those with dissenting views), respected, and participatory in decision making and agrees to uphold mutual responsibilities when implementing a plan.[10]

Summary

Considerations of locus of authority and shared agency are important features to attend to in a shared moral community. The goal in both considerations is to achieve an outcome consistent with a caring response.

Two Prototypes of Ethical Problems

Now that you have acquainted yourself with the common features of all prototypes, you are ready to learn more about the prototypes themselves: moral distress and ethical dilemmas.

Moral Distress: Confronting Barriers to Moral Agency

Moral distress focuses on the agents (A) themselves when a situation blocks them from doing what is right. Moral distress as a term came into the ethics literature primarily through nursing ethics and has become more generalized because of its usefulness in understanding ethical problems that all health professionals experience. Moral distress reflects that you, the moral agent, experience appropriate emotional or cognitive discomfort, or both, because of a barrier from being the kind of professional you know you should be or from doing what you conclude is right. Your emotional response and feelings play a major role in the recognition that you have moved from striding confidently along in your moral life to experiencing that something is wrong. You can see that your response to the situation comes from an awareness that your integrity is threatened because a threat to integrity arises when you cannot be the person you know you should be in your professional role or cannot do what you know for certain is right. Health professionals find that these emotional signals give rise to physical expressions that warn something is wrong: a knot in the pit of their stomach, a catch in the otherwise confident stride, or an awakening in the early hours of the morning with the haunting feeling that something is awry. It can also manifest as frustration, anger, and anxiety. Again, we are reminded that emotions and feelings are critical data of the moral life, trying to say, "Stop! Wait! Don't! Think twice!"

Moral agents in the health professions encounter two types of barriers that create moral distress: type A and type B.

Type A: You Cannot Do What You Know Is Right

A common problem today is the barrier to adequate care of individual patients created by the mechanisms for the delivery and financing of healthcare, although other sources also exist. Recent studies have found that high percentages of moral distress occur over resource allocation and reimbursement constraints, goal setting, maintaining confidentiality, limiting autonomy, withdrawing and withholding care, prenatal testing, and balancing institutional needs versus what is best for the client.[3,11–13] For example, a hospital policy may be to refuse admission of patients who do not have insurance to fully cover the cost of their treatment or to discharge patients who the interprofessional care team judges to be unsuited for the rigors of transition to the home environment. Here, the morally right course of action (C) that would lead to the desired outcome (O) is blocked by policies and practices, resulting in moral distress. Type A barrier is illustrated in Fig. 3.2. The moral distress comes precisely because of the repercussions the professionals believe they may have to endure. Institutional and traditional role barriers keep them from exercising their moral agency for the good of patients.

This does not mean that you will never take into account the larger social context in which you are practicing. As you learned in Chapter 2, sociocultural determinants of a caring response sometimes do alter the course of action you would otherwise take. For instance, health professionals must always attend to the larger public health considerations in the case of a patient with a highly contagious and infectious disease. The patient may

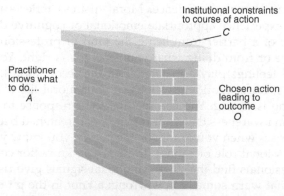

Institutional constraints
to course of action
C

Practitioner
knows what
to do....
A

Chosen action
leading to
outcome
O

Fig. 3.2. Moral distress: type A.

experience forced quarantine or be placed in strict isolation. The health professional's emotional discomfort in such a situation that requires acting for the good of many other individuals is not an example of moral distress. The patient still can be the recipient of the best care possible. Only when you are quite sure you cannot be faithful to the basic well-being of the patient is there legitimate reason for moral distress.

Another powerful barrier to doing what is right is suggested in the previous paragraph but all too often fails to be included in discussions of moral distress. Moral distress often occurs because of internal barriers such as the fear of repercussion of one kind or another—real or imagined—that looms in the professional's awareness, blocking action. Wanting to do the right thing and not having the knowledge, skill, or inner strength to do it while under the weight of anxieties and fears often results in heightened moral distress rather than leading to freedom through action (Fig. 3.3). Unresolved moral distress, with accompanying feelings of depletion or powerlessness, can compromise healthcare providers' ability to uphold their ethical standards and diminish the physical and emotional energy needed to fully attend to patients' needs.[14] This process, faced time after time, can result in *moral residue*, an accumulation of compromises that takes a heavy toll on one's integrity.[15]

To face those uncomfortable feelings and emotions and remain motivated to do the right thing requires that each and every one of us receive support from others to step up, speak out, or stand firm as the occasion calls for it. In some other parts of this book, you will be introduced to team and institutional supports that can help you navigate the burden of these internal barriers.

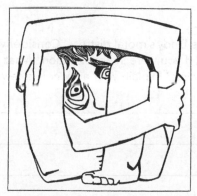

Fig. 3.3. **Internal barriers.** *(From Purtilo R, Haddad A: Respect: the difference it makes. In: Health professional and patient interaction, ed 7, Philadelphia, 2002, Saunders, p 12.)*

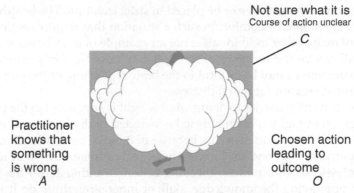

Fig. 3.4. Moral distress: type B.

Type B: You Know Something Is Wrong But Are Not Sure What
Often the barrier may not be policies and practices or internal anxieties and fear, but it may be that the situation is new or extremely complex. Your only certainty is an acknowledgment that something is wrong; the rest is a big question mark. You may question how to arrive at the morally correct course of action (C) or how to work toward a specific outcome (O) that is consistent with your professional goal of achieving a caring response in this instance. The type B barrier is illustrated in Fig. 3.4. The ethical challenge is to remove the barrier of doubt or uncertainty as much as possible, sometimes through probing deeper into the facts of the situation. When there is high uncertainty, doubt requires that the moral agent must seek advice and critically problem solve through the situation to better understand how to address its complexity. As you can readily see, emotions often play a major role in this type of situation, too.

Reflection
Think about Kate Lindy's moral distress. Consider why you might feel uneasy, too, if you were in her situation. What subtype of moral distress is she facing? Explain your answer in a few words here.

_____

_____

_____

_____

Kate's discomfort likely stems from wanting to do what is best for Bill Boyd but being unsure what that is because she likely has not been faced with this set of issues before. She wants to show a caring response that befits a health professional, but she is not sure how to do that under the circumstances. Understandably, she also wants to honor the rules and policies of her workplace but is distressed about charging for Bill's missed treatments given that his lack of adherence is likely associated with his clinical condition. Her moral distress is more of type B.

> ### Summary
>
> Moral distress occurs when the moral agent knows what the morally appropriate course of action is but meets external barriers, internal resistance, or a high level of uncertainty.

As she analyzes the situation, Kate thinks about whether her distress also is related to the fact that she is facing an ethical dilemma. So, join her now in that reflection, as we turn to the second type of prototypical ethical problem: the *ethical dilemma*.

Ethical Dilemma: Two Courses Diverging

Many people call all ethical problems ethical dilemmas. More correctly, an ethical dilemma is a common type of situation that involves two (or more) morally correct courses of action that cannot both be followed; that is, to take course C_1 precludes you from taking course C_2. As a result, you (the agent, the responsible one) are doing something right and also wrong (by not doing the other thing that is also right). You are between a rock and a hard place, between the devil and the deep blue sea (Fig. 3.5).[16]

Ethical dilemmas involve both ethical conflict and conduct. Suppose that Kate Lindy has just read the previous paragraph and realizes that she had an ethical dilemma but did not recognize it at the time. She was aware of her moral distress and that further analysis was needed. Here is why she now knows she had a dilemma.

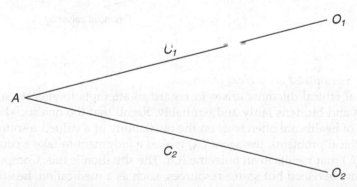

Fig. 3.5. Ethical dilemma. A, Moral agent (or agents); C, Course of action; O, Outcome.

On the one hand, Kate is an agent (A) who has a professional duty to look after her patient Bill Boyd and to take the course of action (C_1) that demonstrates her attempt to give Bill the best treatment possible. The desired outcome (O_1) is psychological well-being and relief of the patient's pain. On the other hand, Kate is an agent (A) who has a duty to abide by the policies of her place of employment. The course of action (C_2) that expresses that duty is to charge for all treatments that are given or are not officially canceled. The desired outcome (O_2) is the financial solvency of the psychotherapy practice. Both outcomes are ethically appropriate, taken alone. However, Kate Lindy probably caused some negative repercussions for Bill in her course of action that included sharing potentially damaging information with Bill's case manager. The case manager did not sound pleased, either by Bill's absenteeism from scheduled treatments or the fact that Bill was being charged for the missed treatments. In charging for the treatments, Kate maintained fidelity to her workplace at the price of protecting Bill Boyd from exposure that may cause him additional problems.

Of course, Kate might have thought that charging for missed appointments is wrong under any circumstance, a position that is periodically examined in the health profession literature.[17]

In subsequent chapters, you will have ample opportunity to work with several types of dilemmas because they are the most commonly confronted type of ethical problem.

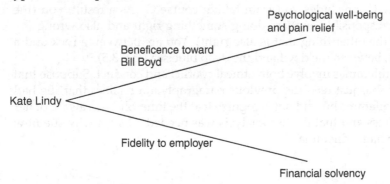

Ethical dilemma in the story of Bill Boyd and Kate Lindy.

Justice Seeking as an Ethical Dilemma

A special ethical dilemma arises in regard to attempts to allocate societal benefits and burdens fairly and equitably. Recall that the one social determinant of healthcare often rests on the availability of a valued resource. As in all ethical problems, the agent (A) makes a judgment to take a course of action (C) that results in an outcome (O). The situation is this: Competition exists for cherished but scarce resources, such as a medication, health professionals' time, money to pay for healthcare, or an organ or other types of lifesaving or quality-of-life–enhancing procedures. The agent's (A) morally right course of action (C) is to give everyone a full measure of the resource to the extent their needs warrant it. In so doing, the outcome (O) is that the patient's legitimate claims are honored and the professional can rest assured in having provided a patient-centered outcome. The scarce supply, however, requires that the agent take difficult, even tragic, courses of action, with the outcome that some claimants get the cherished goods and others do not, or they get less than an clinically optimal share.[18] In short, it is morally right to give your own patients everything they need to benefit from your interventions. It is also morally right to spread resources around to the benefit of others. The question of how to treat each person fairly and to treat groups equitably becomes a challenge that involves a dilemma of justice, a problem that, in an important study of the meaning of caring, was found increasingly difficult in a healthcare system that values cost control and a high margin of profit.[19] This dilemma is a common theme in the health profession literature and society today. You will study this and how you can optimize your efforts in the face of contemporary justice dilemmas more extensively in later chapters of this book.

 Reflection
Describe an example in your chosen field of how you might become involved in a dilemma that requires you to make tough decisions because of scarce resources. One way to approach this is to think of the setting in which you are likely to work and the special, sometimes expensive, procedures that may be available to a range of patients. Another is to imagine conditions under which your worksite is short staffed and you must make difficult choices about where to cut corners.

_____

_____

_____

_____

 Summary

An ethical dilemma occurs when a moral agent is faced with two or more conflicting courses of action but only one can be chosen as the agent attempts to bring about an outcome consistent with a caring response. A special case of a dilemma involves justice issues when a needed resource or service is in limited supply.

Summary

This completes the introduction to your role as a moral agent, the components of any ethical problem, and the two prototypes of ethical problems that will help you to be ready to act ethically. The prototypes of moral distress and ethical dilemmas, along with locus of authority and shared agency considerations, will guide you as you analyze and decide which course of action is most likely to achieve an intended outcome consistent with honoring your professional responsibility.

Questions for Thought and Discussion

1. Jane is a health professions student who is pregnant and does not want to treat a patient admitted to the inpatient medicine service from a local prison for management of end-stage renal disease. Her clinical supervisor thinks her reluctance is because of her pregnant condition and assures her that she is safe because the prisoner is nonviolent and has a one-on-one guard assigned to his room. Jane still hesitates and says, "I know it's irrational, but I'm afraid I will not be effective." She pauses and then adds, "To be honest, I also feel it is God's will when bad people get sick."

   Is Jane's reason sufficiently compelling to warrant her being excused from assignment to this patient? Why or why not? What type of ethical problem faces her clinical supervisor? Describe how you have arrived at this conclusion with use of the three features of any ethical problem.

2. Loretta is a physical therapist specialized in diabetic foot care. She sees Mary monthly. Mary is quite down when she hobbles into the clinic today, with her ankles bandaged and blood oozing through the gauze. She tells Loretta, "I'm sure my feet are much worse this month. I haven't been so good about my sugar, and it didn't help that my husband hit my ankles with his cane twice last week. I think he is upset about my taxi fare to get here. I should stop coming." She begins to cry.

   What are the clinical, legal, and ethical questions that face Loretta in this case? What should she do?

3. Describe an ethical dilemma that you or someone you know has faced. This dilemma does not have to be a problem that arose within the healthcare context. What did you have to take into consideration as you moved toward a decision about which of the two or more courses of action available to you should be taken? Did your decision result in a good outcome?

References

1. Lakoff G: *Women, fire and dangerous things: what categories reveal about the mind*, Chicago, 1987, University of Chicago Press, p 12.

2. Taylor CR: Right relationships: foundation for health care ethics. In Pinch WJE, Haddad AM, editors: *Nursing and health care ethics: a legacy and a vision*, Silver Spring, MD, 2008, American Nurses Association, pp 163–164.

3. Lutzen K, Ewalds-Kvist B: Moral distress and its interconnection with moral sensitivity and moral resilience: viewed from the philosophy of Viktor E. Frankl, *J Bioeth Inq* 10:317–324, 2013.

4. Sherman N: Emotions, ed 4. In Post S, editor: *Encyclopedia of bioethics*, vol 2, New York, 2014, Thomson Gale, pp 740–748.

5. Purtilo R: Moral courage: unsung resource for health professional as friend and healer. In Thomasm D, Kissell J, editors: *The health professional as friend and healer*, Washington, DC, 2000, Georgetown University Press, pp 106–112.

6. Molewijk B, Kleinlugtenbelt D, Widdershoven G: The role of emotions in moral case deliberation: theory, practice and methodology, *Bioethics* 25(7):383–393, 2011.

7. Bechara A: The role of emotion in decision-making: evidence from neurological patients with orbitofrontal damage, *Brain Cogn* 55:30–40, 2004.

8. Xing C: Effects of anger and sadness on attentional patterns in decision making: an eye-tracking study, *Psychol Rep* 114(1):50–67, 2014.

9. Epstein R: *Attending: medicine, mindfulness, and humanity*, New York, 2017, Simon & Schuster, Inc.

10. Bratman M: *Shared agency: a planning theory of acting together*, Oxford, England, 2014, Oxford University Press.

11. Cantu R: therapists' ethical dilemmas in treatment, coding, and billing for rehabilitation services in skilled nursing facilities a mixed method pilot study, *J Am Med Dir Assoc.* 20(11):1458–1461, 2019.

12. Slater DY, Brandt LC: Combating moral distress. In Slater DY, editor: *Reference guide to the occupational therapy code of ethics 2015 Edition*, Bethesda, MD, 2016, AOTA Press, pp 117–124.

13. Bushby K, Chan J, Druif S, et al: Ethical tensions in occupational therapy practice: a scoping review, *Br J Occup Ther* 78(4):212–221, 2015.

14. Rivard AM, Brown CA: Moral distress and resilience in the occupational therapy workplace, *Safety* (1):10, 2019. doi: 10.3390/safety5010010.

15. Hardingham LB: Integrity and moral residue: nurses as participants in a moral community, *Nurs Philos* 5(2):127–134, 2004.

16. Beauchamp TL, Childress JF: *Professional-patient relationships, principles of biomedical ethics*, ed 7, New York, 2012, Oxford University Press, pp 288–331.

17. Knapp S, VandeCreek L: The ethics of advertising, billing, and finances in psychotherapy, *J Clin Psychol* 64(5):613–625, 2008. doi: 10.1002/jcl.20475.

18. Freeman JM, McDonnell K: Making moral decisions: a process approach, ed 2, *In Tough decisions: cases in medical ethics*. New York, 2001, Oxford University Press, pp 241–246.

19. Greenfield BH: The meaning of caring in five experienced physical therapists, *Physiother Theory Pract* 22(4):175–187, 2006.

4

Ethical Theories and Approaches: Conceptual Tools for Ethical Decision Making

Objectives

The reader should be able to:

- Distinguish between an ethical theory and an ethical approach.
- Understand the process of clinical reasoning used by health professionals.
- Distinguish the different modes of clinical reasoning.
- Differentiate ethical reasoning as a distinct mode of clinical reasoning.
- Describe the usefulness of the basic ethics theories and approaches as tools in analyzing ethical problems and attempting to resolve problems by arriving at the most caring response.
- Name five types of ethical theories and approaches that help illuminate what a caring response entails.
- Describe a narrative and what it means to take a narrative approach to an ethical issue or problem.
- Assess the contribution of psychologist Carol Gilligan and others who stress the moral significance of relationships.
- Relate the basic features of an ethic of care to a caring response, introduced in Chapter 2.
- Explain the role of moral character or virtue in the realization of a good life and its significance for health professionals faced with the goal of arriving at a caring response.
- Describe ways the various story or case approaches help one understand what a caring response involves.
- Describe the function of a principle (norm, element) in ethical analysis and conduct.
- Identify six principles often encountered in professional ethics that can help guide one in trying to arrive at a caring response to a professional situation.
- Discuss the meaning of autonomy in Kant's and Mill's theories and the relevance of each to ethical conduct.
- Recognize five reasonable expectations a patient or client has because of the health professional's responsibility to act with fidelity.

- Describe the principle of veracity as it applies in the professional context.
- Recognize the basic difference between deontological and utilitarian ethical theories of conduct and the role of each in the health professional's goal of acting in accordance with what a caring response requires.

New terms and ideas you will encounter in this chapter

clinical reasoning	principle-based	deontology
ethical reasoning	approach	deontological theories
theories and approaches	nonmaleficence	teleology
story or case approaches	beneficence	absolute duties
narrative approaches	autonomy	prima facie duties
ethics of care approach	self-determination	conditional duties
virtue theory	paternalism	teleological theories
character trait	fidelity	utilitarianism
moral character	veracity	rule utilitarians
principles	justice	

Topics in this chapter introduced in earlier chapters

Topic	Introduced In chapter
Moral duty and character	1
Codes of ethics	1
Interprofessional care team	1
A caring response	2
Patient-centered care	2
Professional responsibility	2
Right(s)	2
Prototypes of ethical problems	3
Moral agency	3
Moral distress	3
Ethical dilemma	3

Introduction

In this chapter, you are introduced to a conceptual "toolbox" of ethical theories and approaches you can use to accomplish your professional goal of arriving at a caring response in the wide variety of challenges you may encounter. An ethical theory is researched and well developed and provides us with an assumption about the very nature of right and wrong. Most theories are historically based and have evolved for current usage according to a society's or group's development and a need for interpreting or addressing current moral challenges. In contrast, an approach does not propose to be a complete system or model but an aid to existing theories. For instance, the principle-based approach introduced in this chapter is more recent and has roots in ancient Western ethical theories. Both ethical theories and approaches provide you with a framework for diagnosing, communicating, and problem solving ethical questions you encounter in your clinical practice.[1]

You probably took a look at how many pages you have ahead of you in this chapter and quickly concluded that this is a very long siege of reading! The idea behind this chapter is to provide you with a "mini book" of ethical theory. Depending on your course of study, your professor may add to these pages with another more theoretic text or may split the chapter into smaller parts. You are encouraged to work through the chapter carefully so that the rest of your study of this book is easier and your preparation in ethics more complete.

In Chapter 1, we suggested three general ways that ethical tools have usefulness in your everyday life: (1) to analyze moral issues, (2) to help resolve moral conflicts, and (3) to move toward action when faced with a problem. In Chapter 2, you learned about the caring response as the goal of professional ethical practice. In Chapter 3, you had an opportunity to learn the basic varieties (i.e., prototypes) of ethical problems you will encounter in your professional career. In this chapter, you will gain more knowledge and tools that will enable you to move skillfully from the identification of a problem, through its analysis, and, hopefully, to its resolution through action that achieves your goal of a caring response. Chapter 5 provides a simple six-step process you can follow as you apply everything discussed in this and the previous chapters. To set the stage for your thinking, consider the story of Elizabeth Kim, Max Diaz, Melinda Diaz, and Michael Leary.

🌿 The Story of Elizabeth Kim, Max Diaz, Melinda Diaz, and Michael Leary

Elizabeth Kim is a speech and language pathologist who works in a large urban school system. She is responsible for performing many student evaluations and interventions each day and takes her job seriously. Elizabeth services the Richards Elementary School and two other schools in the Lakeview district. Students and parents who meet Elizabeth quickly learn that she is a bright spot in the otherwise anxiety-producing process of navigating services for children with learning disabilities. Elizabeth prides herself on being thorough and always explains everything to both the students and the parents in language they can understand.

Two weeks ago, Elizabeth had an experience that upset her, and she is not sure what to do about it. A young student, Max Diaz, had met Elizabeth for his speech and language pathology evaluation at Richards Elementary School. Max has an expressive language disorder, and Elizabeth felt strongly that he would benefit from an augmentative communication device. She has used these devices in the past and has seen great success with them. Elizabeth had her quarterly supervision meeting with Michael Leary, the school principal, that afternoon. She talked about Max in the meeting because she was intrigued by his case. She told Principal Leary her evaluation results and that she would be recommending the augmentative device. Principal Leary told Elizabeth, "Please do not put that recommendation in your written report. Max's mother has not been overly involved in advocating for his needs. If we can hold off on meeting with her for Max's education plan until the end of the school year, I won't have to buy the device until the next academic year. Those devices are really expensive, and I don't know if we have the money right now. Besides, who knows if it will really even work for him, given English is his second language." Elizabeth left the meeting feeling uncomfortable.

The speech and language pathology evaluation report was completed and submitted to the administration. Elizabeth did include the recommendation for the augmentative device in the report because she knew that it was in Max's best interest. She was eager to train Max in how to use this type of device. All that was needed now was administrative and parental approval. As soon as the individualized education plan (IEP) could be scheduled, they could move forward. A copy was sent to Principal Leary, Max's homeroom teacher, and his mother, and one was placed in his academic record in the administrative office.

Several weeks later, Elizabeth asked Principal Leary when Max's IEP would take place. She wanted to get his mother's and the team's approval to move forward with various interventions, including the augmentative device. The principal told Elizabeth that Melinda, Max's mom, had been slow to respond to the school's request for a meeting and said, "We offered her a date, but she could not make it. Since then, we have not been able to coordinate with a Spanish interpreter. I may just try to schedule her without one. Actually, the longer it is put off, the better, as we won't have to bear the cost of the device you recommended on this year's school budget."

Elizabeth knew that the longer the meeting took to arrange, the longer Max would go without service; she wanted to say, "Aren't you going to follow up and encourage her to get in soon?" but she did not. She knew Principal Leary would have to schedule the meeting and was also afraid he may be insulted by such a question.

Today, 3 months after the evaluation was completed, Elizabeth is walking another student to the after-school program when she sees Max with his mom, Melinda Diaz, in the corridor. Melinda says, "Oh, you must be the speech therapist. Thanks for the papers you sent to me about Max. It's too bad that you and the teacher couldn't meet a couple months ago. I was looking forward to talking with you all. I can't read English that well, so I had a hard time understanding the papers."

"Oh. Did Principal Leary talk with you about setting another meeting time sooner rather than later?" Elizabeth asks, feeling tense.

"No, he didn't. He just keeps saying, 'Don't worry.'"

"Well," Elizabeth says. "You have the right to set another meeting time sooner rather than later and to have an interpreter there if you want to."

Melinda immediately looks concerned. Elizabeth wants to say something to reassure her, but the words fail her. The school bell rings, and Elizabeth says a hurried good-bye. She feels a gnawing in the pit of her stomach, but she cannot immediately figure out what, if anything, she should do next.

That Elizabeth Kim is distressed is not surprising because something definitely is wrong. In fact, one might wonder about a health professional who felt no emotion at all about this situation: a young child with a learning disorder who is not performing to his potential, and communication between his mother and the school staff that appears to have broken down. Maybe Elizabeth has said too much—or too little—to help this family and school, both of whom have had some difficult discussions to confront. She is not sure how far she should go in advocating for her client and taking on the system.

Reflection

What is a caring, morally responsible action in this type of situation?

_____

_____

_____

_____

We return to this story throughout the chapter, so keep your response in mind.

Ethical Reasoning: A Guide for Ethical Reflection

Clinical Reasoning

As a health professional, you must learn to blend your knowledge, skills, and attitudes in response to varying clinical situations that require your professional judgment.[2] As you have read in the previous chapters, health professionals must learn to be responsible for their actions on others, both clients and the public. So, before we highlight theoretical parts of ethical study that take you deeper into addressing situations, we must discuss clinical reasoning. You may be familiar with the terms critical thinking or practical reasoning. These terms are similar to clinical or professional reasoning.

Clinical reasoning is the complex thought process that health professionals use during therapeutic interactions. Schell defines this process well by stating that clinical reasoning is used by practitioners to "plan, direct, perform and reflect on [client] care."[3] Health professionals use clinical reasoning to analyze and synthesize the information they gather when caring for (or preparing to care for) a patient. Clinical reasoning informs decisions and guides actions in the context of professional ethics and community expectations.[4]

You have likely already been trained to develop your clinical reasoning. During your educational process, has a professor, clinical instructor, or supervisor ever asked you "why" when you gave an answer to a clinical question? If so, they are trying to understand your reasoning. They want to ensure that you not only know the answer to the question but that you have thought about and analyzed the situation from a broad perspective. The process of clinical reasoning is important because it guides your decision making in the care of the patient. The more complex the clinical case, the more demands placed on your reasoning.

Modes of Reasoning

Health professionals use different modes of reasoning in response to particular features of a clinical case (Table 4.1).[5-7] Many modes of clinical reasoning are used simultaneously to solve a clinical problem. For a caring response to be actualized, health professionals must use clinical reasoning to ensure that their decisions have meaning for the client. At various points in your clinical practice, you should stop and ask yourself, "Why am I doing what I am doing?" This helps you reflect on your clinical reasoning. Your reasoning is one of the strongest foundations you can have as a professional. It must continue to grow throughout your career to meet the demands and challenges of our ever-changing patient population and service delivery environment.

Ethical Reasoning

Ethical reasoning is a mode of reasoning used to recognize, analyze, and clarify ethical problems. It is an essential component of clinical reasoning. You use ethical reasoning when you ask yourself, "What is the morally correct action to take for this client?" Ethical reasoning helps guide the provision of professional care with an emphasis primarily on conduct. When you recognize the morally significant features of a clinical scenario, you are using your ethical reasoning. Ethical reasoning requires that you be able to gather relevant information and correctly apply your ethical knowledge and skills in the process of ethical reflection. This requires great attention to the details of each case. Ethical reasoning not only is concerned with recognizing, gathering, and applying ethical knowledge but also emphasizes the process one

Table 4.1 Forms of Clinical Reasoning

Forms of clinical reasoning	Description
Scientific reasoning	A framework for understanding the impact of illness or disease on the patient. Involves the use of scientific methods, such as hypothesis testing, cue and pattern identification, and evidence as related to a diagnosis. Scientific reasoning includes both diagnostic and procedural reasoning. The focus is generally on the diagnosis, procedures, and interventions for a specific condition. Data are systematically gathered, and knowledge is compared.
Narrative reasoning	A framework for understanding the patient's "life story" or illness experience. This type of reasoning helps clinicians make sense of the patient's past, present, and future. Includes an appreciation of how the patient's life story is influenced by culture, condition, and experiences.
Pragmatic reasoning	A framework for consideration of the practical issues that impact care. Such issues include treatment environments, equipment, availability of resources (including training of individual providers), and other realities associated with service delivery.
Interactive reasoning	A mode of reasoning that is used to help clinicians better interact with and understand their patient as a person. Highlights the interpersonal nature of the therapeutic relationship (e.g., the use of empathy, nonverbal communication, therapeutic use of self).
Conditional reasoning	A blending of reasoning that involves the moment-to-moment treatment revision based on the patient's current and future context. Used to anticipate outcomes over short or long periods of time.
Ethical reasoning	A mode of reasoning used to recognize, analyze, and clarify ethical problems that arise. Helps clinicians make decisions regarding the right thing to do in a particular case. The moral basis for professional behaviors and actions. The focus is not on what could be done for the patient; rather, it is focused on what should be done.

Modified from Schell BAB, Schell JW: Clinical and professional reasoning in occupational therapy, ed 2, Philadelphia, 2019, Wolters Kluwer/Lippincott Williams and Wilkins; Mattingly C, Fleming M: Clinical reasoning: forms of inquiry in therapeutic practice, Philadelphia, 1994, FA Davis; and Leicht SB, Dickerson A: Clinical reasoning, looking back. Occup Ther Healthcare 14(3/4):105–130, 2001.

goes through when reasoning about the situation. We successfully engage ethical reasoning when we not only recognize that x is good and y is bad but when we also articulate reasons for *why* x is good and y is bad.[8] Some *theories and approaches* to ethics today use the modes of reasoning outlined in Table 4.1 (e.g., narrative or interactive reasoning) that complement strictly ethical reasoning. Even the theories that focus mostly on character traits, narratives, or relationships must be reflected on. More is said about this as the chapter unfolds.

---

⑤ Summary

Clinical reasoning requires that you be able to gather relevant information and correctly apply your knowledge and skills in a way that meets your desired goal of a caring response. Ethical reasoning is a component of reasoning focused on the ethical dimensions of the situation.

The Caring Response: Using Theories and Approaches to Guide You

You have already learned that the goal of ethical deliberation is to answer the question: "What does it mean to provide a caring response in this situation?" You also have learned that although you will be faced with legitimate competing loyalties as a health professional, your primary loyalty must always be patient centered. All these insights beg for further description about how to actually arrive at the ethically appropriate caring response in a particular situation.

Several ethics theories and approaches are relevant to your work of putting together this caring response. Your ethics work differs from an academic philosopher's because you must not only apply clear thinking to ethical problems, which a philosopher must do (as you learned in Chapter 3), but you must also decide on purposive action. You will not use all the theories or approaches covered in this chapter for any one situation; however, understanding key ethical theories and principles will help build your ethics literacy and guide you through the complex ethical problems you encounter in clinical practice.

The first two types, story-driven or case-driven approaches and virtue theories, emphasize the importance of the kind of person you should strive to be (i.e., your attitudes and dispositions) so that you are well positioned to enact a caring response. Together, the several varieties share the common themes of attending to the details of stories for their moral content, awareness of one's emotions in relation to what is happening in the story, and development of character traits that allow one to be prepared to act in a caring manner. Collectively, they also stress the moral relevance of relationships, both between individuals and within the institutional structures of society.

The last three approaches and theories, principle-based approaches, deontological theories, and teleological theories, are geared to forms of ethical conduct itself. Principle-based approaches have been developed to help people understand general action guides for ethical behavior, some of which are related to duties or rights and others that are related to consequences. Deontological and teleological theories can be broken down into more digestible pieces with a look at their roots: the root word *deonto* means duty; the root word *telos* means end. Already you can see a distinction developing. Deontological theories delineate duties (actually duties, rights, or other forms of action), whereas teleological ones rely on an assessment of the ends or consequences to determine right or wrong. You have heard the expression, "Do the ends justify the means?" Deontologists would say "no"; teleologists would say "yes." As noted previously, some principles guide you toward duty, others toward the "telos" or consequences. Are you ready to delve into these five theories or approaches in more detail?

Story or Case Approaches

In professional ethics, the story is the inevitable beginning point of ethical reflection because you encounter ethical problems in everyday life with everyday patients (or others). In *story or case approaches*, the assumption is that morally relevant information is embedded in the story.

In professional ethics, you also are equipped with foundation stones of ethical codes, a tradition, and societal expectations of how you will respond to legitimate requests for your professional services. Therefore, although the appropriate starting place for ethical analysis is the story, there are standards, principles, and other moral guides against which your opinion must be tested when you are deciding on a caring response. The answer is not simply, "You hold your view and I hold mine, and they are on equal footing, morally speaking." Therefore professional ethics also is foundationalist based by nature.

Narrative Approaches

Narrative is the technical term applied to the story's characters, events, and ordering of events (e.g., the plot), although in healthcare ethics and legal circles you more often see the term *case*. *Narrative approaches* are based on the observation that humans pass on information, impute and explore meaning in theirs and others' lives, commemorate and celebrate, denounce, clarify, get affirmation, and, overall, become a part of a community through the hearing and telling of stories. Stories help us make sense of experiences. Interprofessional care teams increasingly use narrative approaches in practice to better communicate with each other about the patient and to focus on the patient as the center of care.[9] Narrative ethicists conclude that good moral judgment must rely on the analysis and understanding of narratives. Kathryn Hunter, a contemporary leader in narrative approaches to ethics within healthcare, reiterates this point and notes that through narratives:

> [W]e spin and untangle explanatory accounts of the way the world works and how we and our fellow human beings act in every conceivable circumstance. Memories of the past and ideas of the future are expressed in narrative accounts of how the world was and how it will, or should, become.[10]

Her emphasis on "should" underscores the narrative ethicists' position that future moral choices of individuals and communities are shaped through understanding and taking seriously the information and lessons embedded in stories.

Elizabeth Kim's situation is revealed to you as a narrative. The fragmented narrative she herself has received is probably disturbing to her. She lacks certain information about the student's mother, the principal, and their exchanges that she needs to be confident of the moral challenges in the situation. Thus not only is she without all the facts and details, but she may feel she lacks pertinent information to make a valid ethical judgment about the real significance and meaning of the events unfolding before her. From the standpoint of ethical problems, Elizabeth is in a situation of moral distress.

Narrative approaches also highlight that in complex situations, not just one but several accounts exist. Suppose this story simply was titled "The Story of Principal Leary." What different concerns might Principal Leary express regarding his role, his relationships with the student Max, Max's mother (and all students and parents), and Elizabeth, or anything else? It may be a different story than the one told by Elizabeth. Or suppose this story was titled "The Story of Melinda Diaz." Surely this mom's account would include details about her personal life and experiences, her response to her son's learning disability, and her hopes, dreams, and fears. These details would alter inexorably what Elizabeth's story taken alone conveys. Elizabeth finds herself in the middle of a story to which she does not know the ending and wonders what to do. By listening to the many differing perspectives, she can begin to link values to action.[11] Ideally, the incorporation of differing perspectives leads to higher order reflection and allows all involved to consider points of view different from their own.[10] This diligent effort to consider as many voices as possible before interpreting the situation for moral significance is key to narrative analysis.

---

⑥ Summary

Narrative ethics requires attention to the details of the story and that all voices be considered before the situation is assessed for its moral significance.

Approaches That Emphasize Relationships

Some ethical approaches rely on a narrative search for the central moral themes of human relationships revealed in the story. You can immediately see the importance of this insight for health professionals because almost all their work involves relationships. In this approach, ethical issues or problems are embedded in the relationships, not just in the individual's situation. Patient-centered understanding of clinical situations is an example of such a relationship. A patient-centered approach in your professional orientation means that you *always* take the patient (and the patient's network of support) deeply into account regarding your ethical decisions. Not surprisingly, this approach has been promoted and refined by psychologists, particularly those who work in the area of moral development.

Carol Gilligan became an important leader in this area in the 1980s; her work was drawn from a widely accepted model of children's moral development advanced by Harvard psychologist Lawrence Kohlberg. Kohlberg hypothesized that children go through stages of moral development similar to cognitive development and that children become more independent and autonomous as they mature as moral beings. His work became a dominant, if not *the* dominant, moral development theory in the early 1980s.[13] At that time, Gilligan, who was working as Kohlberg's graduate student, noted that his work depended on studies of boys and young men. She repeated some of the work with girls and young women and discovered that her subjects conceptualized ethical issues and problems differently than did their male counterparts. Girls had a high sensitivity to how various actions would affect their important relationships (i.e., with parents, friends, teachers, or other authority figures); Gilligan concluded that girls' "awareness of the connection between people gives rise to a recognition of responsibility for another."[14] Moral maturity was not characterized by an increasing independence from everyone else but rather by decisions that would result in deeper and more effective connections and relationships to significant others and the larger community.[14]

Gilligan's work has become one vital basis for ethicists to emphasize how relationships figure into morality. Many have worked to refine our understanding of the ways relationships are central within various social settings, including professional relationships. Moreover, further examination has shown that, although girls and women may be socialized to think in terms of sustaining relationships, the significance of Gilligan's findings is by no means gender specific. All health professionals enter into a relationship with the patient, and through these relational networks, moral agents have responsibilities toward particular patients with whom they are connected and who in turn are affected by the moral agent's action.[15]

Institutional and other social arrangements of a society influence individual action and relationships, too. Ethical reflection requires recognition of the powerful influence of each player's and some groups' socially assigned "place" in society and how relationships are affected by the assumptions regarding social status.

If you noted the difference in power between Elizabeth Kim and Melinda Diaz or between Elizabeth Kim and Principal Leary because of their relative power and status within the delivery of care, you were correctly paying attention to social or institutional influences on relationships as relevant considerations in ethical analysis.

In summary, in story-driven approaches, the first major task is to be attentive to the details of the situation. How is this accomplished? You must be not only humble in the face of rich diversity but also respectful of deep differences and, to the extent possible, show respect for those differences in your relationships with others. You also must take seriously the larger social and institutional forces that influence relationships, a topic covered in more detail in Chapter 6.

Ethics of Care Approach

So far you have been introduced to ethical approaches you can use to:
- discover the areas of moral relevance by paying attention to the details of a narrative;
- highlight the moral significance of relationships in the situation;
- remember to be attentive to deep differences among persons or groups; and
- appreciate the power of institutional and other social arrangements to influence a situation.

In this subsection, you have an opportunity to examine some ethical approaches that take the idea of care itself as their central feature. Many varieties of a "care ethic" exist at this time, but generally speaking, in an *ethics of care approach*, the major question is "What is required of a health professional to be best able to express, 'I care'?" As you noted in Chapter 2, taken in its richness, care is the language adopted in the health professions ethical literature to emphasize the imperative that professionals must keep a focus on the well-being of the whole person. Within this context, we have emphasized the goal of professional ethics as being a caring response. Bishop and Scudder described the core of an ethic of care as residing in the health professional's "caring presence" as follows:

> Caring presence does not mean an emotive, sentimental, or maudlin expression of feeling toward patients. It is a personal presence that assures others of another's concern for their well-being. This way-of-being fosters trust, mutual concern, and positive attitudes that promote good health. When caring presence pervades a health care setting, the whole atmosphere of that setting is transformed so that not only is sound therapy fostered, but patients appreciate, take pride in, and feel part of the health care endeavor.[16]

At least two aspects of a care ethic approach are implied. First, the approach is dependent on real contact with the patient as a person; that is, it is deeply relational. Second, the approach fosters trust. Trust is a central notion for an ethics approach that derives from a perspective of care. That, in turn, suggests that you as the health professional must bring trustworthiness and empathetic involvement to the relationship,[17] a notion that is discussed in greater detail subsequently in this chapter.

In an ethics of care approach, the caring relationship serves as a frame to evaluate ethical issues. Good care is a process that involves the caregiver's attentiveness, competence, and responsiveness. An emphasis on connectedness, dependency, and vulnerability as essential features provides a focus on humans as relational beings, who need interpersonal relationships to flourish.[18,19]

 Summary

Good care is a process that involves the caregiver's attentiveness, competence, and responsiveness. In an ethics of care approach, the caring relationship serves as a frame to evaluate ethical issues.

Story and Ethics of Care Approaches and a Caring Response

Story or case approaches combine to illuminate several facets of the overall picture of care. For instance, the vigilance directed to the details of the story and its narrator, the emphasis on relationships that shape the story, and a deep respect for the differences that exist among peoples and cultures all are important tools in understanding what it means "to care." You are encouraged to embrace opportunities to refine your own interpretation of what a full theory of an ethics of care involves in your relationships with patients. Not only are these approaches tied to the development of one's professional identity, but they have become increasingly important in fostering the kinds of self-reflection and interpersonal communication essential to interprofessional practice.

We turn now to *virtue theory*. The appropriateness of giving your attention to this theory is expressed by a health professional who, in thinking about their profession, said, "caring behavior involves the integration of virtue and expert activity of… [professional] practice."[20] Virtue ethics focuses on the cultivation of virtues, that when taken together dispose an individual to act justly.[21] In other words, "being" and "doing" are both involved and deeply related. An understanding of virtue theory provides an important link between the motivation to find a caring response and the ethical acts or behaviors that follow from the character traits we cultivate.

Virtue Theory

Many varieties of virtue theory have been developed over the ages. The basic threads that have created the general tapestry of varieties, called virtue ethics, are provided here. In a look back on the early Western development of those theories, Aristotle can be credited with providing a basic framework for this thinking.[22] Within the Judeo-Christian theological tradition that has deeply influenced Western ethics, the virtue dimensions of Thomas Aquinas's theories have had a profound impact on the shaping of virtue theory.[23] Within the health professions and early medical ethics writings, the idea of virtue also was dominant. For example, authors of the Hippocratic School wrote approximately 70 essays on healthcare in addition to the Oath, several of which discussed character traits. For example, The Decorum enjoins that a physician "should be modest, sober, patient, prompt, and conduct himself [sic] with propriety in professional and personal life."[24] In short, the professional caregiver will have the moral fiber necessary to perform the duties outlined in the Oath.

Maimonides was a highly respected and renowned philosopher of the 13th century who wrote extensively about the relationship of medical issues to Jewish law. The prayer of Maimonides is based directly on the belief that the development of certain character traits enables the caregiver to exhibit appropriate moral behavior. In making this promise, the physician calls on God for help to have the right motives worthy of this high calling:

> May neither avarice nor miserliness nor thirst for glory nor for great reputation engage my mind, or the enemies of truth and philanthropy could easily deceive me and make me forgetful of my lofty aim of doing good to my patients. May I never see in a patient anything but a fellow creature of pain.[25]

Maimonides believed that important character traits of the health professional are sympathy for the patient's plight, humility, and a devoted commitment to helping others.

From those early influences, many versions of virtue theory have evolved so that the tapestry of thought today is splendid indeed. The easiest way into the understanding of virtue theory is through the basic idea of character traits and moral character.

Character Traits and Moral Character

A *character trait* is a disposition or a readiness to act in certain ways. Some character traits are moral character traits because they are supportive of high ethical standards. Persons who habitually act in a manner that can be praised by others because their conduct upholds high ethical standards are said to be persons of high *moral character*. To some extent, our society is measured by the type of people in it, and professionals are judged on this basis more than on any other criterion. Your oaths, codes, and standards of practice declare it. Your state licensing laws require it of you.

Certain character traits enable you to be the kind of person you want to be as a caregiver.[26] For example, honesty manifests itself in your trying to refrain from deceiving others for your own comfort or protection. Courage may be needed to speak out against injustice or other wrongdoing. Courage combined with honesty is needed for health professionals to admit that they mistakenly took the wrong treatment approach. Compassion can help motivate you to take action, and help relieve another's pain or suffering despite the circumstance. We will talk more about compassion as a virtue in Chapter 13.

Recall the health professionals involved in Max Diaz's case. Honesty taken alone would dispose you to encourage Elizabeth Kim to tell his mother about the intentional delay in her son's individualized education plan (IEP). Honesty and courage together would dispose you to telling her but also to take every step to ensure that she actually receives the correct information. This may involve some risk-taking conduct if Elizabeth believes an intentional misappropriation is going on. In other words, the two virtues together will drive her to take measures that ensure Principal Leary is held accountable. These two character traits combined with compassion would motivate her to make sure the information is transmitted in a way that shows respect for everyone involved. Together, the habitual practice of exercising these traits would create a high moral character that prompts her to do everything possible to diminish harm and foster a morally healthy work environment, not only in this situation but also in others she encounters.

 Reflection

Patients are very different in their responses to personality types of health professionals. But more fundamentally, they almost all have strong feelings about the kind of person you as a health professional are. Character traits of respect, compassion, and honesty are high on the list of character traits that most patients want to be able to count on. What other character traits do you feel are necessary for health professionals?

_____

_____

_____

_____

The most widely esteemed traits are those that convey an attitude of respect for individuals who come to you as patients. The underlying ideal is that individuals should be treated as ends, not as means to some other end.

Individual, interprofessional, and institutional virtues are important within the health professions. In this respect, one can speak of the moral character of an individual health professional, a team of healthcare providers, or the moral character of healthcare institutions. In addition to the elaboration of specific virtues that should be cultivated, you need to know several other points about the cultivation of virtue.

First, experience is extremely important. Only through experience can we ultimately learn exactly what contributes to a morally good life (the goal of exercising virtue in the first place).

Second, because the cultivation of virtue depends on experience, we cannot simply think ourselves into being virtuous or knowing what virtue consists of. We must add feelings. Emotions must be attended to; as you learned in Chapter 3, they are the motivators toward certain kinds of actions and not others.

Third, in the process of experiencing and feeling what is happening in the situation, we ourselves become transformed. When one follows the inclination of virtue, one is working at becoming more virtuous. We grow into virtue by acting in accordance with what virtue counsels us to do.

Fourth, a community of persons is vital for discerning virtue in a situation. In this regard, the health professions are one community in which such discernment takes place.[27] Keep these four points on cultivation of virtue in mind as you will explore them further in Chapter 6.

Character Traits and a Caring Response

Several positive character traits may be called into play at one time or another to prepare you attitudinally for the action you will have to take to achieve a caring response. Understandably, the development of habits that allow you to move easily into a caring response will serve you well. The ability to live a life of moral excellence requires exercise, but as Aristotle duly notes, high moral character is the key component to a good life overall. Morality is about the pursuit of good; along the way, we all struggle with the balance. We must understand our duties as moral agents and uphold these duties for the right reasons. In addition, because healthcare is increasingly delivered by interprofessional care teams, we have a shared moral obligation to work together to improve care. Acting with honesty and integrity demonstrates commitment to these virtues. Good character traits help us build good moral character and foster a stronger moral culture for the many uncertain tasks we face.

Summary

The early crafters of the idea that professionals must exert high moral character through the cultivation of virtues make good common sense when viewed through the lens of the professional's moral task of achieving an outcome consistent with a caring response.

You already have come a considerable distance in this chapter. Although the professional ethic takes the story and your attitudes to what you learn from it as the fundamental starting point, the ethical challenge does not end there. You must now link virtue with conduct. The caring response requires that you become a certain type of person (i.e., of high moral character) for a purpose—that is, to do what is right. Therefore, because professional ethics require action, dispositions, and character traits, we turn now to ethical theories and approaches collectively termed *action theories*. They include principle-based approaches, deontology, and teleology.

Principle-Based Approach

When you move to purposive action, it is helpful to be able to say, "Toward what end?" Moral agent Elizabeth Kim will ask, "What guidelines can I use to help know if my course of action is in the (morally) right direction to achieve the right outcome?" This concern, and the recognition that guidelines are needed, led to the development of methods that emphasize ethical *principles* and therefore are termed a *principle-based approach*. In most professional ethics literature (and modern social ethics writings), these methods are called principles, but one can also think of them as elements because they do for ethical theory what the basic chemical elements do for chemistry theory: They provide a way to see something concretely that is quite abstract. As you know, a chemical element can be combined with other elements. Sometimes, they combine to form a new compound that looks and acts differently than each of the units taken individually. Sometimes, they clash. Often, two or more elements have different relative weights so that one is heavier than the other. Key principles are shown in Table 4.2 for your future reference.

Table 4.2   Ethical Principles

Principle	When applicable
Nonmaleficence (refraining from potentially harming myself or another)	I am in a position to harm someone else.
Beneficence (bringing about good)	I am in a position to benefit someone else.
Fidelity	I have made a promise, explicit or implicit, to someone else.
Autonomy	I have an opportunity to exercise my self-determination, say-so.
Veracity	I am in a position to tell the truth or to deceive someone.
Justice	I am in a position to distribute benefits and burdens among individuals or groups in society who have legitimate claims on the benefits.
Paternalism	I am in a position to decide for someone else.

There is more to the story than Table 4.2 indicates because "I" may be a person, a group, or even an institution. Principles can help you know how an individual, group, or institution stands in relationship to others, morally speaking. These principles, or shared moral beliefs, guide action and serve to act as standards for moral behavior.[28] The British philosopher David Hume[29] justified this position in his belief that we incur obligations to act in certain ways because we have received positive responses to our own needs to be treated humanely: "I have benefitted from society, and therefore ought to promote its interests." Some philosophers argue that principles help to identify what we should do in special relationships regardless of whether we have received benefits from the other person (or from society). Some such relationships, Hume says, are between parent and child, spouses, faculty and student, or citizen and society. The health professions are another source of special relationship: with patients.

Several principles are extremely important in the healthcare context. For example, the principle of nonmaleficence, or "above all, do no harm," was an explicit theme in the ancient Hippocratic Oath and ever since has been viewed as an overriding moral principle that guides health professionals' conduct toward patients. Because of the importance of these principles, you have this opportunity to examine several in more detail.

Nonmaleficence and Beneficence

Primum non nocere ("first, do no harm") is thought to be at the nexus of traditional healthcare ethics and often is attributed to the authors of the Hippocratic Oath. It is at the very heart of what is meant by a caring response! The principle of *nonmaleficence* is used today to talk about this type of action. The general meaning of the term can be found by breaking it into its prefix, *non,* and the root, *maleficence* ("mal, bad, or evil"). The difference in power between professional and patient alone helps support the instinctive wisdom of this strong call to refrain from abuse. Furthermore, Western societies in general usually attribute greater significance to a harmful act done out of deliberate intent than out of neglect or ignorance. It is difficult to believe that a society could survive if people went around trying to harm each other, and the laws of our land take seriously the necessity of stemming the potential for harm to go unchecked. The early purveyors of professional ethics left nothing to chance and warned health professionals that there was no room whatsoever for acting in ways designed to bring about harm.

In professional ethics, not harming and acting to benefit another *(beneficence)* are treated as separate duties. Sometimes, philosophers treat them as different levels of the same principle or element. When duties are thought of in this latter fashion, at least four types fall along the continuum of the same principle:

- Do no harm.
- Prevent harm.

- Remove harm when it is being inflicted.
- Bring about positive good.
  Professional ethics limits beneficence to the last three on the list.
  Because these two principles are so pervasive in the everyday decision making by health professionals, you are well advised to think about their relevance in every new situation you encounter.

Reflection

Consider the principles of nonmaleficence and beneficence in relation to the story in this chapter. Elizabeth is worried about the direction of Max Diaz's care. She believes his learning and academic progress are being delayed, which is causing harm to his overall success at school. Is Elizabeth following the principle of nonmaleficence by her actions so far? The principle of beneficence?

_____

_____

_____

_____

What evidence do you have that she is or is not?

_____

_____

_____

In your opinion, what would she have to do to be beneficent in this case, given the level of her authority and her knowledge, skills, and compassion?

_____

_____

_____

_____

What members of the interprofessional education team are likely to co-construct this narrative and serve as resources to Elizabeth?

_____

_____

_____

_____

Autonomy

The principle of *autonomy* is the capacity to have the say-so about your own well-being, "the capacity to act on your decisions freely and independently."[30] Some call this the principle of *self-determination*. Obviously, the principle applies to you whether you are acting in your professional role (professional autonomy) or as a citizen (social autonomy) or have become a patient (patient autonomy). Professional autonomy points out that a health professional must be free of encumbrances to act in the best judgment on behalf of patients. Much of the discussion that follows focuses on the important arena of patient autonomy.

A patient's basic healthcare needs have not changed significantly over the decades, but the idea of what fully constitutes a caring response has changed. Today, so many clinical interventions are possible that the type and number of interventions alone may lead to suffering. A few years ago, the health professional who did everything clinically possible for a patient was seen as beneficent. Today, that same professional could find that the process leads to moral regret; the patient or patient's family may charge that harm has resulted because the interventions have gone beyond what the patient wanted or could tolerate.

In light of this situation, the last several decades have seen the emergence of the patient as a more active participant and negotiator of healthcare decisions. The patient's autonomy—say-so or self-governance—has come to be accepted as a legitimate moral claim to be placed in the balance with the health professional's independent judgment about what is beneficent. Again, one is reminded that the emphasis today on patient-centered care is dependent on shared decision making in the relationship. Some suggest that in the United States and many other Western countries, autonomy has too much emphasis and creates a monopoly on our moral attention.

The principle of autonomy (or self-determination) and its role in morality have been developed from the views of diverse and colorful figures in philosophy. Two who have been especially influential are the deontologist, Immanuel Kant, and one of the crafters of a consequence-oriented theory, John Stuart Mill (they are discussed subsequently in this chapter). Both of their interpretations of the principle of autonomy have been adopted in health professions usage. Kant[31] emphasized the role of being in control of one's own choices in accord with a moral standard that could be willed valid for everyone. Therefore his main contribution was his discussion of self-legislation, the reasons for actions. Conversely, Mill[32] focused his thought more on the context of the freedom of action, with the argument that an individual's actions legitimately can be restricted only when they promise to harm someone else. Up to that point, he contends, each person should be permitted to act according to his or her own convictions. Therefore his main contribution was to highlight the social and political context in which the exercise of autonomy can thrive.[32] The two interpretations together point to our assumption today that a patient's input can be rational and that the context of decision making must be conducive to the patient's exercise of real and informed wishes. Anything less fails to meet the criterion of a caring response (Fig. 4.1).

Gilligan, whose studies were introduced previously in this chapter, is among those who criticize a focus on autonomy because it requires that a person be treated as an isolated unit standing alone, over and against all other people, whereas, as you recall, she is among those who emphasize the importance of relationships for the moral life.[33] Hers is a serious

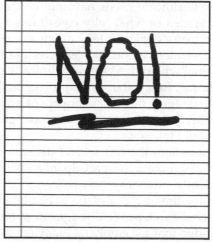

Fig. 4.1. This statement was written on a pad of paper by a 27-year-old hospitalized woman with metastatic ovarian/breast cancer. She could not communicate verbally because she had a tracheostomy and therefore could not speak. The physician had explained that he wanted to reimplement chemotherapy for a tumor that had appeared in her remaining ovary. She had already undergone an oophorectomy and hysterectomy and had received radiotherapy and chemotherapy for the previous tumors before their removal.

criticism. She is correct in her observation that we understand ourselves as moral beings largely within the context of our relationships. Be that as it may, we also live in a society that is highly individualistic in its behavior and laws. The principle of autonomy provides direction in those situations in which individuals are in a position to make a claim on others to respect their selfhood.

Conditions and Considerations in Autonomy

For true autonomy, two conditions are necessary. The individual must have liberty (freedom from controlling influences) and agency (capacity for intentional action). These conditions for autonomy are discussed subsequently in this text as they relate to specific ethical dimensions of practice. For example, much discussion currently is ongoing about autonomy in regard to decisions about the timing and type of death one will have, a topic you will encounter again in Chapter 13. Underlying the idea of a right to die is the more fundamental belief in the right to autonomy or self-determination, but the principle of autonomy has much broader applications than end-of-life situations.

Although autonomy is highly valued in American society in general, this value varies across individuals, communities, and cultures. Given our global and growing national diversity, communal or familial decision making is a consideration that often presents in clinical scenarios. Race, gender, age, ethnicity, socioeconomic status, occupation and place of residence, religion, and sexual identity and orientation are among the most frequently cited socio cultural characteristics. Because culture itself has a broad impact on health and health-related issues, these differences must be appreciated to achieve a caring response. You will explore sociocultural aspects more fully in Section V; however, regardless of the patient's background and beliefs, the act of approaching each patient with respect itself upholds the moral principle of autonomy, even though their decision making may be influenced by specific values that may lead to communal or other forms of decision making that vary from the self-determination associated with patient autonomy.[34]

Paternalism. At times, the patient's deep preferences conflict with the health professional's judgment of what is best for the patient on the basis of the professional's values, which are not necessarily those of the patient. In other words, the conflict is between the patient's choice and the professional's (or interprofessional care team's) judgment of what is best for the patient. In this situation, the principle of *paternalism* or *parentalism* may come into play. Paternalistic or parentalistic decisions are those in which a health professional acts as a parent, with all of the negative and positive connotations. Paternalism is in play when relevant information regarding an individual's medical condition is withheld, defended by the claim that the person interfered with is better off or protected from harm.[35] Paternalism limits patient autonomy; when evoked, the health professional makes a decision *for* the client instead of *with* the client. Considerations of paternalism also arise with respect to the implementation of public health policies and laws (e.g., mandatory seat belt use).

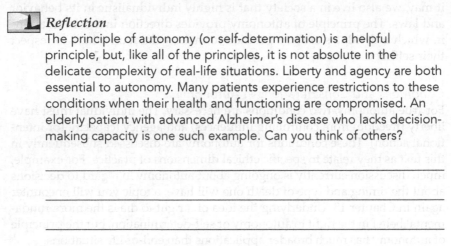

Reflection

The principle of autonomy (or self-determination) is a helpful principle, but, like all of the principles, it is not absolute in the delicate complexity of real-life situations. Liberty and agency are both essential to autonomy. Many patients experience restrictions to these conditions when their health and functioning are compromised. An elderly patient with advanced Alzheimer's disease who lacks decision-making capacity is one such example. Can you think of others?

_____

_____

_____

You will revisit the principle of autonomy several times later in this book. Watch for it.

Fidelity

The principle of *fidelity* comes from the Latin root *fides*, which means faithfulness. Fidelity is about being faithful to one's commitments. Being faithful to the patient entails meeting the patient's reasonable expectations. Patients come with all kinds of expectations. What can be counted as a reasonable expectation?

First is a reasonable expectation that basic respect will be shown to anyone, anywhere. Sometimes, health professionals have been criticized for failing to show basic respect, such as respecting the modesty of a patient.

Second, the patient has reason to expect that you will be competent in what you do.

Third is the patient's reasonable expectation that you will adhere to statements you have subscribed to as a member of a profession. The most public of these statements is your code of ethics.

Fourth, the patient has a good basis for believing you will follow the policies and statements adopted by your place of employment and the laws that are designed to protect patient well-being.

Finally, the patient has good reason to expect that you will honor what the two of you have agreed to, such as the promises involved in any informed consent form the patient has signed, verbal agreements, and serious conversations.

Can you think of others? A caring response cannot be affected if you fail to meet the reasonable expectations of your patients and others.

Veracity

The ethical principle of *veracity* binds you to honesty. Veracity means that you will tell the truth. This principle is more specific than, say, beneficence or fidelity. For this reason, some call it a second-level principle that directs you to engage in a specific type of behavior, which in turn can support your intent to be beneficent or to maintain your fidelity in relationships with patients and others. Kant gave veracity a central role, with the position that veracity is an absolute to which no exception can be made. The lie, he argues in one place, always is wrong because the practice of lying is something that weakens the entire human fabric.[36] Most others weigh veracity heavily regarding its potential for benefiting others but do not make it the absolute or governing duty above all others.

In our story, Elizabeth Kim understandably seemed disappointed about the possibility that Melinda, Max's mom, was not being told the truth about Max's status and the IEP process. The situation was made more complex by the different professional roles of the principal and the speech and language pathologist.

Justice

Patients do not always get all the treatment and attention they deserve or need because of a lack of resources, or access to resources, and anyone who worries about that is worrying about the principle of justice. Discrimination, stigma, bias, and structural inequalities against some individuals or groups may appear to shortchange them, and anyone who worries about that is worrying about the justice of the situation. A lack of due process regarding who receives priority in situations of conflict may cause concern, and anyone who worries about that also is worrying about the justice of the situation. In general, the concern is that all similarly situated individuals receive their fair share of benefits and assume their fair share of burdens. The caring response is achieved when individuals or groups are treated fairly and equitably.

Justice can be thought of as an arbiter. It serves to ensure a proper distribution of burdens and benefits when there are competing claims, not all of which always can be met fully. As you recall, a dilemma of justice is one variety of an ethical dilemma problem. The principle is called on with problems regarding what is rightfully due a person, institution, or society. Several types of justice have particular importance in professional ethics situations: distributive, compensatory, social, and procedural. The complex issues of justice are discussed more fully in Chapters 14 and 15.

Principles and a Caring Response

As you can see, the ethical principles you will encounter most often in your professional roles are very general, but they do serve as guidelines to move you in the direction of action. In their particularity, they are instrumental in helping you further delineate the conditions that must be met if you are to show a caring response toward the patient. For instance, you know that you must honor the patient's reasonable expectations, you must do it truthfully, and so on. In short, the principles themselves force you to consider who the patient is as an individual different from all others.

 Summary

Principles provide general moral guidelines in the search for a course of action that will result in an outcome consistent with a caring response.

You may have noticed that some principles are oriented more toward a conduct or duty-driven ethic. They include fidelity, autonomy, veracity, and justice. Others, namely beneficence and nonmaleficence, require you to weigh the most favorable (or least damaging) consequences in a situation. Both deontologists and teleologists express the need for individual or group actions to be guided according to principles. However, you have not yet had the opportunity to look more closely at these two major theories that have been highly influential in traditional professional ethics approaches. Let's turn to them now.

Deontological and Teleological Theories

Taking Duties Seriously: Deontology

Elizabeth Kim faces a perplexing situation regarding balancing loyalty and honesty. One approach is to identify whether she has a duty that can help her decide what to do. In her search for a duty (or duties), she is appealing to *deontology* and *deontological theories*.

One place where duties are codified is in codes of professional ethics. For example, currently you can find statements such as "respect a patient's dignity" or "honor the patient's [or client's] right to consent to a potential treatment." When you look more closely, the statements imply fundamental ideas about humans—namely, that we stand in relation to each other in a number of morally significant ways. In this regard, deontologists agree with Gilligan and others discussed in this chapter who emphasize the central-ity of relationship and the importance of paying attention to the details of a patient's (or another's) story. Deontologists hold that the basic concepts that individuals and societies recognize and agree on give rise to a shared sense of duty or right. These could be arrived at through reasoning about such things or, others might argue, we intuit them. Although a narrative approach correctly helps focus attention on particular details of a story, the deontologist goes further to say that a concept of duty informs (or is at least available to) all individuals.

Deontological theories hold that you are acting rightly when you act according to duties and rights. In other words, duties and rights are the correct measuring rods for evaluating a course of action and its outcome. Many versions of deontology exist. The person most often identified with deontological approaches is Immanuel Kant, whose philosophies were introduced in the discussion of the principle of autonomy. His basic premises still figure strongly in arguments within healthcare ethics today. He held that every person has an inherent dignity and on that basis alone is entitled to respect. Respect is shown by never using people to achieve other goals or consequences that do not benefit them. He thought that duties help to determine how respect toward others can best be expressed. It follows that the morally correct thing is always to be guided by moral duties. He concluded that some actions are intrinsically immoral, no matter how positive and beneficial one might judge the consequences to be, and that other actions are intrinsically moral, no matter how negative the consequences might be. In short, he said that one cannot judge the moral rightness or wrongness of an act on the basis of its consequences alone.[35] Whatever Elizabeth's conclusion about what Melinda Diaz or Principal Leary should do, Kant would arrive at his decision by a process of determining what their duty should be, not simply whether a better consequence overall would be achieved by one type of act or another. Professional responsibility would be guided by accountability more than responsiveness in the range of consequences.

Reflection

Do you think that this appeal to duties is the correct moral tool to use in the situation in which Elizabeth Kim and Principal Leary find themselves?

Yes_____ No_____

What important moral considerations are taken into account in this approach?

_____

_____

_____

_____

What could be overlooked if they appealed to their sense of duty alone?

_____

_____

_____

_____

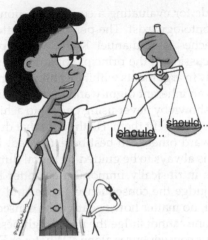

Fig. 4.2. Weighing duties.

As you can begin to see, there are some challenges to applying the deontological approach in its "pure" form. For instance, the idea that one ought to do the right thing, informed by duty, is general. How to show respect for individuals still needs further interpretation in any situation. What should one do when duties or rights themselves come into conflict? Deontological theories require that a method of weighing be available to determine what to do when conflicts arise, and critics charge that there is no obvious way to weigh them (Fig. 4.2). Such a process is not self-evident. Thus the appeal to principles discussed in the previous section is one attempt to provide further detail and interpretation to the general idea of duty and order, or to give varying weight to conflicting duties and rights.

Absolute, Prima Facie, and Conditional Duties

From a deontological viewpoint, principles can assist in interpreting one's duty. Principles that carry the weight of duties may be absolute, prima facie, or conditional. *Absolute duties* are binding under all circumstances. They can never give way to another compelling duty or right. *Prima facie duties* or rights allow you to make choices among conflicting principles. For instance, the prima facie duty of veracity is actually binding if it conflicts with no other duties, or rights, that carry more weight in a given situation. But it is not an element that is absolute either because other elements may be more compelling. In the discussion of the primacy of "do no harm" over "beneficence" in the clinical ethics context, we suggested that each is being treated as a prima facie principle, and the mandate not to harm is more compelling than the mandate to bring about some positive good. A *conditional duty* is a commitment that comes into being only after certain conditions are met. For example, the Americans with Disabilities Act outlines certain duties and rights that apply solely to individuals who have disabilities.[37]

However binding a principle or element is deemed to be, it has the role of providing a marker to guide the conduct of individuals and groups wanting to live a good moral life.

Paying Attention to Outcomes: Teleology

Partially because of some of the criticisms of deontology, *teleology* and *teleological theories* emerged and placed the focus on the ends brought about and the consequences of actions. The most important teleological theory for our consideration of healthcare ethics is *utilitarianism*. This word takes its root from the idea of utility or usefulness.

Utilitarianism

In utilitarianism, an act is right if it helps bring about the best balance of benefits over burdens—in other words, the best "utility" or consequences overall. The original approach was developed first by two English philosophers, Jeremy Bentham (1748–1832)[38] and John Stuart Mill (1806–1873).[39] Note that they are roughly contemporaries of Kant. In fact, they were vigorous opponents of Kant's position.

From a utilitarian point of view, as a moral agent, you must consider what several different courses of action could accomplish, the goal being to fit the action to the outcome that brings about the most good or least harm overall, all things considered. In the case of Elizabeth Kim, you might say, "The goal is to treat Max Diaz in such a way that everyone else will be able to have the same type of care he gets" or "The goal is to be able to live with my own conscience." If both of these goals can be attained by taking one single course of action, it should be taken. If this is not possible, the course of action you believe will bring about the best consequences or "outcomes" overall should take priority.

One important task of this approach is to distinguish alternate paths of action and then predict as accurately as possible the consequences of each path. *Rule utilitarians* are sometimes thought of as a hybrid of deontological and utilitarian approaches. Pure utilitarians weigh the consequences solely in the specific details of each situation. A rule utilitarian holds that you will always bring about more good consequences by following certain "rules" or duties. What the rules should be then becomes the task for these theorists.

Duties, Consequences, and a Caring Response

Deontological and teleological ethics theories have been helpful tools for health professionals because they set a general framework for thinking about specific moral issues and problems in healthcare settings with a focus on the action that needs to take place. Probably as you were reading you were thinking, "Well, both the idea of courses of action consistent with duties and rights and the idea of consequences or outcomes are important in my attempt to arrive at a caring response." In fact, most of us do draw

Table 4.3 Theories of Deontology Versus Teleology

Deontology	Teleology
Duty driven	Goal driven
Means count	Ends count
Kant (deontologist)	Bentham, Mill (utilitarians)

on both to make practical everyday moral decisions. Only occasionally does it make a big difference in what you judge to be right if you follow solely a deontological line of reasoning or appeal to consequences only. Fortunately, most of the time you can take action that is in line with your sense of duty, honor others' rights, and consider the outcomes you are bringing about without any conflict among the three. But it is in the occasional moment during which the means and the ends seem to be competing that it may become necessary to plant your feet firmly in one theory or the other and be able to justify why. See Table 4.3 for a brief summary of deontology and teleology.

Summary

This chapter introduced you to ethical theories and approaches, the conceptual tools that help you the most when faced with ethical problems in your role as a health professional. The ability to absorb a narrative for its moral content and the development of moral character help you to be ready for the hard times when no answers seem to be forthcoming or when you are confronted with something that is not easy to face. You also have learned the most important principles, or norms of ethics, that you need to understand the ethical aspects of your life as a professional. Duties and rights are tools for recognizing and working to resolve problems that arise in your everyday practice. They must be balanced with values so that a caring response can be achieved. Although traditionally much of the language of healthcare ethics has been that of what is owed the patient (i.e., the language of duties), the importance of character traits and attitudes and, more recently, the ideas of patient (and professional and society) rights have enriched the understanding of professional ethics with its goal of ascertaining a caring response. With these basic frameworks at your disposal, you are well positioned to engage in the six-step process of ethical analysis and decision making introduced in the next chapter.

Questions for Thought and Discussion

1. This is an opportunity for the class to create a narrative of a patient, Esther Korn. This group exercise is about a healthcare situation that came to the attention of the hospital ethics committee. (If you have forgotten

what an ethics committee is, go back to Chapter 1.) The entire class can participate in the discussion as members of the ethics committee, and five people can assume various important roles.

- The ethics committee has been asked to give advice on whether Esther Korn should be sent back home or to a nursing home.
- Esther Korn, a 72-year-old woman, has been admitted to the hospital with a diagnosis of dehydration and serious bruises from a fall sustained in her home. She was found by a neighbor, Anna Knight, who says she stops by Esther's home daily because Ms. Korn has lived alone with her eight cats since being discharged from a state hospital with a diagnosis of paranoid schizophrenia, which is believed to be under control with medications. From the degree of dehydration, the health professionals believe that Ms. Korn was very dehydrated before she fell and that she had been lying on the floor for at least a day. The emergency medical technicians who brought her to the hospital described her home as "filthy, full of dirty dishes and clothes strung all over, with cat droppings everywhere."
- Now, 5 days later, Ms. Korn seems confused about where she is, but she does know her own name. She says over and over, "Let me out of here! I want to go home!" Her sister, whom she has not seen "for several years" (according to Anna Knight), does not return the nurses' calls or voice messages. The nurses are not in complete agreement, but most of the staff believe that Esther would be better off placed in a supervised setting for her own safety. Anna Knight and the local priest, who visits her regularly, also have strong opinions about where Esther should live.
- Five people will be "storytellers" to provide some missing parts to her story: one will be Esther, and the other four will be significant others in her life. Together the class can create a fictional story that fills in information about who she is and what may, in fact, be in her best interest in this difficult question facing the ethics committee.
- Person A: Write a few paragraphs about Esther from her neighbor Anna's perspective and what Anna thinks should be done.
- Person B: Write about her from the Episcopal priest's perspective and what she would recommend.
- Person C: Write about her from the perspective of her long-lost sister and what she would recommend.
- Person D: Write a report from the point of view of the primary nurse and what he thinks.
- Person E: Speaking as Esther, give some background as to what kind of person she believes herself to be, what is important to her, and so on.
- When each of the five storytellers has completed this part of the exercise, read the notes aloud to the ethics committee (i.e., rest of the group). After everyone has heard the "bigger picture," answer the following questions:
  - What should be done?

- What ethical approaches or theories influence your thinking the most?
- Which values do you think are the most prominent in this discussion?
- Did anything that was said in these stories change your mind about your initial thoughts regarding what should be done? If so, explain.
- Discuss what the health professionals must do to show caring in their relationship with Esther Korn.

2. Elva, a 370-lb, 62-year-old woman, is in a nursing home after complications of diabetes and several small strokes. Although she has been overweight all her life, she now is at a weight where it is unsafe to transfer her without a bariatric lift. Elva, however, refuses to be moved with it, claiming, "I'm not a piece of meat."

   She can be transferred to a chair with the assistance of four or five staff members. The administration, however, is worried that the staff could be injured physically while moving her. Her daughter insists that it is a violation of Elva's dignity and an unnecessary compromise of her autonomy to submit her to "the indignity of the mechanical lift."

   You are the supervisor of the unit. What ethical principles presented in this chapter can help you to assess what to do in this situation? What should you do?

3. Walter is a resident in the same nursing home with Elva. He is a 78-year-old widower who has been taking antidepressants since the sudden death of his wife 5 years ago. He, too, is visited often by his daughter. The staff of the nursing home inadvertently threw out his dentures with the sheets while making his bed. He had a habit of leaving them on the bed, and, although the staff usually noticed them, a new employee failed to do so.

   Since then, Walter has adamantly refused to have his teeth replaced. The nursing home administration is more than willing to fit him with a new set of dentures and to pay all costs. His daughter is very much in agreement with the administration that he should have his teeth replaced. They are all aware that his nutrition is suffering as is his ability to be understood when he tries to talk.

   Should Walter be allowed to continue without his dentures? What principles and other considerations of ethics should you, as a nursing home administrator, bring to bear on your decision on how to proceed in this situation? What should you do? Use your understanding of the different ethical theories and principles to add to the depth of your ethical thought and proposed action.

References

1. Doherty RF: Ethical practice. In Schell BAB, Gillen G, editors: *Willard and Spackman's occupational therapy*, ed 13, Philadelphia, 2019, Wolters Kluwer, pp 513–526.

2. Sullivan WM, Rosin MS, Shulman LS: *A new agenda for higher education: shaping the life of the mind for practice*, New York, 2009, Wiley.
3. Schell BAB: Professional reasoning in practice. In Schell BAB, Gillen G, editors: *Willard and Spackman's occupational therapy*, ed 13, Philadelphia, 2019, Wolters Kluwer, pp 482–497.
4. Higgs J, Jones M: Multiple spaces of choice, engagement, and influence in clinical decision making. In Higgs J, Jensen G, Loftus S, et al, editors: *Clinical reasoning in the health professions*, ed 4, St. Louis, 2018, Elsevier, pp 33–44.
5. Schell BAB, Schell JW: *Clinical and professional reasoning in occupational therapy*, ed 2, Philadelphia, 2019, Lippincott Williams and Wilkins.
6. Mattingly C, Fleming M: *Clinical reasoning: forms of inquiry in therapeutic practice*, Philadelphia, 1994, FA Davis.
7. Leicht SB, Dickerson A: Clinical reasoning, looking back, *Occupational Ther Healthcare* 14(3/4):105–130, 2001.
8. Devettere RJ: *Practical decision making in health care ethics*, ed 4, Washington, DC, 2016, Georgetown University Press.
9. Clark PG: Narrative in interprofessional education and practice: implications for professional identity, provider-patient communication and teamwork, *J Interprof Care* 28(1):34–39, 2014.
10. Hunter K: Narrative. In Post SG, editor: *Encyclopedia of bioethics*, ed 3, New York, 2004, Macmillan, pp 1875–1876.
11. Brody H, Clark M: Narrative ethics: a narrative, *Hastings Cent Rep* 44(1): S7–S11, 2014.
12. Deleted in review.
13. Kohlberg L: *The philosophy of moral development: moral stages and the idea of justice*, San Francisco, 1981, Harper and Row.
14. Gilligan C: *A different voice: psychological theory and women's development*, Cambridge, MA, 1982, Harvard University Press.
15. Nortvedt P, Hem MH, Skirbekk H: The ethics of care: role obligations and moderate partiality in healthcare, *Nurs Ethics* 18(2):192–200, 2011.
16. Bishop A, Scudder J Jr: Caring presence. *Nursing ethics: holistic caring practice*, ed 2, Sudbury, MA, 2001, Jones and Bartlett Publishers, pp 41–65.
17. Schuchter P, Heller A: The Care Dialog: the "ethics of care" approach and its importance for clinical ethics consultation, *Med, Health Care Philos* 21(1):51–62, 2018.
18. Nortvedt P, Hem MH, Skirbekk H: The ethics of care: role obligations and moderate partiality in healthcare, *Nurs Ethics* 18(2):192–200, 2011.
19. Ludovica De Panfilis, Silvia Di Leo, Carlo Peruselli et al, "I go into crisis when …": ethics of care and moral dilemmas in palliative care, *BMC Palliative Care* 18(1):1–8, 2019. doi: 10.1186/s12904-019-0453-2.
20. Bradshaw A: The virtue of nursing: the covenant of care, *J Med Ethics* 25:477–481, 1999.
21. Hawking M, Curling FA, Yoon JD: Courage and compassion: virtues in caring for so called "difficulty patients", *AMA J Ethics* 19(4):357–363, 2017.

22. Aristotle: Nichomachean ethics. In Barnes J, editor: *The complete works of Aristotle*, vol 2, Princeton, 1984, Princeton University Press, p 1729.

23. Aquinas T: Summa theologica. In Pegis AG, editor: *Basic writings of St. Thomas Aquinas*, New York, 1945, Random House.

24. Hippocrates: Decorum. In Jones WHS, editor: *Hippocrates II*, Cambridge, MA, 1923, Harvard University Press, pp 267–302, Loeb Classical Library.

25. Maimonides: Prayers of Moses Maimonides (H. Friedenwald, Trans.), *Bull Johns Hopkins Hosp* 28:260–261, 1927.

26. Rushton CH: Integrity: the anchor for moral resilience. In Rushton CH, editor: *Moral resilience: transforming moral suffering in healthcare*, New York, 2018, Oxford University Press.

27. Marton M: *Personal communication*. In National Endowment for the Humanities Seminar on "Justice, equality and the challenge of disability." Bronxville, NY, June 24, 2002.

28. Doherty RF, Peterson E: Responsible participation in a profession: fostering professionalism and leading for moral action. In Braveman B, editor: *An evidence-based approach to leading & managing occupational therapy services*, ed 2, Philadelphia, 2016, FA Davis.

29. Hume D: On suicide. In Gorowitz S, Macklin R, Jameton A, editors: *Moral problems in medicine*, Englewood Cliffs, NJ, 1976, Prentice Hall, p 356.

30. Beauchamp T, Childress JF: *Principles of biomedical ethics*, ed 8, New York, 2019, Oxford University Press.

31. Kant I: *Lectures on ethics (L. Infield, translator)*, New York, 1963, Harper and Row, pp 147–154.

32. Mill JS: On liberty. In Burtt EA, editor: *The English philosophers from Bacon to Mill*, New York, 1939, Random House, pp 1042–1060.

33. Gilligan C: *Psychological theory and women's development*, Cambridge, MA, 1982, Harvard University Press.

34. Haddad AM, Doherty RF, Purtilo RD: Respect in a diverse society. *Health professional and patient interaction*, ed 9, St. Louis, 2019, Saunders, pp 60–76.

35. Dworkin G: Paternalism. In Zalta EN, editor: *The Stanford encyclopedia of philosophy*, 2019. Available at https://plato.stanford.edu/archives/fall2019/entries/paternalism/.

36. Kant I: In Beck LW, editor: *Critique of practical reason and other writings in moral philosophy*, Chicago, 1949, University of Chicago Press, pp 346–350.

37. *Americans with Disabilities Act*, H.R. Rep. No. 485 (II), 101st Congress, 2nd Sess. at 22 12, 1990.

38. Bentham J: An enquiry concerning human understanding. In Burtt EA, editor: *The English philosophers from Bacon to Mill*, New York, 1939, Random House, pp 792–856.

39. Mill JS: Utilitarianism. In Burtt EA, editor: *The English philosophers from Bacon to Mill*, New York, 1939, Random House, pp 895–1041.

● 5

The Six-Step Process of Ethical Decision Making

Objectives

The reader should be able to:
- Identify six steps in the analysis of ethical problems encountered in everyday professional life and how each plays a part in arriving at a caring response.
- Describe the central role of narrative and virtue theories in gathering relevant information to achieve a caring response.
- Understand how the application of evidence-based practice supports the ethical decision-making process.
- List four areas of inquiry that will be useful when gathering relevant information to make sure you have the story straight.
- Describe the role of conduct-related ethical theories and approaches in arriving at a caring response.
- Describe why imagination is an essential aspect of seeking out the practical alternatives in an ethically challenging situation.
- Discuss how courage assists you in the ethical decision-making process.
- Recognize two benefits of taking time to reflect on and evaluate a chosen moral action.

New terms and ideas you will encounter in this chapter

six-step process of ethical decision making	chemical restraints evidence-based practice	time-limited trial rounds

Topics in this chapter introduced in earlier chapters

Topic	Introduced in chapter
Ethics	1
A caring response	2, 3, 4
Moral agency	3
Moral distress	3
Ethical dilemma	3
Ethical reasoning	4
The importance of story or narrative	4
Paternalism	4
Deontology	4
Utilitarianism	4
Character traits	4

Introduction

You have come a long way in your search for resolution of ethical problems consistent with a caring response. Distinguishing prototypes of ethical problems and understanding ethical theories and approaches provide you with a necessary foundation to support your ethical reasoning. In this chapter, you have an opportunity to apply the conceptual tools you have learned using a problem-solving method to analyze and move toward resolution of ethical problems. The story of Michael Halloran and Amrou Croteau is a good starting point for this discussion.

 The Story of Michael Halloran and Amrou Croteau

Amrou Croteau, a physical therapist, has just begun working in a municipal group home. The facility has a reputation for maintaining high standards of care. When Amrou interviewed for the position, she made a thorough tour of the home and talked with several employees and residents. Everything seemed "in order," and she took the job.

Amrou is now ending her second week of work. She goes to the group home office to read the medical record of a resident who may be transferred to another facility because of his worsening mental status. She learns that Mr. Michael Halloran is a 46-year-old man with cerebral palsy, insulin-dependent diabetes mellitus, renal hypertension, and a history of depression. Mr. Halloran has been a resident at the home for almost 2 weeks. He was admitted because of his inability to safely care for himself after a recent hospitalization for a fall and renal insufficiency. According to the record, he is "confused" most of the time and has required heavy sedation to "keep him from becoming violent." Mr. Halloran is almost blind as a result of diabetic retinopathy. No neurologist's report is found in the record.

Amrou decides to introduce herself to Mr. Halloran before she goes to lunch. When she finds Mr. Halloran's room, she is surprised to see a frail-looking middle-aged man slumped over in a wheelchair and struggling to read the sports section of the newspaper. Amrou introduces herself and tells Mr. Halloran that she is the physical therapist on staff and that she will be coming back to treat him in the afternoon.

Mr. Halloran squints in an effort to see Amrou. Abruptly he raises up on one elbow and says, "Maybe you'll listen to me. I'm scared! They keep giving me shots and pills that make me crazy here! Can you get them to stop?"

Just at that moment, a nurse comes into the room with a syringe on a tray. "Hi, Mr. Halloran," she says in a firm, loud voice. "Lift your johnny, please. It's time for your shot!"

Mr. Halloran protests that the shots are making him "crazy as a hoot owl." But the nurse has exposed his loose-skinned thigh and is deftly injecting the solution before Mr. Halloran succeeds in resisting. He tries to take a swipe at her, but she backs off quickly. She pats his bony hip and says, "There now, you're okay, Mike," and leaves immediately. Mr. Halloran leans back in the wheelchair and sighs. He looks toward Amrou and says, "See what I mean! I may have a disability, but I am not stupid. I know these places dope people like me so we stay quiet." Amrou struggles with what to say to Mr. Halloran; he seems to be in genuine anguish. She reaches out to pat his hand, but he pulls it away, motioning her away with his paper.

Amrou is upset and confused. She has a gnawing feeling in her stomach that something is wrong in the way Mr. Halloran is being treated. At lunch, she shares her concern with Brenda Rendazzo, the nursing supervisor for the residence. Brenda is highly respected by residents and staff alike. Amrou tells Brenda it seems that Mr. Halloran is not being treated with the dignity that the residents deserve. She doubts that Mr. Halloran is "violent" but cannot put her finger on why she felt so much anger at the nurse who efficiently and without undue harshness gave him the injection. Maybe it is because she believes the medication is being used to "sedate" Mr. Halloran unnecessarily. As she recounts what happened, she can feel a seething rage rising up in her. She decides, on the spot, that she will talk to the group home administrator and announces that intention to Brenda.

Brenda listens attentively. When Amrou pauses for a few disinterested bites of her sandwich, she says, "Amrou, you have been here only 2 weeks. I can understand your uneasiness at what you thought you saw happening. And maybe you are right—maybe Mr. Halloran is not being treated with the respect he deserves. But remember, you are new here, and there is much that you don't know. We are doing for him what we think is best and trying to protect our staff from his dangerously aggressive behavior. He was worse before we started him on the benzodiazepines."

Amrou does not feel any better after lunch. She wants to talk to someone and decides to call a colleague from graduate school who works as a social worker in another residential home.

As in most actual situations, Amrou's first encounter with what appears to be an ethical problem has left many questions unanswered. The path from Amrou's first perception to possible action consistent with a caring response traverses the *six-step process of ethical decision making*.

The Six-Step Process

Ethical decision making requires your thoughtful reflection and logical judgment (i.e., ethical reasoning, discussed in Chapter 4), although the situation usually presents itself in a "mumbo jumbo" of partial facts and strong reactions. The six-step process of ethical decision making provides a framework for working through ethical questions like the one Amrou is facing. The steps serve as practical tools to guide you through the intertwining of emotion, cognition, application, and action toward decision making. They allow you to take the situation apart and critically reflect on competing view points, looking at it in a more organized, coolheaded way.

In Chapter 1, you learned that ethics is reflection on and analysis of morality. The six-step process is, overall, a formalized approach to both. In the context of healthcare, your professional ethics dictates that your reflection is directed toward arriving at a caring response in a particular situation. As a moral agent, your reflection and ensuing judgment are geared toward action.

Step 1: Gather Relevant Information

The first step in informed decision making is to gather as much information as possible. Anyone viewing this situation might ask the following questions:
- What clinical practice guidelines or research evidence support (or contradict) the use of benzodiazepines for clients with aggressive behavior?
- Does Mr. Halloran have cognitive changes from organic brain disease or other central nervous system dysfunction that might explain his agitation and aggressive behavior?
- What tests have been conducted to confirm the type and degree of neurological involvement?
- What does his "violent" behavior consist of?
- Is he at risk of injuring himself or others?
- What might have happened in Mr. Halloran's history to make him afraid of the nursing staff or the whole setting and therefore to react in a hostile manner?
- Has the medical director been made aware of Mr. Halloran's complaints about the effects of the medication?
- What is the recent history of the exchanges between Mr. Halloran and the staff?
- What other approaches (along with medication) to Mr. Halloran's ostensibly violent behavior have been, or could be, attempted?

- What resources/protections are in place for Mr. Halloran, given that he is a vulnerable client transitioning to residential care?
- What evidence is there that approaching the group home administration will create problems for Amrou, Ms. Rendazzo, or others?
- What other information about physical and *chemical restraints* (i.e., medicines that sedate the patient) in group residential settings should Amrou seek?

Reflection
Did you think of other questions as you read the story?

_____

_____

_____

_____

The necessity for close attention to details takes you back to Chapter 4, which introduced the importance of the story or narrative. Without knowledge of as much as possible about the story, the attitudes, values, and duties embedded in it are impossible to ascertain. As you probably recall, the theories and approaches to ethics have important clues about how each of these is an important consideration in arriving at a caring response. The fact-finding mission is absolutely essential as a safeguard against setting off on a false course from the beginning.

Some of the benefits of seeking out the facts in the situation described previously are that you may be able to determine whether Amrou's perception of Mr. Halloran's treatment is accurate and you may understand why the various players in this drama are acting as they are. Although Brenda Rendazzo's comments are difficult to interpret, she may be implying that Amrou's response would be tempered by more knowledge of the situation. Often, what initially appears to be a "wrong" act is, after all, a right or acceptable one once more of the story is known.

Fact finding also could help Amrou identify the focus of her anger more specifically. What triggered the response? Was it Mr. Halloran's apparent helplessness in the situation? The nurse's actions? What Amrou has read about the evidence surrounding the use and misuse of chemical restraints?[1-3] Why has Mr. Halloran been labeled as "confused" and "violent" when Amrou believes he showed no signs of being either? Is Mr. Halloran's assertion correct, that the staff are treating him differently because he is a disabled adult? Fact finding is an essential step in Amrou's ethical reasoning process. She must clarify the known facts of the case—what could she be assuming that might not be true? Facts are things that are true. They can be tested or proven. Opinions are things that are believed. Some beliefs are true, others are not. Some beliefs are backed by evidence, others are not.[4] All of the facts are needed to make a judicious and well-reasoned decision.

Attending to Evidence-Based Practice in Ethical Decision Making

Health professionals today are morally obligated to ensure their clinical decisions are informed and reflect best practice.[5] Sound clinical reasoning integrates *evidence-based practice* with clinical expertise and the client's preferences, beliefs, and values. Clinical research (reviews of data, meta-analyses, position papers) can lend substantial evidence to support ethical reasoning. Catlin puts this well when stating that "good ethics are based on good evidence."[6] Collecting all levels of evidence, from empirical studies to consultations with subject matter experts, is a key part of the gathering relevant information process to problem solve through step 1 of the ethical decision-making process.

The following general checklist for data gathering will help you organize your thoughts around your specific situation. The list is adapted from a handbook designed for clinicians.[7]

1. Clinical Indications
    A. What is the diagnosis or prognosis?
    B. Is the illness or condition reversible?
    C. What are the patient's symptoms?
    D. What is the present treatment regimen?
    E. What evidence supports this treatment regime? Does any evidence contradict it?
    F. What is the usual and customary treatment for this type of condition?
    G. What is needed to relieve suffering or to provide comfort?
    H. Who are the primary caregivers?
    I. What can you learn about this patient's medical and social history?
    J. Who are the members of the interprofessional care team who are treating this patient, and what are the results of their evaluations and treatments to date?
2. Preference of the Patient
    A. What outcome does the patient want in this situation?
    B. Who has communicated the realistic options to the patient?
    C. What was the patient actually told?
    D. What evidence do you have that the patient's needs, wants, and fears have been heard by key decision makers?
    E. Is the patient competent to make decisions about this situation?
    F. Do any family or other cultural influences need to be taken into account? If the patient is not competent, is another person speaking as a legitimate legal substitute for the patient?

3. Quality of Life
  A. What are the patient's beliefs and values that make up his or her personal value system?
  B. What quality-of-life considerations are professional and family caregivers bringing to this situation, and how are their biases influencing the decision processes?
  C. Is there any hope for improvement in the patient's quality of life?
  D. Are there any biases that might prejudice the interprofessional care team's evaluation of the patient's quality of life?
4. Contextual Factors
  A. What institutional policies may influence what can be done?
  B. What are the legal implications (court cases, statutes, and so on) regarding this issue?
  C. Are scarce resources an issue?
  D. How will these services be paid?
  E. Are there family caregiver issues that may influence the plan of care?

Reflection
This general checklist is extensive but not exhaustive. Jot down some other types of information you think will help Amrou to accurately analyze this situation.

_____

_____

_____

_____

Summary
Gathering as much relevant information as possible sets the essential groundwork for analysis and action consistent with arriving at a caring response.

When you have searched out the information you and others deem relevant or when you are convinced no additional helpful information is forthcoming, you are ready to proceed to the next step.

Step 2: Identify the Type of Ethical Problem
Even while the initial fact finding is taking place, Amrou can begin to determine the type of ethical problem (or problems) she is facing and in that

regard make significant progress toward arriving at a caring response. In the beginning, her worry was the following.

Mr. Halloran is a human, and the gold standard of care (as introduced in Chapter 1) is that humans always should be treated with dignity. Part of being treated with dignity includes patients taking part in their own treatment decisions whenever possible; in Mr. Halloran's case, this includes, at the very least, being treated with sensitivity to the anguish that he appears to be experiencing. To ignore his distress shows a lack of compassion, if not outright cruelty, and reduces him to the status of an object. Mr. Halloran is not being treated as a person ought to be treated, which blocks the goal of achieving a professional caring response.

This is where the prototypes of ethical problems you encountered in Chapter 3 begin to work for you.

Moral Distress

You know that Amrou is experiencing emotional distress. She has witnessed a scene that baffled her, and she finds herself unable to forget about it. Our guess about the fundamental basis of Amrou's distress is her perception that Mr. Halloran is not being treated with the dignity he deserves as a human. The distress, then, is consistent with Amrou's role as a professional with a moral responsibility to help uphold human dignity. In other words, she is a moral agent in a situation that she surmises involves morality, and that, because it is worrying her, merits further attention. If she tries but fails to put more information in place, she may confirm that her distress is, in fact, moral distress type B. You also can presume that she has the virtues of a compassionate person, otherwise she would not be worried about what she witnessed.

Ethical Dilemma

Goaded by her emotional responses, character traits, and the awareness that she is experiencing moral distress, Amrou is well positioned to assess whether she also has an ethical dilemma (or dilemmas). Do you think there is an ethical dilemma here?

Amrou learns that quite a few of the staff (but not all) believe the medications are being used disproportionately to the amount of "violence" Mr. Halloran has been demonstrating. In fact, some of the staff confide that they believe he is being sedated not to benefit him but to keep him more in line with the conduct of the other more docile and cooperative residents. Mr. Halloran has seemed very agitated and suspicious at times, and the medication has helped to improve his feeling of security, so that raises the possibility that it *is* benefiting him in that way. Of course, the group home is shorthanded, and the administrator points this out when Amrou finally goes to talk with her. Her argument is that if everyone took as much time and extra attention as Mr. Halloran did (when not medicated), no one would receive a fair amount of treatment. The principle of justice introduced in Chapter 4, and addressed more thoroughly in Chapter 14, is an issue.

Finally, the administrator mentions that some of the staff are afraid of Mr. Halloran and that she has a responsibility for their safety too. There are several issues here in which Amrou, as an employee and interprofessional care team member, may be implicated as partial agent. Foremost of these is whether the employees, as a team, are acting ethically in the use of restraints under any circumstances. The one ethical dilemma that falls squarely on Amrou's shoulders at the moment, however, is this: Amrou's dilemma arises from the fact that she has become more persuaded that she was right about what she saw happening to Mr. Halloran. She believes the principle of beneficence to him is being compromised. But she can also agree with the points made by the administration and some of the staff regarding fairness to other residents. She is experiencing difficulty in deciding what to do to honor the several principles that guide professional action in this situation. In summary, she has an ethical dilemma.

Moral Agency

If Amrou decides that someone other than herself, the administration, or the other team members should be making decisions regarding any aspects of Mr. Halloran's treatment (or the group home policies regarding treatment), she may face a locus of authority conflict. For instance, although the story does not give you the benefit of knowing whether Mr. Halloran's input is being included in the decision, Amrou could decide that the authority for this decision should rest with Mr. Halloran. From what we have been told, we can assume that the staff and medical director have determined that the patient is not competent to make such a decision, and therefore they are acting paternalistically. Regardless, it is important to remember that all members of the interprofessional care team share agency in ensuring that Mr. Halloran receives the care he deserves. They must work together, with the patient and the administration, to navigate conflict and execute a safe, efficient, effective, and compassionate plan of care.

◎ Summary

An essential step in analysis is to identify the type or types of ethical problems that you face.

Step 3: Use Ethics Theories or Approaches to Analyze the Problem

In Chapter 4, you were introduced to ethical theories and approaches. You have seen in the preceding pages that the narrative approach, which keeps relevant details of the story at the center of Amrou's deliberation, is the most crucial for her eventual decision to be consistent with professional ethics.

She also needs certain basic attitudes to help guide her on the path of a caring response as she deals with her own anger about what she observes. Therefore virtues such as compassion are among her most fundamental resources. You learned that situations that require the health professional to be an agent (i.e., take action for which she or he is morally accountable) draw on ethical theories that focus on principles, duties and rights, and/or consequences. In other words, they are the tools for action.

Take a minute to review these action theories:

1. Utilitarianism
   Focuses on the overall consequences
2. Deontology
   Focuses on duty

Amrou's story may make comparison of the two theories easier than when they were presented in Chapter 4.

If agent (A), Amrou, is like most health professionals and is guided by the principles of duty and rights in her professional role, she probably will decide that her weightier (i.e., more compelling) responsibility is to Mr. Halloran.

If agent (A), Amrou, approaches the dilemma from a utilitarian standpoint, she will spend less time thinking about duties to Mr. Halloran and will be guided by the desire to bring about the overall best consequences in this situation. The overall best consequences may be to ensure the safety of the other residents and her coworkers.

Reflection
Which approach do you find yourself leaning toward in Amrou's and Mr. Halloran's situation? Why?

_____

_____

_____

Recall the ethical principles you learned in Chapter 4. Which principles can be balanced when considering the use of chemical restraints for Mr. Halloran?

_____

_____

_____

Summary

In step 3, you use ethical theories and approaches as the foundation for your ethical reasoning, which moves you toward resolution and action that is consistent with a caring response.

Step 4: Explore the Practical Alternatives

Amrou has decided what she should do. The next step is to determine what she can do in this situation. She must exercise her ingenuity and confer with her colleagues regarding the actual strategies and options available to her. Suppose she decides that her initial perceptions were correct and that she must act on behalf of Mr. Halloran, even though the staff sees no problem?

At this juncture, many people oversimplify the range of options available. They tend to fall back on old alternatives when under stress, a behavioral pattern you can probably recognize from your own stressful situations. Therefore imaginative pursuit of options is not only a big challenge, but also an invaluable resource in resolving ethical problems. In recounting Amrou's story, we learned that she believed her range of options was to confront the group home administrator or do nothing. A diligent search for other options can now make the difference between her doing the right thing or allowing a moral wrong to go unchecked.

 Reflection
Apply your own thinking to Amrou's situation and list all the alternatives you believe she has. Try to identify a minimum of four.

1. _____

2. _____

3. _____

4. _____

After listing the alternatives, which one do you think is the best? Why?

Often, a good idea is to try out some of the more far-fetched alternatives with a colleague whom you trust and with whom you can share the situation without breaching the patient's confidentiality. Amrou did this with the nursing supervisor. We do not know how the supervisor's counsel helped in the end, but we are sure that her words led Amrou to further examination of what her next step should be.

It is also important not to limit your range of alternatives based on time. In some situations, an alternative is proposed as a *time-limited trial*. This allows the provider or interprofessional care team the opportunity to both negotiate and think innovatively about solutions that support a caring response. A time-limited trial must be aligned with the patient's goals of care and be weighed for its benefits and burdens. Time-limited trials are further discussed in Chapters 12 and 13, when we explore ethical dimensions in chronic and end-of-life care.

 Summary

Imagination enhances ethical decision making by allowing you to think more creatively and expansively about the alternatives.

Step 5: Complete the Action

Think of all the work Amrou has already done. She responded to her initial feeling that something was wrong, followed her compassionate disposition that motivated her to not let the matter go unnoticed, thought about and decided on the type of ethical problem(s) she was encountering, applied one or more ethical theories and approaches to support her reasoning, and exercised her imagination to identify practical options needed to effect a caring response. She also shared her worry with at least one other person she knew commands her respect and that of others. Now she has one more task, but it is the crucial one, and that is to act.

If Amrou fails to go ahead and act, the entire process so far is reduced to the level of an interesting but inconsequential philosophic exercise; worse, it may result in harm to Mr. Halloran. Of course, Amrou may consciously decide not to pursue the situation any further, but insofar as it involved her deliberate intent, it is different than simply failing to follow what seems a correct course of action. If harm comes to Mr. Halloran or others because of Amrou's inaction or unnecessarily narrow focus, she is an agent of harm by her own omission or neglect. The solid ethical foundation she laid in steps 1 to 4 will have been of no avail.

Why would anyone fail to act in this type of circumstance? Mainly because it is sobering to be an agent in such important matters of meaning and value in others' lives.

 Summary

The goal of your analysis is finally to act!

Some decisions are literally life-and-death decisions, but all are of deep significance to the people who face the particular situation. Although the previous step required imagination, this final step requires courage and the strength of will to go ahead, with the knowledge that there may be risks or backlash. As Amrou becomes more experienced, she will be increasingly aware that her integrity of purpose must be supported by her sound ethical reasoning, compassion, and courage.

Step 6: Evaluate the Process and Outcome

Once she has acted, it behooved Amrou to pause and engage in a reflective examination of the situation. The practical goal of ethics is to resolve ethical problems, upholding important moral values and duties. The extent to which Amrou's decision led to action that upheld morality, however, is knowable only by reexamining what happened in the actual situation. This evaluation is germane to her growth and development as an ethical professional and is essential if the outcome she hoped for was not realized.

In the traditional medical model, a widespread mechanism for addressing interventions that go awry in the clinical setting is morbidity and mortality ("m and m") rounds. If you have not yet been in the clinical setting, the term *rounds* may be new to you. *Rounds* is the general term used for meetings of clinicians. Some rounds are held sitting in a room (sit-down rounds), and others are held walking from patient to patient (walking rounds). Rounds are a means for reflective discernment. They are an explicit way for the interprofessional care team to integrate diverse expertise, reflect on practice, solve problems, and innovate together.[8] Morbidity and mortality rounds allow health professionals whose interventions did not yield the hoped-for results to present the case to their peers for further evaluation. Sometimes ethical committees or your own unit staff meetings conduct ethics morbidity and mortality rounds to have a group review of a particularly difficult situation that seemed not to meet the ethical goal of a caring response. This type of activity not only leads to improved patient outcomes, it promotes ethical reasoning, supports interprofessional communication, and helps ensure that care is individualized, just, and benevolent.[9–12]

Amrou's case is not unique. Studies have shown that the topics of conflict around goal setting and dual obligations are among the most frequently cited ethical issues encountered by rehabilitation practitioners.[13–16] Given this, suppose you, like Amrou, have just been through the process of arriving at a difficult ethical decision and have acted on it. Some questions you might ask yourself are the following:

- What went well?
- What were the most challenging aspects of this situation?
- How did this situation compare with others you have encountered or read about?
- To what other kinds of situations will your experience with this one apply?
- Who was the most help?

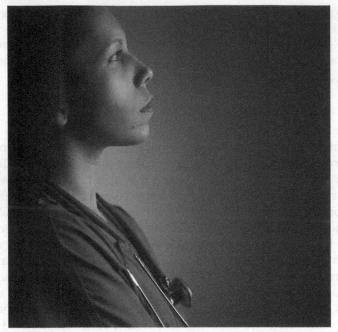

Fig. 5.1. Critical reflection = clinical growth. *(Copyright iStockphoto.com/ MarilynNieves.)*

- What do the patient, family, and/or others have to say about your course of action?
- Overall, what did you learn?
- Do you think in retrospect that you failed to give adequate attention to anything?
- Did you miss the mark at one or more times? In what regard?
- What would you do differently if you were faced with the same situation again?

All of these questions will serve you well in your preparation for the next opportunity to decide what a caring response entails in that new situation. When you reflect, you advance your ethical reasoning and are better prepared for the next time you are faced with a challenging situation (Fig. 5.1).

Summary

Reflection is the link to critical thinking. It allows you to reframe problems, extract meaning from experiences, and engage in lifelong learning to bring about best practice in a variety of settings.

Summary

If you studied this chapter carefully, you have identified the six-step process that anyone faced with an ethical question can apply in searching for a caring response.

1. Get the Story Straight
   Gather as much relevant information as possible to get the facts straight.
2. Identify the Type of Ethical Problem
   If step 1 confirms that there is one.
3. Use Ethics Theories or Approaches to Analyze the Problem
   Decide on the ethics approach that will best get at the heart of the problem identified in step 2.
4. Explore the Practical Alternatives
   Decide what should be done and how it can best be done (explore the widest range of options possible).
5. Complete the Action
   Call upon your strength of will and moral courage to act.
6. Evaluate the Process and Outcome
   Reflect on your experience to better prepare yourself for future situations.

Questions for Thought and Discussion

1. The first step in ethical decision making is to gather as much relevant information as possible. The information-gathering process, however, can become so extensive that it could become an end in itself and could actually deter one from proceeding to action at all. What types of guidelines would you use to decide that you have as much information as you need or can obtain?
2. A necessary step in ethical decision making is to act on one's own conclusions about what ought to be done. Under what conditions, if any, would you decide not to act according to your own best moral insights and judgment? That is, what, if any, are the limits to your willingness to act ethically?
3. What type of reflective practices will you integrate into your professional work to ensure that you think critically about both the art and science of your patient care delivery? Who has served as a resource to you in the past to help you advance your thinking and level of reflection? Will that person continue to help you evaluate your decision-making process? If not, what structure will you need to ensure that you continually improve your practice through the reflective cycle?

References

1. Maust DT, Lin LA, Blow FC: Benzodiazepine use and misuse among adults in the United States, *Psychiatr Serv* 70(2):97–106, 2019.
2. McCreedy EM, Yang X, Baier RR, et al Measuring effects of nondrug interventions on behaviors: music & memory pilot study, *J Am Geriatr Soc* 67(10):2134–2138, 2019. doi: 10.1111/jgs.16069.
3. Manthorpe J, Wilkinson A, Chinn D, et al: Changes and sticking points in adult safegaurding: a discussion, *Br J Community Nurs* 17(7):334–339, 2012.
4. McBrayer, JP Why our children don't think there are moral facts. *NY Times*: Opinionator. March 2, 2015. Available at https://opinionator.blogs.nytimes.com/2015/03/02/why-our-children-dont-think-there-are-moral-facts/.
5. Christiansen C, Lou JQ: Evidence-based practice forum: ethical considerations related to evidence-based practice, *Am J Occup Ther* 55:345–349, 2001.
6. Catlin A: Doing the right thing by incorporating evidence and professional goals in the ethics consult, *J Obstet Gynecol Neonatal Nurs* 42:478–484, 2013.
7. Jonsen A, Siegler M, Winslade W: *Clinical ethics: a practical approach to ethical decisions in clinical medicine*, ed 5, New York, 2002, McGraw Hill, pp 1–12.
8. Doherty RF: Building effective teams. In Jacobs K, editor: *Occupational therapy manager*, ed 6, Bethesda, MD, 2019, AOTA Press.
9. Hepp SL, Suter E, Jackson K, et al: Using an interprofessional competency framework to examine collaborative practice, *J Interprof Care* 29(2):131–137, 2015.
10. Schmitz D, Groß D, Frierson C, et al Ethics rounds: affecting ethics quality at all organisational levels, *J Med Ethics*. 44(12):805–809, 2018.
11. Beaird G, Dent JM, Keim-Malpass J, et al Perceptions of teamwork in the interprofessional bedside rounding process, *J Healthc Qual* 39:95–106, 2017.
12. Kadivar Z, English A, Marx BD: Understanding the relationship between physical therapist participation in interdisciplinary rounds and hospital readmission rates: preliminary study, *Phys Ther* 96:1705–1713, 2016.
13. Foye SJ, Kirschner KL, Brady Wagner LC, et al: Ethical issues in rehabilitation: a qualitative analysis of dilemmas identified by occupational therapists, *Top Stroke Rehabil* 9(3):89–101, 2002.
14. Doherty RF, Dellinger A, Gately M, et al: *Ethical issues in occupational therapy: a survey of practicioners*. Poster presented at the American Occupational Therapy Association 2012 Annual Conference, Indianapolis, 2012.
15. Slater DY, Brandt LC: Combating moral distress. In Slater DY, editor: *Reference guide to the occupational therapy code of ethics and ethics standards*, ed 2015, Bethesda, MD, 2016, AOTA Press, pp 117–124.
16. Bushby K, Chan J, Druif S, et al Ethical tensions in occupational therapy practice: a scoping review, *Br J Occup Ther* 78:212–221, 2015.

Ethical Dimensions of Professional Roles

6

Ethical Life as a Health Professional: Integrity, Resilience, and Courage

The reader should be able to:

- Identify several ethical themes that run through the continuum of professional life from that of student to licensed professional.
- Describe academic integrity and its relationship to professional integrity.
- Recognize the importance of moral courage as a virtue of health professionals.
- Define moral resilience, and reflect on how it can fuel our intentions to act ethically.
- Explain what a caring response entails when the object of care is oneself.
- Identify the three hallmarks of burnout in health professionals.
- Discuss the place of self-respect in one's ability to survive professional life ethically.
- Describe a personal values system and its relationship to caring for oneself.
- Identify two types of threats to personal values encountered in the health professions and some strategies for meeting them ethically.
- Evaluate the professional continuum, and reflect on goals to support health professionals' well-being and resilience.
- Discuss mindfulness and other healthy self-care practices.
- Describe the idea of a reflection group and its function in helping to maintain personal and professional integrity.

New terms and ideas you will encounter in this chapter

academic integrity	self-care	conscience
professional integrity	clinician well-being	conscientious objection
legal fraud	self-respect	cooperation with
moral courage	personal values system	wrongdoing
moral resilience	professional values	principle of material
the professional	duties to yourself	cooperation
continuum	aspiration	mindfulness
burnout	responsibilities to yourself	reflection group

Topics in this chapter introduced in earlier chapters	
Topic	*Introduced in chapter*
Integrity	1
Caring response	2
Moral distress (types A and B)	3
Ethical dilemma	3
Moral agency	3
Utilitarianism	4, 5
Ethical principles	4
Six-step process of ethical decision making	5
Reflection	5

Introduction

The ethics foundation presented in Section I of this book will serve you well during your student days and throughout your career as a health pro fessional. This chapter focuses on moral development and the opportunity to exercise appropriate ethical decision making throughout your career, beginning with your time as a student. Your role as a student and some of the particular opportunities and stresses of this period are especially important to include because no matter your age, the student years are when your approach to ethical decision making in your professional role takes shape.

Special Challenges of Student Life

As a student, or novice clinician, you have the advantage of coming into a situation with a fresh perspective in which you can raise issues that more seasoned professionals could miss or might gloss over. At the same time, a situation sometimes is misjudged solely because some students do not have the advantage of having served in a professional role or in a particular set-ting for a long time.[1] Your professional judgment is developing in your early clinical experiences.

The story in this chapter highlights some ethical problems inherent in your role as a student.

 The Story of Mitch Rice, Gail Campis, the Belangers, and the Botched Home Visit

Mitch Rice is a nursing student in his last year of professional education. He has enjoyed his professional training, especially in the actual patient care environment. Today, however, he went to bed discouraged and wondering whether he had made the correct career choice.

Mitch is on a home healthcare rotation. He has an excellent supervisor, Gail Campis, who has tried to provide a wide range of learning experiences and proper supervision during his time with her. This has not been an easy task; the census for the home care association is high, and with major cutbacks in professional staff, she has been busier than usual. He is sorry to learn that she is going on vacation tomorrow and that his supervision will be turned over to another nurse, Eugenia Cripke.

Today, Ms. Campis asked Mitch if he would open the case on Mr. Belanger while she went to do follow-up diabetes training with another patient in the same elderly housing complex. She told Mitch, "I should not be that long; it's a follow-up session, and once it's done, I will be right down to join you. I will have my phone on if you need me." He was somewhat uncomfortable about going alone to see a patient he had not seen before. He also remembered being told by his academic clinical coordinator at school that under no circumstances should he go into a patient's home unsupervised. But he agreed to do so, not feeling free to question Ms. Campis about whether that was correct procedure. Instead, he assured her that he had done this type of intake enough times under her supervision that he felt he could do it. She agreed.

When he knocked at the Belangers' door, a large woman in a filthy housedress peered through a crack in the door. At first, she did not want to let him in, but he showed her his name tag as identification and she admitted him. He gave her his name and introduced himself as a student nurse. Mrs. Belanger was already walking laboriously across the room toward the other occupant, an equally large man who appeared unable to comprehend what was going on. The man strained to peer at Mitch from a large armchair set up in the midst of the clutter in the small living room. Mitch knew the man's name was Tom, but he was unprepared for the greasy-skinned and ill-groomed person drooling onto the front of a mucus-stained shirt.

When Mitch told the patient what he had come to do, the man grunted. The woman said, "I don't know why everyone insists we need a home nurse; we are doing just fine." Mitch replied that his role was to ensure that Mr. Belanger safely transitioned back home and that they were able to manage his medications after his recent hospitalization. He said, "I see that the doctor ordered that Mr. Belanger use his inhaler three times a day. Did he already use it this morning?" Mrs. Belanger reported that he did not. She could not remember how to help him use it, and Mr. Belanger had been too tired to do anything. Mitch was getting more and more worried. Mr. Belanger had questionable safety, and Mrs. Belanger did not appear to be effectively supporting him in his care. "Okay," Mitch said to Mr. Belanger. "Let's just start by taking your vital signs." Mitch set up his stethoscope and oximeter.

Mr. Belanger's blood pressure was 139/94 mm Hg, and his oxygen saturation was 85%. Mitch immediately knew that Mr. Belanger was in the danger zone. He wished his supervisor were there. Mitch said, "Mrs. Belanger, I need you to go get me the inhaler. Let's see if we can help Tom breathe better." Mitch worked with Tom on some deep breathing exercises, and with those, in addition to the inhaler treatment, he was able to increase Tom's oxygen saturation to 89%. Mitch completed the nursing intake and reinforced with Mrs. Belanger that she needed to assist Tom with another inhaler treatment in 4 hours. He also reviewed all of Tom's prescribed medications and had him take his blood pressure medicines (which also had not yet been taken). Ms. Campis had not joined Mitch, so he completed the visit and told Mrs. Belanger that someone would return tomorrow morning to check on them. In the meantime, he let her know that he would contact Tom's primary care team to let them know how the visit went. Mrs. Belanger told Mitch, "Just make sure you don't tell them that I forgot to give him the inhaler. They'll be all over me for that." Mitch left the Belangers' house and called Gail to let her know he had completed the visit, but the call went right to her voice mail.

When he returned to the office, Gail Campis was there, clearing off her desk. "How did it go?" she asked. "Awful," Mitch said. "I have serious concerns about Mrs. Belanger's ability to support Tom in his care. He is not saturating well, and we will need to call it in to his primary care team because it looks like they have been trying to document these lapses more consistently to better help this patient and family." "Oh dear," Gail replied. "We can't do that today. I will get in so much trouble with the agency if they find out that I let you do that encounter on your own. Hopefully he will be okay tonight, and you can follow up with Eugenia tomorrow."

Mitch had meant to try to persuade Gail otherwise, but for some reason, her comments unnerved him. He said, "Okay. I guess Mr. Belanger will be fine for one night."

Gail came over to Mitch. "Thanks so much for getting me through that squeeze. I knew you could handle that." She continued, "I will just place a holder note in his record, and you can follow up tomorrow with Eugenia." Gail pulled up Tom Belanger's record on the home agency laptop computer and wrote, "Initial nursing evaluation and intake with student nurse and family. Full note to follow." She hurriedly gathered her things, saying, "Mitch, I have enjoyed working with you as a student. You will make a fine nurse. And you will enjoy working with Eugenia Cripke." Mitch now is completely turned about and is wondering with dread what tomorrow will bring.

Almost everyone would agree that both Ms. Campis and Mitch Rice exercised poor ethical judgment.

Reflection

As you look at the story through Mitch's eyes, what are the reasons he is feeling discomfort after the day's events? Jot them down here.

_____

_____

_____

_____

During Mitch's clinical education experience, he faces an ethical problem and clinical and legal ones that have features very similar to those he will encounter in his eventual career as a licensed professional. Many times, health professionals are faced with unexpected situations that are unsettling for one reason or another. However, the opportunities to use his ethics knowledge and skills have presented themselves from the time he set foot in his educational program.

The Goal: A Caring Response

You have already learned in Chapter 3 that for a person to be held responsible for her or his actions the person must be the moral agent in the situation. The health professional's agency revolves around being able and willing to provide a caring response in a variety of health-related situations. The conduct and attitudes for realizing this goal are embedded in the classroom experience. When you entered your program, you may have signed a student honor code or a statement of *academic integrity*. Many universities have such codes and other ethical guidelines that detail the range and scope of moral agency and responsibility and the responsibilities of the faculty toward the student. If you study the guidelines carefully, you see that the items together are designed for the positive outcome of the ability to maintain your integrity and the integrity of your profession. When integrity is honored in the classroom setting, then the student has exercised academic integrity. When integrity is honored in the clinical setting, one has exercised *professional integrity*.

Professional education program honor codes, modeling by professionals, and other guidelines allow you to fully appreciate the opportunities for refining the character traits and ethical conduct consistent with a caring response. The stakes grow higher when students enter the environment of their future professional activities. This environment is where Mitch Rice's ethical challenge takes place—in this instance, in a home care visit as a student. Some factors in his degree of moral agency are the nature of his role as a student, the character of the student–professor relationship, and his inexperience regarding some types of life situations more generally.[2]

Reflection

Consider Mitch Rice's experience, and write down some areas in which he has moral agency as a student.

What is he ethically responsible for?

What is the minimum he would have had to do to constitute a caring response? This answer will give you a good basis for comparing your judgments about a student's moral agency with the suggestions in the paragraphs that follow.

_____

_____

_____

Overall, you have an ethical responsibility to take full advantage of your student role to refine your ethical decision making with supervision. Most of Mitch's experience was characterized by this type of situation. Until their last day together, Gail Campis gave him ample opportunity to practice his skills with her supervision in a variety of settings. He had the benefit of continual discourse and feedback from her. Once you graduate, you no longer have the formal clinical, ethical, and legal supervision that you have as a student to help protect you from making poor judgments.

The Six-Step Process as a Student

As Mitch's experience illustrates, things do not always go smoothly. In the next few paragraphs, the six steps of ethical decision making are highlighted so you can see what is involved in each step and where moral agency resides in your role as a student. Together, these examples can be summarized as follows. You have a moral responsibility to:

1. Gather relevant information from the patient or family, the patient's clinical record, and your supervisor. Include any doubts about your qualifications if you have been given the authority by your supervisor to act independently and you feel ill equipped to do so.
2. Openly share what you know about the patient and other aspects of the situation with the healthcare team in an attempt to identify clinical symptoms and ethical problems.

3. Use the knowledge and skills you do have, including ethical theory and approaches, to participate in arriving at a caring response. Refrain from acts that are wrong for anyone to commit.
4. Be ready to help identify the best alternatives possible for patients and others who are faced with ethical problems.
5. Remain faithful to your own convictions, and exercise the will and courage to act on them.
6. Give yourself the opportunity to reflect on your action with your supervisor and others.

With these six guidelines, let us go back to the story to give you an opportunity to move step by step through Mitch's situation.

Step 1: Gather Relevant Information

The first step in ethical decision making is to gather all of the relevant facts. Students practice with supervision because they are assumed to have little knowledge gained from experience and also partial classroom knowledge and skills. You probably have had some training in what to look for and how to interview, and you also have had an opportunity to observe others' conduct. But if you have doubts about either your knowledge or your skills, your responsibility is to express these doubts at the outset.

In retrospect, Ms. Campis used poor judgment in sending Mitch Rice to the Belanger home alone. Although she thought he was capable of completing the technical procedures competently and independently, she had not thought through all the ramifications of the situation he might encounter. For instance, she was not responsive to the literature on barriers to recovery for vulnerable adults and opportunities to prevent readmissions and adverse events.[3,4] She had a responsibility, especially in her role as supervisor, and in that respect, she failed. In fact, if Mitch's actions (or in this case, failure to act) led to litigation against the caregivers, she would be held legally responsible for what "her" student did or did not do.

Nonetheless, that does not leave Mitch Rice in a position of having no ethical responsibility. Students have a moral obligation to tell a supervisor if they feel a serious lack of knowledge or capabilities. Likely this awareness is also one of the reasons Mitch feels so disquieted at the end of the day. Moreover, by the time he completed his first visit, Mitch Rice knew how Mrs. Belanger feels about students. He knows the difficulties other students will have with the Belanger home and their ability to do what is needed for Tom. During this one visit, what other information did Mitch gain that you consider relevant to good patient care for the patient? For other patients?

Step 2: Identify the Type of Ethical Problem

The second step in ethical decision making is to be alert for ethical problems in the situation. Students have a responsibility to share what they know with others who are accountable for and must be responsive to the patient's well-being. Sometimes students are great reservoirs of information. Although some patients may be hesitant to let students treat them, the converse often is true as well. And some patients feel safer telling a student what they do not want to say to a professional. In such moments, you are a key member of the interprofessional care team in regard to planning optimal treatment approaches, including providing insight into ethical issues.

This is your opportunity to identify some ways in which Mitch's situation fits the prototypical ethical problem of moral distress.

One structural barrier that keeps Mitch from doing the right thing is that he does not feel at liberty to question his supervisor's request to withhold the details of the visit to the primary care team. This external situation is accompanied by the interior barrier of anxiety. But why? Ms. Campis has not presented the situation in such a way that he has reason to fear her disfavor; she does not appear to be motivated to wield her power unfairly or to be punitive. His anxiety and subsequent behavior may be at least partially explained by the nature of the student–teacher relationship in which the imbalance of power between the two is built into the structure. Mitch's situation is an example of why some of the approaches you encountered in Chapter 4 place so much stress on imbalances of power within institutional structures themselves. This explanation fits the prototype of moral distress type A in which a "structural" barrier keeps Mitch from doing what his better moral judgment dictates.

Mitch also may be experiencing moral distress type B. He knows a lot but is still in training. Understandably, the limited professional experience Mitch brings to the setting leaves some unknowns. He knows how to interview a client, triage vital signs, and administer a breathing treatment, but the larger narrative of the story leaves many gaps for him to fill in as he goes along. For instance, perhaps he has had limited experience talking with people like the Belangers. He may never have seen a person with the degree of cognitive impairment Tom Belanger manifests and may not know the best way to treat the Belangers as a couple (patient and caregiver, with all the additional dynamics of the husband–wife relationship). He is not sure how to instill enough confidence in either of them to ensure they are safe at home and compliant with their plan of care. He also is forced to reckon with his new realization that with home care, a professional goes into the private "sanctuary" of a person's home and must adapt to the home environment to make a caring response possible.[5] In Chapter 3, you studied the role of emotion in ethical decision making and how emotion can be both helpful and a barrier to moving ahead. Mitch is frustrated, afraid, and angry, but those responses do not indicate that he is uncaring. He is overwhelmed by the enormity of the unknown and insecure in his judgment about what to do, which are not unusual student responses. As a student yourself, you may recognize a tendency to discredit your own feelings, intuitions, and judgments. Students often are reticent to show their clinical supervisor their emotions for fear that they will be judged as weak. The worst outcome of this student-related stress is that you may assume you are completely unable to evaluate a situation correctly or even to get enough information to make a sound ethical assessment of it.

In contrast, the best outcome is to use emotion as an opportunity for support and discussion. The student years are the time to embrace vulnerability as a path to become as well prepared as possible. Vulnerability is not weakness; it is the willingness and courage to engage in a difficult conversation. It serves as a source of accountability and authenticity and prepares us to be lifelong learners.[6]

Summary

As a student, you may be faced with moral distress and not affect an adequate caring response because of structural and knowledge barriers to acting on what is right, compounded by anxiety and other emotions. At the same time, you have an opportunity to prepare for situations in which you are the one fully responsible for the outcome.

Step 3: Use Ethics Theories or Approaches to Analyze the Problem

The third step in ethical decision making is to apply the principles and other ethical guidelines available to you in your role. Again, as a student, you may not be sure how to apply them in your new role. At the same time, if you look closely at Mitch's situation, you can conclude that his actions include morally wrong or illegal acts. A bottom line regarding your moral agency as a student is that you have a responsibility to refrain from acts that are wrong for anyone to commit.

Reflection

What are examples of Mitch's failure to exercise his moral agency and take responsibility for his actions that are similar to any relationship in which one person has an ethical responsibility not to harm the other? Jot your examples down here.

_____

_____

_____

_____

You may have found several places where you think this happened. Presumably, you agree that one occasion was his silence. The more glaring example of his dishonesty was his decision to not communicate Tom Belanger's status to the primary care team, a lapse that, in retrospect, may lead to an adverse event or unsafe outcome for Mr. Belanger. Mitch's inaction is not applicable only in the health professional–patient relationship; intentional omission of care provision causes harm by undermining trust and misleading the client and family in ways that diminish their right to autonomy. He has ignored the duty to do no harm. The principle of veracity is supportive of the duty to be truthful, too. No circumstance excuses him from these important principles of ethical decision making.

As is common in situations that pose ethical distress, one ethical problem often leads to another. You may be asking yourself, so how are Mitch and his supervisor going to document the care Mitch provided? How will they bill for the visit if the supervisor was not present for Mitch's session? Mitch knows that entering false statements on a medical record is illegal. He and Ms. Campis both would be committing *legal fraud* if they billed for an evaluation that the licensed nurse did not perform. This act could cost him his professional career and lead to criminal sanctions. What are some of the reasons this breach of professional responsibility is viewed as so serious by society as a whole?

If you are reasoning about this as a utilitarian, you are on the path to legitimating his course of action on the basis of the overall good consequences you may believe will result. Within professional ethics, however, the ethical principles not to harm (nonmaleficence) and truth telling (veracity) in regard to the patient take on the strength of duties. They are vital as means of honoring that in the role of professional the patient's interests take priority. A caring response requires unequivocally that the decisions be patient centered. Not unlike breaches of academic integrity, breaches in professional integrity often occur when professionals attempt to "cut corners" and they lose focus on the patient. This is where the concept of intent comes into play. Intent is a part of misconduct because it means that a person has set his or her sites on wrongdoing. Therefore, to the extent that Mitch understands his role as a health professional, he cannot justify withholding key information or making false statements in the record without understanding that he is engaged in wrongdoing.

---

⑥ Summary

As a student, your role as a moral agent means that you are not protected from ethical distress and that you must participate in deciding how to arrive at a caring response in a specific situation.

During your formative years as a student, you have an opportunity to refine your ethics skills, although at times they make you uncomfortable.

Step 4: Explore the Practical Alternatives

Step 4 in ethical decision making is to seek the viable alternatives and find the one that most fully approximates or achieves a caring response.

One of the reasons health professionals enjoy working with students is that students often provide creative approaches to old problems. Professionals who have been facing similar issues for years get bogged down in habit or become discouraged because attempted solutions have not been successful in the past. (How many times have you heard, "We've tried that before, and it didn't work"?)

Your unwillingness to offer suggestions is not a morally neutral act. Sheer robustness, arrogance, or ill-placed criticisms are not welcome. At the same time, as a student, you are a moral agent whose scope extends to your readiness to voice your thoughtful opinion when you are invited to do so and to taking a posture of readiness to contribute such ideas rather than standing by passively and keeping your insights to yourself.

Although Mitch has seriously breached the responsibilities consistent with his role as a moral agent, he can still offer suggestions from the perspective of what he observed in the Belanger family. Of course, he also has a moral responsibility to contribute his thoughtful ideas regarding all the other situations he has had the opportunity to witness and participate in during his tenure in this clinical setting.

⊙ Summary

You have a moral duty to participate with others in seeking practical alternatives for patients faced with difficult ethical decisions. You have a right to receive support and guidance for this from your faculty in both the classroom and the clinic.

Step 5: Complete the Action

Step 5 in ethical decision making is to act. A student's responsibilities include the four forms that are described in the following paragraphs.

Act Within the Limits of Competence and Self-Confidence

Always seek to balance your knowledge, skills, and abilities with the need for supervision. This balance helps ensure that the patient is the beneficiary at all times. With this overriding guideline in mind, the next three forms are simply logical complements.

Act According to Convictions

Some general protections for health professionals to honor their integrity and therefore avoid moral compromise were introduced in Chapter 1. Similar protections should apply to students. For instance, during your student experience, you have a responsibility to make your convictions known so that you are never placed under pressure to participate in a procedure that undermines your values or your profession's code of ethics; and you have the responsibility to inform your educational program administrators and supervisors in advance of any such situation so that patient care is never compromised. Whenever possible, you should leave plenty of lead-in time for your request to be heard and considered in a timely manner.

Right Any Wrongdoing

Another dimension of living according to your convictions is to right any wrongs you yourself have done in regard to a patient or other situation within your student professional role. No one enjoys having to do damage control after wrongdoing, but Mitch needs to engage in self-care that will serve him well in the future when he errs. Health professionals who cultivate the virtue of humility are able to better maintain integrity and cultivate this character trait in themselves and others. There is no better investment than taking care of yourself by keeping your conscience clear. His admission will also ensure that Tom is spared any additional harm as a result of a missed medication or poorly coordinated care. Tom's cognitive disability places him at risk of neglectful care and health complications. As the caregiver, Mitch's duty is to honor the principle of nonmaleficence.

Reflection

If you were Mitch, how would you go about correcting this serious error in ethical judgment?

_____

_____

_____

_____

You must begin to practice during your student years if you are going to be able to admit shortcomings and mistakes throughout your career. Nothing is more harmful to you professionally and personally than to get into the habit of "covering up" your mistakes or deceits. When approached thoughtfully, professors and supervisors almost always are forgiving of student missteps and stand ready to discuss and help prevent such breaches from happening again.

Address Others' Wrongdoing Constructively

The arduous moral task of constructively addressing the wrongdoing of others is also a part of everyone's responsibility in the healthcare environment, including yourself and your fellow students. Quiet, diligent observation is a reliable guidepost in your assessment of wrongdoing by your fellow students or by professionals. As noted, a legitimate worry about expressing your concern arises because, as a student, you may be aware that you do not have full knowledge of the situation. In his study, Branch[7] noted that medical students tend to question their own moral judgment when faced with differing values expressed by authority figures. That said, your innate ethical sense can only strengthen if, during the student years, you take advantage of the opportunities to engage in ethical dialogue with your mentors.[8]

In the end, these challenges should not keep you from addressing ethical wrongdoing. For instance, Mitch knows with certainty that Ms. Campis acted wrongly in sending him to the Belangers' home alone, no matter her rationale. Mitch, however, did not challenge that act, so he also acted with poor judgment. Rather than the two of them maintaining a conspiracy of silence, he can help report his own wrongdoing in the context of acknowledging that she, too, was a partner in the way this situation unfolded.

Moral Courage

As you learned in Chapter 1, one of the most essential resources in your professional life is your own integrity. At times, maintaining that integrity requires *moral courage*. Moral courage is an essential virtue for all health professionals. It is the individual's capacity to overcome fear and stand up for core values and ethical obligations.[9] Central to moral courage is knowledge of the situation, rational control of one's emotions, and the ability to manage the fear and risk involved in putting ethical principles into action.[10,11] Mitch will need moral courage to right his wrongs and act on behalf of Mr. Belanger. He must prepare to face tough decisions and confront the uncertainties associated with his resolve to right this wrong. Through trusting that his perspective counts and voicing his concerns, Mitch can overcome the sense of moral powerlessness that is so often associated with moral distress.[12] Speaking up cultivates moral courage and translates our intention, values, and behaviors into integrity-preserving actions.[13]

Step 6: Evaluate the Process and Outcome

In the sixth and final step of ethical decision making, the moral agent steps back from the heat of action and goes over the process to think about what can be learned about a truly caring response, how it might be done better next time, or how it applies to other situations. Only through this conscious process is your own moral development enhanced.[14] By now you are aware that a caring response in regard to present or future patients should ultimately drive your motivation at all times. If any action or inaction flies in the face of this basic core of your professional identity, that path should not be taken again.

Your reflection also should include an acknowledgment that you are "in it together" with your clinical faculty; their job is to guide you in ways that encourage you, not discourage you. A study of 272 nursing students in a baccalaureate educational program showed that when clinical faculty as individuals were themselves "caring [toward students], gave encouragement and positive feedback, demonstrated…new procedures, encouraged critical thinking, clearly stated faculty expectation of students, and conducted pre- and post conferences,"[15] students learned the important dimensions of their clinical role more effectively. If, on reflection, you are experiencing that type of treatment, you will want to model your own behavior toward others in your work situation in the future on how you yourself were treated.

Given Mitch's situation, he certainly owes it to himself to reflect on what happened and why. He has a moral obligation to work with Ms. Campis, the home care agency, his academic program, and other stakeholders to ensure the delivery of efficient, effective, and safe care. He also has a responsibility to future patients not to let this negligence happen again. He has a moral responsibility to himself to regain his self-respect by gaining more insight into the incident.

Summary

If you reflect back over steps 1 through 6, you see that a student's moral agency applies at every step of ethical decision making.

The Professional Continuum

The development of professional expertise occurs along a continuum. *The professional continuum* begins in the student years when you begin to build the knowledge, skills, and attitudes necessary for entry-level competence in your chosen field. This process then continues into your career as a licensed professional. Many factors contribute to the progression of expertise; however, research has shown that most individuals transition from slower (novice) problem solving to faster, more automated problem solving (expert).[16] Schon,[17] Dreyfus and Dreyfus,[18] and Benner[19] have all made substantive contributions to the field of professional inquiry, learning, and thinking. In her seminal 1984 work, Patricia Benner applied the skill acquisition work of Dreyfus and Dreyfus to the practice of nursing. Benner described five levels of proficiency: novice (no experience), advanced beginner (marginally acceptable performance), competent (moderate, specific performance), proficient (moderate, broad experience), and expert (extensive experience, intuitive). If you think about your own development of skills, these levels of competence make sense. For example, if you have reached the point of having on-site experience in your future work environment, recall the first time you looked at or maneuvered a hospital bed or used a stethoscope.

What you saw then is different from what you see now because you have experienced many trials with this equipment. Through these trials, you have learned to more quickly manipulate, calibrate, interpret, and problem solve the application of this equipment into your daily practice.

A professional goal for all health professionals should be to become an expert in the full scope of one's practice, and to help others do the same.[20] The progression along the novice to expert continuum is a journey that requires you to integrate a combination of formal knowledge, know-how, expertise, experience, and skills.[21] While reading this, you may be thinking "Well then, I guess the only thing that will make me an expert is more time and experience." Not so. Reflecting on shared experiences and constructing knowledge with your faculty, preceptors, and colleagues is key to the advancement of your ethical reasoning and progression along the professional continuum. As you recall from Chapter 5, critical reflection leads to clinical growth.

Responsibilities of Self-Care

You have come a long way in thinking about the ethical dimensions of professional practice in a general way. Next we offer you an opportunity to think about the essential task of *self-care* as you assume your professional role and throughout your professional life. Honoring your own deep personal values and needs is extremely important because as a professional you are always expected to think about others. How can you also take care of yourself in ways that prepare you to flourish in your professional role in all kinds of situations you will encounter? Janice K.'s story helps focus this discussion.

 The Story of Janice K., Her Personal Values, and the Policies of Her Workplace

Janice K. is a dietician employed by a community health clinic affiliated with a large multihospital health plan. Part of the mission of the clinic is to provide nutritional counseling and services for people in an underserved area of her community. She loves working in this setting and believes that her professional responsibility includes helping to ensure that people in such areas have the same access to healthcare benefits as everyone else. Until now, she has told many of her friends and family how delighted she is to have found this position in a town where she can be close to her family. But recently, everything has changed. Janice is distressed because she has learned that the health plan has designated her clinic as a site where abortion counseling and services will be added to its family planning programs. Janice has strong religious convictions that abortion is murder and that this practice should be stopped by whatever means possible. In her words, "Whenever an abortion is performed, two patients, mother and child, are harmed, and the latter is murdered. This is against any interpretation of professional ethics that I can imagine. It's against life."

She realizes that her personal morality is bumping up against society's legal acceptance of abortion procedures in medically competent settings. But this is no comfort. She is anxious, has been experiencing sleeplessness, and is feeling vulnerable and angry about this turn of events, just when everything seemed to be falling into place.

This story could lead to many interesting and important ethical discussions, but in this chapter, we focus on the prime importance of your personal values and needs as foundational wellsprings of survival in your professional career. Many of your values have a moral component that may comprise your personal morality. You have had some opportunities to think about your personal morality already in the course of studying this text. In Chapter 1, you were introduced to the ideas of personal morality and integrity and some ways that society tries to protect these in professionals. So far, every story in this text has posed an ethical problem to you as you try to put yourself in the shoes of the person who is the moral agent searching for a caring response. Now you have an opportunity to step back and focus on yourself.

In Janice's situation, her beliefs and the values that inform those beliefs are powerful forces that guide her thinking about her duties and what kind of character traits she should strive to develop so that she can flourish as a human in any situation, including her workplace. That is the challenge each of us faces. The next section turns the lens from your quest for a caring response solely focused on the well-being of the patient to considering what you can do to act in a way that takes good care of yourself too.

The Goal: A Caring Response

At the center of finding a caring response to yourself is the development of deep *self-respect*. Respect comes from a Latin root that means to hold something or someone in high regard. Respect for the dignity of individuals is an overriding virtue in professional ethics, and, as we noted in Chapter 1, it can be thought of as the gold standard against which we can measure our attempts to achieve a caring response. But respect is almost always understood as referring to the deference one pays to another person, particularly the patient. Where in professional ethics is the encouragement to cultivate and incorporate respect for oneself?

Traditionally, very little about self-respect has been found in the professional ethics literature. An understanding of modern moral psychology has been necessary to bring it together with respect for others. An American moral philosopher, John Rawls, relied heavily on psychology to help clarify the relationship of respect for self and respect for others.[22] As adults, he notes, one source of self-respect is the awareness that we are contributing to society's well-being. Professionals have an opportunity for almost daily feedback about how their contributions to patients' lives are helping society. This supports the idea that their own needs also deserve to be respected. And so, unlike other analyses that make respect solely a virtue about how to respond to others, Rawls interprets the development of self-respect as an engine that can drive our daily activities toward human flourishing. True self-respect allows us to flourish as selves and, in turn, allows us to have high regard for the societal tasks we assume to do our part in supporting human flourishing for others as well.

Your understanding of self-respect will result in the recognition that if you do not respect yourself, your ability to enjoy deep job satisfaction in your professional task of caring for others will be undermined.[23] Research has found that professionals who find meaning in their professional activities view their work as being deeply connected to their core values and moral orientation.[24] Their self-respect partially is tied up with having basic values from which to draw and is reinforced by acting according to those values. In short, the often overlooked attention to building self-respect is an extremely important dimension of exercising a caring response toward yourself.

Moral Resilience
Addressing ethical tensions while attending to self-respect requires moral resilience. *Moral resilience* is defined as "the capacity of an individual to sustain or restore their integrity in response to moral complexity, confusion, distress, or setbacks."[25] Effective self-care is one way to build your moral resilience. The other is something you are doing right know—building your ethical competence! Studies show that ethics education, and engaging in ethical reflection, ethical decision making, and ethical behavior helps build individual resilience.[26–28] We will continue to explore self-care strategies later in this chapter.

Information Gained From Identifying Your Personal Values
As health professionals, we must reflect on our own needs and values and begin early in our careers to analyze the influence that they have on our practice. A *personal values system* is the set of values you have reflected on

and chosen that helps you lead a good life. Usually people adopt personal values that partially overlap with societal values and that are in harmony with them.[29] Personal values are imparted, taught, reinforced, and internalized. Many values are moral values, and in this case, you can readily discern their relation to the personal, group, and societal moralities presented in Chapter 1.

Reflection
Name some personal values that help to give meaning and enjoyment to your life. Include at least one that you identify as a moral value, such as honesty or justice.

_____

_____

_____

_____

As you become a professional, you will also incorporate *professional values* into your values system. Professional values help explain the reasonable expectations that society can count on regarding what a profession promises to do or not do. As mentioned in Chapter 1, these values usually are outlined in ethics standards or core values statements. Most health profession organizations articulate these values (e.g., altruism, equality, compassion, dignity) to demonstrate the core beliefs associated with their identity. Take the time to find and reflect on the values your own professional organization has generated. In addition, some core values are shared across many professions, which creates a value set for the moral community made up of professionals who can depend on each other to be working according to the same mindset. We talk about these values more in Chapter 7. The upshot is that while we emphasize self-care in this chapter, the integrity that allows you to go forward with clarity and job satisfaction requires that your professional values be taken deeply into account in every decision you make.

Summary
Your personal values system gives you the foundation for decisions that support self-care. When faced with an ethical issue that involves how to honor yourself, this system allows you to act on your own convictions in a meaningful way that best protects your personal moral integrity. Your professional values must be included in this deliberation for you to maintain professional moral integrity.

The idea of what self-care entails has been conceptualized in several related ways. Some of them are shared here, including self-care as a duty, an aspiration, and a responsibility. In addition, valuable emphasis has been placed on the role of conscience in maintaining self-care.

The Duty of Self-Care

In Chapter 2, care was included as a duty in our deliberation about the meaning of a caring response. It is usually interpreted as a duty of caring for others, but it applies equally to oneself. In Chapter 4, duties were placed under the usual umbrella of expectations of moral conduct between individuals. Duties usually describe commitments that individuals make to other people or groups to act in certain ways that are believed to uphold the moral life. Therefore it is unusual to talk about *duties to yourself;* however, just as one has a duty to respect patients in virtue of their rational nature, one has a duty to respect oneself as a health professional. One philosopher, among others who made a compelling case to do so, is W.D. Ross, a 20th-century British moral philosopher influential in developing the idea of moral obligation who included the duty of self-care and a commitment to improving yourself among his list of duties. He believed that the duty of beneficence (doing good toward others) and doing good toward yourself arise because each of us should produce as much good as possible. Only in honoring the claims on your own health and welfare and in responding to claims from others can a complete picture of the overall good being produced be expressed. In other words, Ross treated self-care as a duty in that it brings about good generally, but, of course, you are the major beneficiary![30] His (rule) utilitarian weighing of benefits depended on everyone keeping these duties or rules. We can expect Janice to find a way forward in her dilemma (Fig. 6.1) that allows her to honor her duty to be faithful to her religious beliefs while weighing the various alternatives she has open to her. Her moral distress will continue to keep her feelings and emotions alive as she works her way through the challenge she faces.

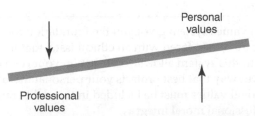

Fig. 6.1. Balancing personal and professional values.

● ⬛ *Reflection*
Can you think of some examples in your everyday life when you were not being "good" to yourself, or even harming yourself? What are reasons you chose to act this way?

_____

_____

_____

_____

The idea of a duty to oneself is seldom reflected in health professions' codes of ethics probably because of the "other directedness" of the professions' orientation. One example that emphasizes one's duty to self is the American Nurses Association Code of Ethics for Nurses, which states, "[T]he nurse owes the same duties to self as others, including the responsibility to promote health and safety, promote wholeness of integrity and character, maintain competence and continue personal and professional growth."[31] Others do emphasize the duty to remain competent and continue to develop professionally, but almost always those duties are cast into the context of professional duties to patients and societies.

Aspirations of Self-Care

Another way to think about self-care is as an aspiration worth achieving. An *aspiration* is an ideal standard of excellence toward which you strive; when you have attained that standard, you have gained a better quality of life. Therefore, even if you do not agree that taking good care of yourself has the full force of a duty, you can embrace it as something worth cultivating. Anytime you realize such an aspiration, you do owe it to yourself to reward the accomplishment. For example, when you have aspired to lose weight or as a student make a high grade in a course and you achieve the goal, you owe it to yourself to acknowledge your success by going out to buy a new pair of jeans or taking time from studying to read a novel. Similarly, in the realm of the moral life, you may aspire to be courageous, to go the second mile, or to set an example of high moral character for others. Has there been a time recently when you experienced this kind of self-satisfaction (Fig. 6.2)? The primary reward in this case is in seeing the good you are capable of bringing about and knowing you have made a stride in developing a high moral character. You owe it to yourself to stop to enjoy the good it has done for others. You owe it to yourself to be aware that next time it will be easier.

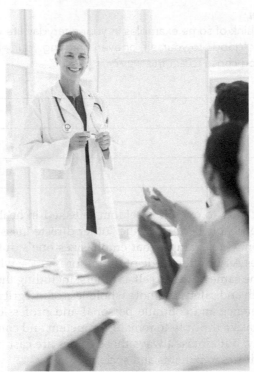

Fig. 6.2. Celebrating professional achievement. *(Copyright iStock.com/ Neustockimages.)*

Summary

Reinforcing in yourself the good that comes about by honoring your duty of self-improvement or aspiring to be good to yourself helps you prepare for healthfulness and a chance to flourish throughout your professional career.

Responsibilities of Self-Care

A third way of conceptualizing what it means to include a caring response to yourself among your professional tasks is to think of *responsibilities to yourself*. As you recall from Chapter 2, responsibility includes accountability but also has the root idea of responsiveness embedded in it. Responsiveness guides you toward being kind and gentle with yourself as you face difficulties. From the student years onward, health professionals can be extremely demanding of themselves, with the belief that they must grin and bear stress quietly. However, research in the health professions now shows that this is

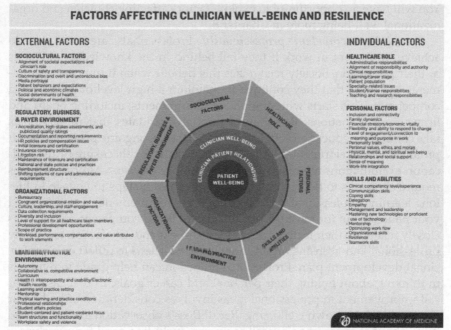

Fig. 6.3. Factors affecting clinician well-being and resilience. Brigham TC, Barden AL, Dopp A, et al: 2018. A journey to construct an all-encompassing conceptual model of factors affecting clinician well being and resilience. NAM Perspectives. Discussion Paper, National Academy of Medicine. Available at https://doi.org/10.31478/201801b. *Reprinted with permission from the National Academy of Sciences, Courtesy of the National Academies Press, Washington, D.C.*

simply not true. The rising rate of *burnout* in the health professions has led many to refer to it as a public health crisis. The thee hallmarks of burnout are emotional exhaustion, (being emotionally depleted or overextended), lack of personal accomplishment (feeling one cannot make a difference), and depersonalization (characterized by difficulty making personal connections).[32] In addition, to burnout, witnessing trauma, disease, injury, suffering, death, disability, and social injustices can lead to psychological stress for health professionals caring for individuals and families with complex needs. This stress includes posttraumatic stress disorder, emotional distress, anxiety, and postsecondary trauma. There are various dimensions impacting *clinician well-being*. Fig. 6.3 highlights how clinician and patient well-being is multifactorial and interconnected. You will note that some of these are individual factors such as personal factors and skills and abilities, whereas others are external factors such as the regulatory and business environment.

You will have an opportunity to explore factors affecting clinician and organizational well-being more in Chapter 8.

Remaining competent professionally. Professionals are not able to achieve fulfillment in work if they fall behind in the knowledge and skills of their profession. Society recognizes this benefit when it imposes requirements to ensure that they continue to maintain a high level of professional competence. This starts with graduation requirements, including board and licensure examinations. It continues through mandates that professionals take continuing education courses and demonstrate ongoing proficiency, and professional development in other ways. Sometimes relicensure or recertification examinations are required after a number of years. Almost all states require clinicians to document that they have taken steps to engage in lifelong learning professionally. One goal of these requirements is to safeguard your patients, but for most people, the idea of being competent on the job is closely related to their feelings of accomplishment and satisfaction too. Many professional and licensing organizations ask clinicians to reflect on a professional development plan. Professional reflection can help guide individuals in thinking about linking their personal and career goals. In that case, your self-improvement in professional areas involves consideration of both your patients' and your own well-being. Recall Ross's observation that we should bring about as much good overall as we can, including good for ourselves.

Improving yourself personally. Beyond improvement in professional areas, responsibilities of self-care include the development of personal health habits, skills, and interests. What efforts do you make to maintain a high quality of physical, mental, and spiritual health? Do you have hobbies or other interests? Well-rounded persons always make better professionals insofar as they have relief from the demanding routine of professional work. One of the best safeguards against becoming bored or burned out is to have outside compelling interests that require concentrated attention and provide delight. Thus many application forms for programs of study or jobs include a question about interests, hobbies, and personal skills unrelated to work. Some health professionals use creative or expressive arts as forms of self-care. Many feel that they provide an outlet for reflection and restoration. Initial research into the benefits of these types of structured self-care is promising.[33]

L *Reflection*

What are some ways you enjoy spending your time outside of your work and study? List them in order of priority.

_____

_____

_____

_____

Let Your Conscience Be Your Guide
Janice surely is struggling with what it entails to let her conscience be her guide. How many times have you heard that phrase when you were about to do something that others had some doubt about? What is a *conscience* anyway? The Oxford English Dictionary describes it as, "The internal acknowledgment or recognition of the moral quality of one's motives and actions, the sense of right and wrong as regarding things for which one is responsible."[34] This is the starting point of deliberation that Janice has chosen, and her alternatives all reflect some measure of the work she has done to examine her own conscience. Already her first reaction has been refined by going through a reflective process of ethical decision making. All of her proposed activities indicate her objection to the proposed service; on that basis, she can be said to be a conscientious objector. However, conscientious objection as a concept has a more specific meaning.

Conscientious objection. *Conscientious objection* is an act of resistance or defiance against existing practices, policies, laws, and other expectations that others in that person's position have agreed to. The objector asks to be an exception. The root idea came from when otherwise eligible inductees refused to serve in the military on the basis of religious or other deeply held objections to war. The burden of proof is on the objector; many democratic nations have allowed alternative service if the person's reasons are accepted as legitimate. In Chapter 1, you encountered the legal concept of moral repugnance designed to protect objectors on religious or other grounds from having to participate in the procedure of abortion. Whether or not her involvement as a dietician will be seen as participation in abortion as a procedure is up to the administration to decide.

Conscientious objection has arisen in situations other than abortion in the healthcare setting. Some issues include the participation by health professionals in capital punishment via lethal injection, force-feeding in prison or military settings, clinician-assisted suicide, stem cell research, genetic testing, and provision of reproductive technologies. In some cultures, situations may include work on religious holidays, touching of dead bodies, or physical examinations of patients of the opposite gender. Refraining from participating in these procedures can be regarded as an individual's effort to protect moral integrity.[35] Increasingly, healthcare institutions recognize the wisdom of policies that spell out the conditions in which conscientious objections are honored.

Commonly in such policies, a conscientious objection is a legitimate position for a person to take but is **not** honored if:
• The objection does not have a plausible moral or religious rationale or the abstention is discriminatory against a patient or group of patients.
• The degree of negative patient impact is too great (e.g., emergency care is compromised, the timing is deleterious to serious patient needs, no substitute is available).

- The cumulative burden on other employees is too great.
- The treatment is considered an essential part of the health professional's work.

The benefit of this type of policy in Janice's workplace is that, as she considers her alternatives, she can go into the situation knowing that she will be treated equitably with other employees and will have an idea of how the institution will be "listening" as she states her case. At the same time, patients who are anticipating or have undergone an abortion and who have nutritional needs that require the dietician's expertise must be given the same high quality of care as all other patients. Therefore, if she asks for abstention from treating these patients (or working with interprofessional care team members more directly involved in the abortion procedure) and another dietician is not found to care for the patient, Janice will be required to place the patient's needs above her own conscientious objection.

One part of the distress Janice is feeling is that at times all of us find ourselves in a situation where we believe there is wrongdoing but are not in complete control to stop it. Furthermore, sometimes opportunities for achieving a good end and avoiding other greater wrongdoing can depend on "cooperating" with wrongdoing in some fashion. A way to think about the justification for *cooperation with wrongdoing* is embodied in the *principle of material cooperation*. Note that the scholars who have developed this moral principle depend on the relationship of intent and the ensuing conduct chosen in such dilemmas. Often ethical principles such as beneficence or nonmaleficence are discussed devoid of the intent behind the action. The idea of material cooperation brings the intent into center focus. They take seriously the truth posited in the introduction to ethical problems in Chapter 3: An ethical dilemma entails acknowledging that sometimes harm is one effect of achieving something more morally compelling, although the goal is to minimize the harm. At the same time, one must never directly intend the harm, overriding the basic purpose of the principle of nonmaleficence, "do no harm."

The principle of material cooperation. The following guidelines are offered in the principle of material cooperation:
- Cooperation with wrongdoing is easier to justify if the wrongdoing will happen with or without one's personal cooperation.
- Cooperation cannot be directly intended by oneself. The cooperation is occasioned solely by one's position as a member of a group, such as employment in an institution in which there is wrongdoing.
- The more remote the personal cooperation, the better.
- The benefit that is attained by the degree and type of cooperation one tolerates must greatly outweigh the wrongdoing that results from other alternatives that attempt to block the wrongdoing.

In a specific situation, this general set of guidelines for when one might justify cooperating with wrongdoing to some extent has to be submitted to further interpretation.

⑥ Summary

As a professional, the starting point of conscientious objection is an examination of personal values and conscious. The burden of proof is on you, as a professional, to be familiar with institutional policies and conditions so that these guidelines can be honored and made available to you as a basic self-care resource.

Strategies for Success as a Moral Agent

Professional practice is rife with opportunities to apply your ethical knowledge and skills in real-life situations and continue to remain competent and happy in your choice of career. The paragraphs that follow offer strategies for building moral resilience and surviving professional life ethically.

Find a Mentor

Mentors serve to help your confidence grow and your experience deepen. Successful health professionals learn early on that finding the right person to mentor oneself as a student, novice, or experienced professional always adds a margin of value to other sources or learning and development. This person may or may not be a professor or one's institutional supervisor. Imagination and gumption help you let the person know how much you can benefit by being in conversation with them.

Practice Moral Courage

Whether you are a student or novice clinician, you can enhance your ability to show moral courage by advancing professional and sociocultural competence, applying ethical reasoning, practicing self-care, and continually reflecting on your own professional goals, learning, and growth. Engaging with our vulnerabilities and practicing standing for what matters most is a way to cultivate courage through lifelong learning.

Implement Resilience-Building Strategies

Building resilience is both an individual and team commitment in today's care delivery environment. Cultivating self-awareness and mindful practice has been shown to have positive outcomes not only for health professionals, but also for patients. *Mindfulness* facilitates greater presence and attention, two skills that help enhance ethical awareness and support moral resilience. One basic mindful practice is purposeful pausing, or taking a mindful moment. Mindful moments provide time to notice, reflect, and gain perspective. They only take a moment, but pausing (even for one breath) creates space to focus on the present, allowing the mind and body to relax, and helping individuals be more present and nonjudgmental.[36,37]

Developing your own personal self-care plan can that includes mindfulness can support professional well-being. Establishing a plan, with specific goals and strategies for achieving goals, can serve as a practical tool at any point along your career trajectory. Activities such as healthy self-care practices (exercise, yoga, outdoor activities) and good social supports can support your personal resilience. Practicing skills of communication and conflict management/negotiation discussed in Chapter 10 will also support your personal development in this area. But you cannot go it alone. Self-care is only one solution to the problem. You will need to call on organizational resources such as ethics committees, peer counselors, critical incident debriefing sessions, and employee assistance programs. These supports, along with other systematic approaches, are discussed further in Chapter 8 in which we will focus on organizational ethics.

Reflection
What is one character trait or skill you would like to develop to build your own moral resilience?

_____

_____

What specific activities will you engage in to develop this skill?

_____

_____

Remember Your Code and Ethics Resources
As you recall from Chapter 1, professional codes of ethics, and consultation with ethicists and ethics committees, can provide guidance in clarifying moral values, duties, and other aspects of morality in specific clinical situations. How the interprofessional care team and organizational structures can support ethical practice is further discussed more specifically in Chapters 7 and 8.

Create and Participate in a Reflection Group
A *reflection group* is one mechanism for assessing prospective and recent decisions involving self-care in the professional role. By sharing concerns and exercising personal vigilance, all professionals can become better equipped to respond more effectively, efficiently, and caringly with each new situation, remaining true to a caring response to oneself. Mitch's and Janice's processes and eventual decisions provide an opportunity to engage other colleagues in what they went through. They, too, have an opportunity to reflect on their own personal values and how and when such values may

present moral distress or an ethical dilemma. It is highly recommended that all places of employment have a mechanism that allows health professionals to gain the insights of others when faced with, or looking back on, a difficult ethical decision; if it does not, you can exercise your leadership by being an agent in creating one. These mechanisms are extremely helpful for ensuring self-care and a high-quality, well-working professional environment. Whether the group is designed to assist in your discernment around decisions you are about to make or in looking back on what happened, it brings the collective wisdom of the group to bear on what can otherwise be an extremely lonely journey.

Summary

Surviving professional life ethically requires self-awareness, experiences (and reflection on them), a commitment to living according to your personal values system, vigilance in maintaining integrity, and strategies for fulfilling responsibilities to yourself. Special ethical challenges during your student years involve both the peculiarities of the student–supervisor relationship and the limits of your own knowledge and experience. From the time you enter your professional program, you are a student-professional and are bound to certain duties and guiding professional values. It is the mutual task of students, classroom faculty, and clinical supervisors working together to ensure that students trust their developing competencies and abilities, understand their role as moral agents, and act appropriately to ensure that a caring response consistent with the demands of professional responsibility is exercised. In fact, the purpose of this book is to you think clearly about a wide variety of ethical situations before you are faced with the weightier responsibilities associated with professional practice after completion of your studies. As you transition from student to licensed professional, self-care is preparation for the most challenging ethical moments with the highest stakes. Acting out of a position of self-respect, taking good care of yourself, and being kind and gentle with yourself will prepare you for confident ethical decision making and a fulfilling professional career. In Chapter 7, you will have an opportunity to further examine how colleagues and the institutional mechanisms for support and accountability in healthcare also are relevant to one's professional integrity and moral resilience.

Questions for Thought and Discussion

1. You are working in a community health center, and one of your colleagues asks you to take over one of her cases for her. She said, "I am having a hard time with this case and don't think I can help them. I think I might be getting burned out. You are so much better with the refugee

families. Can you take the case over for me?" How should you respond? Why?

2. You overhear one of the rehabilitation aides say to another colleague, "I just pretended to treat her. She was sleeping and will never know the difference. It's such a drag to treat someone who is so out of it." This provider has cheated a patient out of her treatment. Is this different from cheating on a classroom test? Is so, why is it? If you observed a classmate cheating, should your response to it be different than if you learned that a patient was not treated? In each case, what should you do?

3. Melissa Y. is a therapist who works in a chronic pain clinic that includes some inpatient beds. She has become distressed in the past month because she is increasingly convinced that one of her longtime nurse colleagues is "siphoning off" some of the narcotic medications intended for the patients. Her personal values and her professional sensitivity dictate that she pursues the issue. If you were Melissa, how would you proceed, exercising your moral courage but also wanting to be prudent in taking this important step?

4. Some of the physicians who participated in the Nazi medical experiments testified that their activities did not run counter to their personal values. When asked how this could be, they stated that they were simply "doing their job." Discuss the limits of using an individual's personal conscience, convictions, or understanding of the professional role as the ultimate standard of moral judgment. What, if any, higher standard is there? What types of checks and balances do you want to have in place to minimize wrongdoing in an institution or society?

References

1. Haddad A, Doherty R, Purtilo R: Respect in the professional role. *Health professional and patient interaction*, ed 9, Philadelphia, 2019, Elsevier Saunders, pp 2–11.
2. Hewko SJ, Cooper SL, Cummings GG: Strengthening moral reasoning through dedicated ethics training in dietetic preparatory programs, *J Nutr Educ Behav* 47(2):156–161, 2015.
3. Greysen SR, Hoi-Cheung D, Garcia V, et al: Missing pieces—functional, social, and environmental barriers to recovery for vulnerable older adults transitioning from hospital to home, *J Am Geriatr Soc* 62:1556–1561, 2014.
4. Ma C, Shang J, Miner S, et al: The prevalence, reasons, and risk factors for hospital readmissions among home health care patients: a systematic review, *Home Health Care Manage Pract* 30(2):83–92, 2018.
5. Garcia T: Ethics in home care, *Home Health Care Manage Pract* 18:133–137, 2006.
6. Brown B: *Daring greatly: how the courage to be vulnerable transforms the way we live, love, parent, and lead*, New York, 2015, AVery.

7. Branch WT Jr: Supporting the moral development of medical students, *J Gen Intern Med* 15(7):503–508, 2000.
8. Yerramilli D: On cultivating the courage to speak up: the critical role of attendings in the moral development of physicians in training, *Hastings Cent Rep* 44(5):30–32, 2014.
9. Lachman VD: Strategies necessary for moral courage, *Online J Issues Nurs* 15(3), 2010, manuscript 3.
10. Purtilo RB: Moral courage in times of change: vision for the future, *J Physical Ther Educ* 14(3):4–6, 2000.
11. Murray JS: Moral courage in healthcare: acting ethically even in the presence of risk, *Online J Issues Nurs* 15(3), 2010, manuscript 2.
12. Carse A, Rushton C: Harnessing the promise of moral distress: a call for reorientation, *J Clin Ethics* 28:15–29, 2017.
13. Rushton CH, editor: *Moral resilience: transforming moral suffering in healthcare*, New York, 2018, Oxford University Press.
14. Garrigan D, Adlam AL, Langdon PE: Moral decision-making and moral development: toward an integrative framework, *Dev Rev* 49:80–100, 2018 Sep 1.
15. Brewer MK: Being encouraged and discouraged: baccalaureate nursing students' experiences of effective and ineffective clinical faculty teaching behaviors, *Int J Hum Caring* 6(1):46–49, 2002.
16. Anderson JR: *Cognitive psychology and its implications*, ed 7, New York, 2010, Worth Publishers.
17. Schon D: *The reflective practitioner: how professionals think in action*, London, 1983, Temple Smith.
18. Dreyfus SE, Dreyfus HL: *A five-stage model of the mental activities involved in directed skill acquisition*, Berkley, CA, 1980, University of California Operations Research Center.
19. Benner P: *From novice to expert: excellence and power in clinical nursing practice*, Menlo Park, CA, 1984, Addison-Wesley Publishing.
20. Ulrich B: From novice to expert, *Nephrol Nurs J* 38(1):9, 2011.
21. Susskind D, Susskind R: *The future of the professions: how technology will transform the work of human experts*, Oxford, UK, 2017, Oxford University Press.
22. Rawls J: *A theory of justice*, ed 2, Cambridge, MA, 1999, Harvard University Press.
23. Purtilo R: New respect for respect in ethics education. In Purtilo RB, Jensen GM, Royeen CB, editors: *Educating for moral action: a sourcebook in health and rehabilitation ethics*, Philadelphia, 2005, FA Davis, pp 1–10.
24. Green BH: The meaning of caring in five experienced physical therapists, *Physiother Theor Pract* 22(4):175–187, 2006.
25. Rushton CH: Moral resilience: a capacity for navigating moral distress in critical care, *AACN Adv Crit Care* 27(1):111–119, 2016.
26. American Nurses Association: *A call to action report: exploring moral resilience toward a culture of ethical practice*, 2019. Available at www.nursingworld.org.

27. T. et al. *A journey to construct an all-encompassing conceptual model of factors af-fecting clinician well-being and resilience.* Discussion Paper, National Academy of Medicine, 2018, Washington, DC. Available at https://nam.edu/journey-constructencompassing-conceptual-model-factors-affectingclinician-well-resilience.

28. Irby DM: *Improving environments for learing in the health professions*, New York, 2018, Josiah Macy Jr. Foundation.

29. Purtilo R, Haddad A, Doherty R: Respect: the difference it makes. *Health pro-fessional and patient interaction*, ed 7, Philadelphia, 2014, Elsevier Saunders, pp 3–15.

30. Ross WD: *The right and the good*, Oxford, England, 1930, Clarendon Press, pp 26–27.

31. American Nurses Association: *Code of ethics for nurses with interpretive state-ments*, Washington, DC, 2015, ANA.

32. Trzeciak S, Mazzarelli A: *Compassionomics: the revolutionary scientific evidences that caring makes a difference*, Pensacola, Florida, 2019, Studer Group, LLC.

33. Nan JKM, Lau BH-P, Szeto MML, et al: Competence enhancemennt program of expressive arts in end-of-life care for health and social care professionals: a mixed method evaluation, *Am J Hosp Paliat Med* 35(9):1207–1214, 2018.

34. *Oxford English dictionary, CD-ROM version 3. 1*, Oxford, England, 2004, Oxford University Press.

35. Lachman VD: Conscientious objection in nursing: definition and criteria for acceptance, *J Medsurg Nurs* 23(3):196–198, 2014.

36. Rushton CH, editor: *Moral resilience: transfoming moral suffering in healthcare*, New York, 2018, Oxford University Press.

37. Lueke A, Gibson B: meditation reduces implicit age and race bias: the role of reduced automaticity of responding, *Soc Psychol Personal Sci* 6(3):284–291, 2014.

●7

Shared Moral Community: Ethical Decision Making in Interprofessional Teams

Objectives

The reader should be able to:
- Describe some major areas of professional life that present ethical challenges to members of an interprofessional care team.
- List five guidelines that are useful in assessment of whether a prospective place of employment supports teamwork and collaborative care delivery.
- Identify how shared moral agency and ethical decision making contribute to interprofessional collaborative practice and development of a shared moral community.
- Recognize the key role effective teamwork plays in improving the quality and safety of healthcare.
- Discuss several reasonable expectations a health professional can have of professional peers.
- Define peer review and assess its usefulness as a mechanism to maintain the high moral standards of a profession.
- List several types of impairment that health professionals may experience that create ethical challenges for the interprofessional care team.
- Outline the appropriate steps to be taken to report unethical conduct.
- Define whistle-blowing, and understand the supports for individuals and teams involved in whistle-blowing situations.
- Develop several alternative strategies for dealing with a colleague who is engaging in incompetent or unethical conduct, and describe the probable outcomes of each line of action.

New terms and ideas you will encounter in this chapter

competencies for interprofessional collaborative practice	preventable adverse event	whistle-blowers/whistle-blowing
dual relationship	peer evaluation	impairments
	peer review	intervention

Topics in this chapter introduced in earlier chapters	
Topic	Introduced in chapter
Interprofessional care team	1
Patient-centered care	2
Responsiveness	2
Ethical distress	3
Shared agency	3
Faithfulness or fidelity	4
Beneficence	4
Nonmaleficence	4
Deontology	4
Utilitarianism	4
Ethical reasoning	4
Six-step process of ethical decision making	5
Moral courage	6
Integrity	1, 6
Moral resilience	6

Introduction

This chapter launches a new focus. Until now, you have mostly considered your moral agency role as an individual student or professional. But you are a moral agent in respect to other roles you assume, too, with one of the most interesting as a member of an interprofessional care team. As introduced in Chapter 1, the interprofessional care team is a group of professionals, sometimes with adjunct staff to assist, that becomes the unit of decision making. A team is designed to meet the same ethical goals of a caring response as individual professionals so that members of a team, working together, accomplish collectively what individual professionals aim to do. You have already seen some examples of professionals working together to provide compassionate, quality care to patients. Now you will observe them as they also participate in other team activities, demonstrating that the search for a caring response to them is as important to quality patient care as is your commitment to finding a caring response toward a patient.

Usually, the two focuses of your care are completely compatible with your ultimate goal of doing what is best for each patient. In fact, team-oriented care was designed to enhance the effectiveness of this goal. Occasionally, however, problems arise within teamwork that threaten to compromise the patient's good, the team's effectiveness, or both. You have an opportunity here to examine both some strengths and some challenges in teamwork. The story of Maureen Gudonis and Isaias Echevarria is one example of how conflict or questions arise about the ethically right thing to do.

The Story of Maureen Gudonis and Isaias Echevarria

Maureen Gudonis is an occupational therapist with 7 years of experience with adult and pediatric patients. She is excited to transition to her new job at Essex Community Health Center (ECHC), an innovative community-based integrated care facility. Maureen has seen the difference a good interprofessional care team can make and embraces the concept of this community-based medical home model to support both adults and children with chronic medical conditions. Maureen's first few weeks at ECHC go very well. She is introduced to various members of the interprofessional care team, including her friend Daniela with whom she worked some time ago in a local acute care hospital and who now is a nurse practitioner in the practice. Maureen consults with the primary care team, participates in rounds, and performs occupational therapy evaluations and interventions with a focus on caregiver education, activities of daily living training, and lifestyle modification to support patients with effective disease and medication management. At Maureen's 1-month evaluation, her supervisor thanks Maureen for the contributions that she has made to the delivery of care at ECHC. She tells her, "In the short time you have been here, your interactions and interventions have helped the team enhance the health and wellness of our patients, decrease disability, and increase medication compliance." Maureen is so pleased. She and her friend Daniela decide to go out for dinner to catch up and celebrate how well things are going.

At dinner, they reminisce about their work at the hospital, and Daniela tells Maureen how happy she is that Maureen has joined ECHC. They worked in the local acute care hospital together years ago and always found it frustrating when care was fragmented between outpatient medical practices, hospitals, and home care agencies. They both feel that they are making a difference in this new model. Daniela says, "Actually, I need to refer a patient that I saw today to you. It's Isaias Echevarria. I think you see his mom, Lourdes, for her diabetes. They are a great family and have been through a lot."

The next day, Maureen gets a referral for Isaias. Isaias is a 16-year-old Guatemalan boy with a history of attention-deficit/hyperactivity disorder (ADHD) and osteosarcoma. He was diagnosed with ADHD at age 13 years and was diagnosed with stage III metastatic osteosarcoma 2 years ago. Isaias was treated with chemotherapy and limb-sparing surgery with grafting, but his postoperative period was complicated by infection and he needed additional surgery, including a below-knee amputation. Isaias has completed his treatment and is referred to Maureen for management of chronic pain and for assistance with school reintegration.

Maureen meets with Isaias. He has all the stressors of a patient managing life with cancer but is also a tenacious teenager. Maureen and Isaias talk about his chronic pain and how it limits his participation in school tasks. Between the Adderall for ADHD and the pain, he is unable to sleep at night, which makes a morning routine for school nearly impossible. He is doing well with basic bathing and dressing, but he has not been wearing his new prosthetic because of pain. Maureen talks about different strategies with Isaias, but he reports, "I have tried all of those things; nothing works. The pain is too bad." Maureen probes more, saying, "Remember your last good day. What made a difference?" Isaias responds, "The only thing that makes a difference is when my mom gives me some of her boyfriend's marijuana to smoke. I haven't really told anyone because we only tried it a few times, but both times I slept through the night. She would kill me if she knew I told you, but I figure soon enough it will be okay because it is legal in a bunch of states now. Plus, what have I got to lose?" Maureen does not know quite how to respond. Isaias's mom did not accompany him to his appointment today. Maureen lets Isaias know that they are going to need to talk about this more and include his mom and the interprofessional care team in the conversation; in the meantime, she advises him to refrain from any additional marijuana use.

Maureen is overwhelmed and walks to Daniela's office to tell her about the visit. Daniela says, "Oh my gosh, Maureen! Dr. Horner is going to be irate. I don't know what she will do. You know she lobbied up at the statehouse against the marijuana bill and feels very strongly about it. We'll have to pull the team together. I'll look up his other medications. We might even have to file on the mom. Ugh. Don't you wish he never told you?" Maureen thinks about what Daniela says. What a way to round out her first month.

You will have an opportunity to reflect on this story throughout the chapter because it highlights several strengths and types of ethical challenges that you could, and probably will, face in your role as a member of the interprofessional care team. The first thing to consider is the importance of providing support to and accepting support from each other as teammates.

The Goal: A Caring Response

No one who works in the healthcare setting day in and day out escapes moments of self-doubt, anger, or utter frustration. As you read in Chapter 6, a great deal is expected of you in regard to taking good care of yourself as a student or professional. Even so, at times, your involvement in the human suffering of illness and disease is intense, the responsibilities arduous, and the challenges monumental. The wear and tear of taxing schedules, patients whose problems seem overwhelming, or a day in which everything that could go wrong does can discourage even the most competent, optimistic person.

The key role that effective teamwork plays in improving the quality and safety of healthcare is increasingly recognized. Several national and international groundbreaking reports argue that team-based, interprofessional care is a key strategy to achieving a safe, efficient, integrated, and cost-effective healthcare

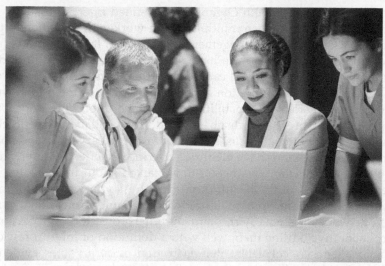

Fig. 7.1. Interprofessional care team. *(Copyright iStock.com/sturti.)*

delivery system.[1-6] Teams are likely to problem solve more effectively than individual providers and together provide more oversight and congruency to the patient's plan of care. But you cannot just put a cadre of providers together and expect them to be an effective team. Teaming toward the common goal of a caring response can be hard work. A team is different from a group because, by definition, a group is a collection of people with something in common, but a team is a collection of people working together toward a common agreed-on goal or outcome.[7] Effective teams improve health outcomes and have been shown to increase quality of care, improve the coordination of care delivery for clients with complex conditions, reduce medical errors, reduce hospitalization time and costs, enhance accessibility for clients, and contribute to improve client satisfaction and workforce well-being (Fig. 7.1).[8]

 Reflection
Think about a recent healthcare experience you may have had. How did the individuals you interacted with work together? Did they talk to each other and work collaboratively? Did they help you navigate the complexities in the healthcare system?

_____

_____

_____

_____

In 2010, the World Health Organization defined interprofessional collaborative practice as "when multiple health workers from different professional backgrounds work together with patients, families, carers [sic], and communities to deliver the highest quality of care."[1] An important feature of the interprofessional care team is that its members see beyond their own professional affiliation and become aware of their contextualized patient care–related capabilities for collaboration. The concept of interprofessional professionalism emerged from collaborative practice, education, and research. It focuses on the competencies, values, and norms that multiple professions have identified as critical to effective interactions in the provision of care.[9] In Chapter 6, we talked about the personal and professional values of the health professional. As you work on an interprofessional care team, you will also incorporate interprofessional values into your values system. Stern[10] and the interprofessional professionalism collaborative outline them well with a definition of interprofessional professionalism as "consistent demonstration of core values evidenced by professionals working together, aspiring to and wisely applying principles of altruism, excellence, caring, ethics, respect, communication, and accountability to achieve optimal health and wellness in individuals and communities." In 2011, the U.S. Interprofessional Education Collaborative defined a set of core *competencies for interprofessional collaborative practice*. Revised in 2016, these competencies are organized into four domains: (1) values and ethics for interprofessional practice, (2) roles and responsibilities, (3) interprofessional communication, and (4) teams and teamwork (Fig. 7.2).[2]

Given these recent trends, many institutions currently recognize the need for team support and collaborative governance. In many organizations there is an effort to hold departmental or interdepartmental meetings so that issues may be addressed in a nonthreatening, supportive setting. This type of arrangement usually improves and sustains good working relationships among team members and provides a refuge in which individuals can receive needed support. They provide opportunities for deliberation, negotiation, and communication clarification to facilitate consensus building in complex situations. In any department, such arrangements can help to humanize the environment for workers and patients alike.[11] In this regard, it makes sense to think of teamwork as the institution's acknowledgment of such stresses and the implementation of actual mechanisms to address them as its caring response to the situation.

Fortunately, it is highly probable that you will find a supportive net of interprofessional care team members in your work setting. Once you are employed, or if you already are, you can help create a greater support network among team members by being attentive to the "blahs and blues" that a colleague seems to be experiencing, by risking sharing your own doubts or discouragements with people you judge to be trustworthy to help you

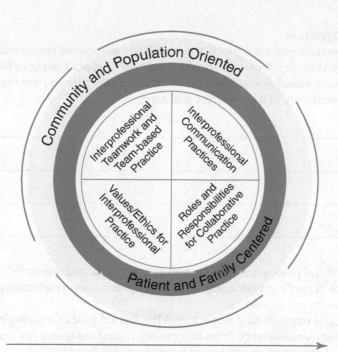

The learning continuum prelicensure through practice trajectory

Fig. 7.2. The learning continuum prelicensure through practice trajectory. *(Redrawn from Core Competencies for Interprofessional Collaborative Practice, sponsored by the Interprofessional Education Collaborative, May 2016. Copyright Association of American Medical Colleges.)*

through them, and by making suggestions regarding the need for mechanisms designed to work through problems as a team. As Maureen's situation implies, friendships may take root in the shared experiences, concerns, and time spent with other members of the interprofessional care team. A friend you meet in a work situation may become the key figure in building a supportive network, and as friends, the two of you can provide support for each other and others. The joy of discovering and cultivating such a friendship is among the most rewarding of the many fringe benefits of a health professional's career.

The ethical components that guide close, convivial working relationships are similar to those in the health professional–patient relationship.[12] Team members also should be recipients of caring responses from you and others. Some ways to achieve these responses include telling the truth, honoring confidences, valuing different contributions, acting with compassion, communicating positively, listening actively, and respecting the dignity of your colleagues.[13,14]

Reflection

Because you are a moral agent with the associated responsibilities, what do you think you should reasonably expect from your fellow teammates? Name some things that indicate that you are the beneficiary of their respect and care.

_____

_____

_____

_____

The ethical principle of fidelity and interprofessional research[14–16] provide guidance regarding reasonable expectations for team relationships. These expectations are as follows:

1. Collegial trust, mutual respect, and the shared goal of a caring response
2. Substantive assistance from teammates regarding questions about good patient care or other matters of professional judgment
3. A willingness by all teammates to be flexible and carry a fair share of the workload
4. Sympathetic understanding regarding work-related stresses
5. An environment conducive to a high level of functioning and one that fosters work satisfaction for everyone involved, not just some members of the team
6. A commitment by everyone to respect differences in values and contributions of other team members and to embrace each person's unique gifts
7. Encouragement to develop both professionally and personally within the work environment
8. A commitment to establishing ways of communicating and working together that includes negotiating and developing roles with each other to support the team's work

As you think of other things you would expect and want to help protect and encourage, be bold in making suggestions to those with whom you work. Sometimes a well-placed word can help to increase everyone's imagination about how the team can work together more effectively.

Ⓢ **Summary**

Good teamwork is based on respect. You can expect respect from others and also must show respect to them in your common quest for an optimal caring response.

With the background established thus far in this chapter, turn to the six-step process of ethical decision making to learn how it applies to team issues.

The Six-Step Process and Team Decisions

Let us take Maureen's situation as an opportunity to apply the process of ethical decision making introduced in Chapter 5. So far, you have applied it to situations that involve the individual health professional's decisions regarding direct patient care. At the same time, interprofessional issues will arise among team members, and those issues lend themselves to analysis and (hopefully) resolution with use of the same process. Some ethical considerations you have not yet encountered must be taken into account in a team peer relationship. The last part of this chapter focuses on the challenges of peer review and the duty to report unacceptable conduct of a teammate.

Step 1: Gather Relevant Information

Maureen has to gather all the relevant information about Isaias's case. What is his current treatment and medication regime? Is there an immediate health and/or safety risk to this patient? What evidence does she have (other than the patient's report) that his mother has been sharing marijuana with him? What do the current state laws dictate regarding cannabis use for medical purposes and beyond? What is the scientific evidence regarding cannabis safety and effectiveness for the treatment of cancer-related pain? Does this literature vary across adult and pediatric populations? Who are the stakeholders in Isaias's care who need to know about the cannabis use? What is the Essex Community Health Center (ECHC) policy on reporting self-disclosed drug use in minors? What is their stance on the use of marijuana for medicinal purposes? Right away you can see that her discovery of Isaias's marijuana use disclosure not only impacts her care, but it also impacts the entire interprofessional care team.

Team Loyalty as Relevant Information

No one questions the importance of support to professional peers; now here is a peer with a need. Little imagination is needed to understand why Maureen's emotional response is to immediately become overwhelmed. She may even be more overwhelmed after talking with Daniela than she was before. Maureen has a responsibility to communicate with her team, and with the patient and family, to ensure that Isaias receives the appropriate care.

The Ethical Challenge of Dual Roles

Not only is Maureen in a health professional–patient relationship with Isaias, she is also in one with his mother. Within healthcare settings, this type of situation is referred to in the literature and ethical guidelines as a *dual role*. Maureen has an obligation to Isaias as a new patient, but she also has an obligation to his mother as a patient and caregiver. She also has a responsibility to uphold her obligations to her personal values and the team's values. Maureen may personally be in favor of medical marijuana use for certain conditions, but her professional practice may be opposed.

The situation of a *dual relationship* is always one occasion for careful reflection about appropriate boundaries in the professional setting.[17] As Maureen tries to sort out her priorities in her role as a health professional treating the patient Isaias, she becomes strikingly aware that she and Isaias's mom are in a new psychological dynamic with each other. In her professional role, if Maureen's unfavorable bias toward Isaias's mom becomes an occasion for allowing an uncaring response, she will be acting unethically.

⊚ Summary

Loyalties to one's teammates and the situation of dual roles create occasions for ethical discernment.

Steps 2 and 3: Identify the Type of Ethical Problem and Use Ethics Theories or Approaches to Analyze It

Maureen is faced with an ethical distress problem. As you recall from Chapter 3, sometimes ethical distress arises when a situation is new or complex. As medicine and technology advance, new treatments are introduced into the clinical setting and bring with them opportunities for ethical reflection regarding how to best balance the benefits and burdens of these interventions. The same holds true when new policies, laws, and regulations are implemented. Because uncertainty is a barrier, Maureen is faced with an ethical distress type B. However, Maureen is not going it alone. She practices in a highly collaborative model, so Maureen and her colleagues share agency for the outcome of this ethical problem. They must critically problem solve through this situation as a team to analyze its varied dimensions to maintain their emphasis on quality of care.

Maureen also needs to attend to the considerations of locus of authority. In her role as an occupational therapist, Maureen does not prescribe; however, she educates patients in medication management and works with the team to determine the best care plan for each individual patient and family. By attending to both locus of authority and shared agency, Maureen can trust that her colleagues are committed to group discussion, collaborative decision making, and mutual trust in the disposition to act on the intentions of the team over the individual. If the team does not stay together in its shared goal of providing good patient care, it will fail in achieving the goal of a caring response. Therefore that Maureen is invested in the well-being of both her patients and her colleagues is not at all morally questionable. Because the medical use of marijuana is relatively new in the United States and the laws that govern its use (and the health professional's involvement in the prescription and education process) vary from state to state, this is one area in which care providers can find themselves intertwined in legal, ethical, and clinical problems. Let us use the literature and societal view of this issue to briefly explore their intertwining.

At the time of publication of this text, thirty-three states and the District of Columbia have some form of legal medical marijuana (i.e., cannabis) use. The parameters that legislate its use vary from state to state in regard to qualifying conditions and dispensing requirements. Despite legislative activity at the state level, marijuana is still an illegal federal substance, and the U.S. Food and Drug Administration classifies it as a Schedule I drug, which means it has no acceptable medical use.[18] This current framework surrounding medical marijuana means that patients and providers cannot be assured of the product's purity, safety, and efficacy. It also means that providers who advise patients regarding medical marijuana use may be prosecuted by the Drug Enforcement Administration for their actions. Maureen has the additional complexity of reasoning through all this information, knowing that her patient is a teenager and that children are impacted differently by marijuana use than adults. Maureen knows limited research is available regarding cannabis use, recent studies have shown benefits for chemotherapy-induced nausea and vomiting, as well as epilepsy, but insufficient evidence is available to support use for neuropathic pain.[19] The literature also strongly warns against its use in teenagers because of the increased risk of schizophrenia and structural changes in the brain.[18,20] As you can see, the interprofessional care team's moral distress is compounded by the lack of research evidence to guide their clinical decisions.

The ECHC care team must balance the rights, duties, and responsibilities of the patient, the family, and themselves as licensed care providers. Although society may greatly value self-determination and individual rights, providers have an ultimate duty to, above all, prevent harm. Maureen and the interprofessional care team need to balance the patient's (and mother's) autonomy with the principle of nonmaleficence. How should Maureen and the interprofessional care team balance the greatest good for this patient and family? She has to further weigh in those utilitarian considerations before making her final decision.

 Reflection

After analyzing the situation this far, what more do you want to know to decide whether Maureen's duties or utilitarian considerations should govern her decision?

_____

_____

_____

_____

What character traits do you want Maureen to have when she makes this decision?

_____

_____

_____

_____

Step 4: Explore the Practical Alternatives

Several options are open to Maureen and the interprofessional care team, including:

1. Call the state Child Protective Services Department to file an unfit parent report.
2. Let it go. Society is changing, and cannabis use is becoming more acceptable. Reevaluate Isaias on his next visit.
3. Document the disclosure, but accept Isaias's mom's actions because she is a well-intentioned person and is doing her best to care for her child.
4. Schedule an immediate appointment or phone conversation with Isaias's mother to discuss Isaias's disclosure. If the sharing of cannabis is verified to have occurred, educate Isaias's mom regarding the potential consequences of her actions, given Isaias is a teenager, including the risk of side effects and possible adverse events as a result of cannabis use.

Can you add others?

It is key that Maureen decided to not go it alone in managing this ethical distress. Interprofessional care teams problem solve more effectively than solo providers and provide more oversight to reduce medical errors that can harm patients.[21] By bringing the disclosure to the team's attention, Maureen can more effectively work with her colleagues to deliver patient-centered care that is timely, safe, effective, and ethical.

In review of the alternatives, consider the first option. Although the team's intention may be to take their duty to report seriously, they should question whether they have all the accurate factual information needed to proceed with such action. Best practices in the care of children and youth dictate that providers ensure due diligence before reporting a caregiver as unfit or calling Child Protective Services. This includes knowledge of state and federal laws related to mandated reporting. For example, federal law defines child abuse and neglect as "any recent act or failure to act on the part of a parent or caretaker, which results in death, serious physical or emotional harm, sexual abuse, or exploitation, or an act or failure to act which presents an imminent risk of serious harm."[22] However, only in certain states is parental substance use included in abuse statutes.

The team needs to balance their dual obligations: to Isaias's mother, who is also a patient in the practice, and to their professional obligations to protect Isaias's well-being. For a caring response to be actualized, fidelity to the patient (and family) must come first, remembering that they are part of the interprofessional care team setting the goals of care for Isaias. Isaias's mother has a reasonable expectation that the ECHC team will seek out and listen to her concerns in caring for Isaias. Conversations regarding risky health behaviors are never easy; conversations that imply possible neglect and abuse are even harder. The team must work together, in close coordination with the social worker, to follow protocols and collectively determine the probability of future harm and necessary steps to ensure Isaias's safety.[23] This generally starts with inquiry, rather than accusation. For this reason, proceeding directly with option 1 is not recommended.

The second option relieves the team of difficult conversations but does not uphold their duty to pursue fully what a caring response requires in this situation. Ignoring a problem never makes it go away. Although the decriminalization of cannabis has led to more social acceptance and therapeutic uses, significant controversy remains. To do nothing is to miss an opportunity for patient and parent education and to protect Isaias from a *preventable adverse event*. Recent studies show that premature death associated with preventable harm to patients was estimated at more than 400,000 deaths per year.[24] Most medical errors result from complexities in the healthcare system, but they also happen when providers and patients have problems communicating. Medical errors are the third leading cause of death in the United States, preceded only by heart disease and cancer. Medical error has been defined as "an unintended act (either of omission or commission) or one that does not achieve its intended outcome, the failure of a planned action to be completed as intended (an error of execution), the use of a wrong plan to achieve an aim (an error of planning), or a deviation from the process of care that may or may not cause harm to the patient."[25] If Maureen and the team do nothing, they may find that on his next visit Isaias is more anxious and depressed or that the cannabis could begin to interact with one of his cancer or attention-deficit/hyperactivity disorder (ADHD) medications. The best way to prevent adverse events is for patients to be active members of their care team and participate in their healthcare decisions. By not letting the conversation go, Maureen and her colleagues ensure that Isaias and his mother stay engaged and use reliable sources of information to evaluate their treatment choices. It also ensures that important details of the case are not missed, paving the way for self-care and self-compassion, which can enable the members of the interprofessional care team to do their job better.

In the third option, you see that documenting the disclosure is some action; however, it falls short of ensuring that Isaias receives the quality care he deserves.

The ethical priority in regard to Maureen's distress is the health and safety of Isaias. This is what makes option 4 the most ethically sound alternative. Assuming that Isaias's mother's intent is to help, not harm, her son, the interprofessional care team must do the following:

- Move beyond their own personal beliefs.
- Remove barriers regarding scope of practice.
- Communicate effectively with special attention to cultural humility.
- Engage Isaias and his mother in the implementation of a safe and effective plan of care.

This starts with educating both Isaias and his mom regarding the evidence related to cannabis use. The ECHC aims to improve the health outcomes of all its patients. Helping patients make informed decisions and building caregiver skills are integral to this mission. You will read more about organizational missions in Chapter 8.

Reflection

Four alternatives have been presented as options. If you listed additional alternatives, this is a good time to take a few minutes to analyze each.

_____

_____

_____

_____

Step 5: Complete the Action

Maureen and the ECHC team must now come to a consensus and act on their chosen alternative. Because all team members have their own professional code and set of values, debate regarding the best course of action can be anticipated. Some may have strong views regarding the societal use of cannabis; others may feel it falls outside the role of the health professional to discuss the use of marijuana because it is an illegal federal drug. That said, successful interprofessional care teams agree to appreciate different viewpoints and support a team decision. This requires that "irreconcilable differences" be ironed out before the team decision involves the patient and the family. In their shared agency, they have shared accountability and responsibility to present as a unified front, ensuring that Isaias and his mother do not receive conflicting information. Effective teams share decisions and take ownership for their practice at the point of care. You will learn more about organizations in the next chapter, but it bears mentioning here that structural factors within organizations can either enhance or impede interprofessional teamwork.

Step 6: Evaluate the Process and Outcome

Once Maureen and the ECHC team have made their decision and acted on it, they are wise to reflect on it from the perspective of individual providers and as an interprofessional care team. Hopefully, their action will have been such that a desire to provide compassionate, patient-centered care will have been successfully balanced with the demands of their moral roles as professionals. The key for Maureen and the interprofessional care team is to reflect on the process they went through in deciding what action to take for this family. They should reflect on what went well and what did not, so that they can be better prepared as an interprofessional care team to deal with the next circumstance that arises. This allows them to face a similar situation in the future with more confidence. The team may also come to a consensus on potential policies that they could implement regarding the reporting of nonprescription drug use in their clients. These policies may serve as guides for future cases and empower the staff through their contributions to the moral community of the workplace. Crocker and colleagues[14] have developed a series of reflective questions to inform the development of collaborative practice. These questions are summarized in Box 7.1.

Summary
Shared moral agency, shared ethical decision making, and shared ethical reflection honor the tenets of interprofessional collaborative practice.

Peer Evaluation Issues

A second category of ethical challenge in team membership arises around the concept of *peer evaluation*. The basic idea is that a professional is asked to evaluate the performance or other qualities of a colleague who is in a similar professional position. Increasingly, members of professional organizations, educational institutions, and treatment facilities are asked to evaluate the quality of their colleagues' work, team skills, and moral character.[26]

The standards against which the evaluation is judged may be set by your professional organization or immediate workplace or may be imposed by governmental or other agencies, and you may find it mandatory to participate in them. We turn our attention now to three varieties of peer evaluation: peer review, reporting unethical behavior, and whistle-blowing.

Peer Review

Peer review is designed primarily to ensure that high standards of professional practice are upheld in your workplace. It may be a resource that the administration uses when salary increases and honors, promotions, or other

Box 7.1 Reflective Questions to Inform the Development of Collaborative Practice

Engaging positively with other people's diversity:
- How willing am I to engage with complexities and the diverse needs of others?
- How do I indicate to others my willingness for such engagement?
- When and how is respect for others' contributions evident in our team?

Entering into the form and feel of the team:
- What is it like for new members entering the team?
- How quickly are they expected to establish understandings?
- What are the implications of this for developing collaborative practice?

Establishing ways of communicating and working together:
- What roles do structured and opportunistic communications play?
- Where do valuable discussions occur?
- What are the key features of these discussions?

Envisioning together frameworks for patients' rehabilitation:
- How does the team establish shared understandings about patients' goals and directions?
- What is the nature and value of my contributions to these goals?
- Can a patient's aspirations, perspectives, and fears be heard in our discussions?

Effecting change in people and situations:
- What outcomes are being sought?
- What organizational constraints do we encounter, and how do we deal with them?

From Crocker A, Trede F, Higgs J: Collaboration: what is it like? Phenomenological interpretation of the experience of collaborating within rehabilitation teams, J Interprof Care 26:13–20, 2012. Reprinted by permission of Taylor & Francis LLC.

work-related distinctions are being determined. Writing letters of recommendation for a colleague who is applying for a new job is a form of peer review that is used by the prospective employer. Another form of peer review is 360-degree feedback or evaluation. Peer review via 360-degree feedback is an evaluation method that includes feedback from one's supervisor, one's colleagues, one's subordinates, and customers, or, in the case of healthcare, patients and or families. The goal is for the individual to gain information regarding performance from multiple perspectives. Although the main emphasis in peer review is on its value as a procedure to ensure that standards and practices remain of high quality in the health professions, it also functions secondarily as a personal profile of a person's progress (or lack of it)

• in attaining professional or leadership stature. Peer review documents often generate data that then become a basis for comparisons among similarly situated colleagues.

With this understanding of peer review, let us consider the case of Susan Sitler and Tom Erwin. Susan and Tom are both respiratory therapists who work in a large teaching hospital. Susan and Tom have not told anyone at work that they are in a romantic relationship and are planning to be married in the autumn. They are both in their early 30s and wish to remain at their current place of employment because of the benefits they have built up by staying there, their favorable opportunities for advancement, and because they enjoy the part of the country where they live.

Although both are about the same age, Susan has worked longer as a respiratory therapist, and everyone agrees that she is exceptionally well qualified as director of the respiratory therapy unit in the intensive care unit (ICU). She has written several articles, engaged in clinical studies, and learned some difficult diagnostic techniques through special training.

News has just come out that Sandra Haynes, the other chief respiratory therapist, has decided to take a position elsewhere. The hospital administration has decided to merge Susan and Sandra's departments into one large unit, and a nationwide search will be conducted to find the best person to be the director. There are two in-house candidates within the institution itself: Susan is one, and the other is a woman who has been in the other department about as long as Susan has been in the ICU and who also seems well qualified.

After the first extensive search is made, four people are still in the running. Both Susan and the other woman are among them. As part of the administration's attempt to make an informed choice, they now ask several people
• to submit peer evaluations of Susan and the other candidate. Tom is among those asked to make this peer evaluation of each of the two candidates.

Susan and Tom are elated at the possibility that Susan may be appointed director of the new department. Tom believes that Susan is well qualified, but he also knows that she very much wants the position. They both are aware that her substantial increase in salary would be helpful for them financially and may even enable them to put a down payment on a house.

Reflection
Should Tom write a letter of recommendation for his future wife? Why or why not?

_____

_____

_____

_____

The following paragraphs share an ethical line of thinking. Do you agree? Why or why not?

Tom may think that whatever he says is not going to make a difference anyway, but that is an avoidance of assuming the responsibility he has been asked to assume. From a moral standpoint, he should try to work out a method of acting responsibly by writing the assessment. At the same time, anyone who finds out about his "other" relationship with Susan will certainly cast doubt on his objectivity and, likely, his intentions.

Because the primary purpose of peer review is to help maintain the standards of professional practice, he must do some soul-searching to assure himself that the high esteem he has for Susan professionally really is based on the high quality of her work and her skills. If he can give a positive response to that issue, he should go ahead; however, he should let the administration know that he and Susan are engaged to be married. He should document his statement with examples of her work and try especially hard to recall areas in which he believes she can continue to grow. The disclosure that he has a vested interest as a friend or fiancé allows the person reading his letter to take into consideration the bias he may introduce. Hopefully, the person reading the review will know that it is difficult enough to comment on one's peers and that an additional emotional challenge is introduced by their intimate personal relationship.

Even when the added component of friendship or a romantic relationship is not present, peer review by team members can be an emotionally taxing situation. Essentially you are being asked to engage in a process of affirming or discrediting your fellow team members in relation to their professional quality and skills. Why is it so difficult? In the first place, all health professionals have some doubt about their own judgments from time to time, simply because the nature of professional practice is fraught with ambiguities. As a result, in most cases, it is not surprising if you are hesitant to pass negative judgment on someone else's activities, knowing that everyone has an Achilles' heel. Second is the fear that if you are too rough on colleagues, the tables may one day be turned on you. Finally, sometimes loyalty to one's profession acts as a deterrent to saying anything negative about one of its members. Whatever the source of the difficulty, the health professional who assumes this responsibility with an honest, fair, and compassionate approach can help to uphold the high standards of professional practice. In the end, this approach benefits the peer, the patients, and the professions themselves.

An advantage of peer review as a mechanism is that this practice usually involves obtaining the considered opinions of several people. When it can be done without compromising confidentiality, this practice helps mitigate biases that might arise from having only superiors conduct the review on their own. The person who reads the reviews (i.e., the administrator, search committee chairperson, or other) looks for areas of congruence among the several reviewers. If one evaluation is radically out of line with the others, further clarification may be sought.

 Summary

The aim of peer review is to uphold the high standards of professional practice. Your participation in such a process is one of your professional responsibilities.

Reporting Unethical or Incompetent Colleagues

Interprofessional care teams rely on trust, collaboration, and shared accountability. From time to time, a team-related ethical challenge arises when evidence shows that a team member is engaging in unethical or incompetent behavior. Professional organizations and government licensing and disciplinary boards acknowledge and report unethical and incompetent behavior by health professionals, clinical investigators, and healthcare administrators. The bases of such behaviors include *impairments* from substance use disorder, the apparent inability to exercise sound professional judgment, and breaches of professional integrity through sexual misconduct/sexual abuse of colleagues and/or patients, theft from patients or institutions, fraudulent billing, illegal business arrangements, and practicing without a license, outside the scope of one's license, or under other false pretenses. You need not watch medical drama shows to know that health care is a business and health professionals include all types of people.

Reporting Wrongdoing

The philosopher Socrates, in the philosophy dialogue "Laches," discusses with his disciples what wisdom is. He concludes that it is "prudent courage." Reporting of unethical or illegal conduct in a colleague or in another requires moral courage, but it is helpful to be wise by engaging in thoughtful ("prudent") reflection before going forward. A well-reasoned concern is a well-respected one because it shows your ability to self-assess and evaluate. An essential rule of thumb is to honor the confidentiality of everyone involved, reporting only information that is relevant to the situation and containing the report to documented evidence. Understandably, if you self-report on an error in judgment you made, you may be asked to justify how it happened and work with your supervisor or others to rectify it.

Whistle-Blowing

To make matters more complicated, usually the knowledge of harm to patients or colleagues gradually comes to the attention of colleagues and often in a form that creates many questions about the legitimacy of the rumor, the witnessed event, the mental stability of the person in question, or other troubling factors. Given the complexity of the healthcare delivery system and the fallibility of humans who practice in it, you may find yourself in a situation in which you need to report an unethical colleague. When such a person is reported to organizational leadership or governmental agencies, the persons who make the report are called *whistle-blowers*, and their action is called *whistle-blowing*. Whistle-blowing is characterized as a prosocial behavior motivated by compassion or concern for others' rights and welfare and intended to benefit others or society at large.[27] Those who report unethical behavior require the support of trusted organizational leadership and mentors to support them in divulging the wrongdoing.

Standards of Conduct and Fitness to Serve Others

Dramatic examples of wrongdoing often hit the newspapers. At the same time, more common problems arise that are not as dramatic but are potentially just as dangerous to patients. For instance, take the case of a health professional who has family problems and copes with excessive lack of sleep or overuse of prescription medications.

Unfortunately, rumors about teammates one works with, side by side, or consults with are more easily dismissed as a curiosity than viewed as an enemy among the ranks. And regrettably, rumors are more easily believed as carrying a kernel of truth when the person is disliked or suspected in the first place. Even so, in almost all cases, this type of rumor is first met with disbelief by most people. Indeed, to base one's judgment solely on such a report is morally indefensible behavior.

What should guide you in your attempt to arrive at a caring response when faced with hearsay information? As in most such situations, the information should not be totally denied or ignored, but a final judgment about the person should never be made on this tenuous ground. The process of gathering relevant information must be taken especially seriously. The characteristics of the person who makes the complaint should be taken into consideration, but this person should never be dismissed as senile, crazy, irrational, or otherwise unable to report accurately what has happened. At the very least, the person making the complaint should be listened to and asked directly for details. An environment of open communication and a no-blame culture help facilitate a commitment to quality and safety. A further step is to ask whether the person is willing to put the complaint in writing. Although this in itself does not render the alleged offender guilty, it is a sign that the person observing the conduct is willing to describe perceptions of the situation in writing and probably is willing to defend the statement before a grievance committee or in a court of law if necessary. Hesitance to report a peer in cases of a serious offense often comes from fear of reprisal from the alleged offender or fear of stigma (e.g., in cases of rape).

Safety is the most immediate concern. If a pattern of alleged abuses or mistakes emerges, it calls into question the health professional's fitness to practice and must be followed up on immediately. Almost all institutions currently have appropriate processes for reporting suspicious or outright improper conduct. These processes are designed to protect the rights of everyone involved and to provide due process under the law and should be followed rigorously. Familiarity with such policies when considering accepting a position, or if already in a position, prepares you to take appropriate action should a situation arise.

The moral decision to blow the whistle on a fellow team member can be among the most agonizing in your career as a health professional.[28] From a psychological viewpoint, there is tremendous potential for your own ego, beliefs, and hopes to take a battering. The loss of an errant colleague also can signal the loss of a friend or the loss of your belief in ideals you thought were shared ideals. Understandably, you may be comforted to believe that you will not be faced with such a dilemma, especially if the offender is a close friend, but to hope for such good fortune does not excuse you from trying to prepare for it. Your moral character is always tested. Knowing when and how to proceed with incriminating evidence when a colleague or friend is implicated takes a full dose of courage, patience, and fortitude; a striving toward justice; much compassion; and a capacity for sympathetic involvement.

 Reflection
Before you read ahead, list some courses of action you could take if you increasingly believed that your colleague had an alcohol or drug dependency that was interfering with patient safety or the overall well-being of the workplace.

_____

_____

_____

_____

One alternative in some situations is to stave off a developing problem before a real offense is committed. Often, the breaking point between a professional's attempt to maintain self-esteem or professional responsibilities and total resignation to the destructive forces at work within is the realization that colleagues have turned their backs. Most people know when they are in trouble. At the point of greatest need and alienation, a direct contact from someone who cares enough to confront the problem tactfully often can provide courage for one to seek help and can be the thin thread back to more sound functioning. An *intervention* is a method that has been developed in which a group confronts a person directly, within a context of ensuring that the person is being held in their care but urging them to take responsibility for change. Trusted members of the team can form such a group. Morag Coate, a British writer quoted in Kay Jamison's book, *Night Falls Fast: Understanding Suicide,* was contemplating suicide but decided not to take her life when she became convinced that her doctor cared. She wrote afterward, "Because the doctors cared, and because one of them still believed in me when I believed in nothing, I have survived to tell the tale."[29]

Unfortunately, rates of depression and suicide in health professionals are on the rise.[30] Cross-sectional studies of physicians have found burnout (discussed in Chapter 6) to be independently associated with 25% increased odds of excessive alcohol use/dependence and 200% increased odds of suicidal ideation.[31,32] Whether it is a patient or a teammate who loses the will to go on because of a serious problem makes no difference. You, the one link, or the team as a whole may be sufficient for the person who is spinning out of control to get his or her bearings.

Whenever possible, you should act to affirm such a person as someone in a struggle and offer your support. This may include recommending that the person not continue to practice, at least until he or she is on more solid footing. The motivation for risking yourself enough to reach out to a fellow team member in distress often arises from a sense that it could be you in a similar situation and that, in some fundamental regard, we all are in the game together and must care for each other as caregivers.

Another possible alternative is to do nothing. The shortcoming of this position is that once the potential problem has come to light, doing nothing also is a course of action. When harm to others or the teammate's self is likely to ensue, your neglect has become complicity. The professional disciplinary committees of most states and the codes of ethics of most professions now count this type of inaction as an offense as serious as committing wrongdoing yourself. Chapter 6 addressed this situation briefly in the discussion of moral agency and resilience.

 Reflection

If you have not already done so, check the code of ethics of your chosen profession to see whether it includes a statement of responsibility to report unethical or incompetent colleagues. Write a few notes about how it would and would not help you.

_____

_____

_____

_____

A third course is to act decisively to remove the teammate from a position in which further harm can be done. This is the appropriate course of action once the relevant information has been gathered and analyzed and is persuasive. A secure rule of thumb is to keep the information as contained as possible with the usual channels of communication and institutional or other disciplinary mechanisms designed for this purpose. It is extremely important to honor the alleged violator's privacy, respect, and legal rights, no matter how grievous a "crime" you may think the person has committed.

Unquestionably, some difficult judgment calls are involved in actually taking the final step of whistle-blowing. Some checkpoints include:

- If possible, you should communicate to the person that you have reached the point at which you plan to call attention to the alleged violation of ethical, competency, or legal standards.
- You should decide whether to talk to anyone else before you act, knowing that sometimes there is strength in numbers and that your own perceptions may be skewed.
- You must give careful attention to whether you have exhausted the other possibilities that may allow you to take a less radical step and still be responsible in your role as a moral agent.

Should you be faced with a whistle-blowing situation, your ability to strike a balance between your sensitivity to the human situation and a commitment to proceed requires moral courage. The attention you have given to it here will serve you well.

As always, any opportunity you have to help prevent such situations is time extremely well spent. An environment conducive to moral acts is one that provides a balanced, safe, and open forum for discussion. Short of that, if your institution has developed guidelines about unethical or incompetent conduct, use them as aids. If not, you and your teammates can contribute greatly to the constructive functioning of the institution by helping to develop policies that will implement whistle-blowing procedures with the following guide posts:

- Promote a culture of speaking up to ensure patient safety at all times.
- Encourage thorough documentation.
- Use state and national professional associations for guidance
- Ensure due process judiciously.
- Provide as much support to everyone involved as possible.
- Require that the institution persevere to the completion of the review and take action consistent with the findings.
- Debrief the process post resolution/completion with a focus on supporting the interprofessional care team and practice milieu.

Completion probably will involve the roles of several others, such as administrators, regulatory board members, compliance officers, risk managers, and designated people in professional associations. The actual personnel and processes vary. Your job in seeing the issue to completion is to work diligently within prescribed professional and other organizational mechanisms.

Summary

Whistle-blowing may involve reporting impaired, unethical, or incompetent colleagues. Health professionals have the right to expect guidelines to ensure protection of all parties involved while the appropriate bodies follow up on reports and the assurance that the investigation will be accompanied by appropriate action.

In the heat of challenging situations regarding peer relationships, certain character traits that dispose you to be thoughtful also will help you to know whether and how to proceed. An acute sensitivity to the various people affected combined with the courage, duty, and resilience to act compassionately is an essential moral tool in such situations.

Summary

This chapter focuses on interprofessional collaborative practice and the key role that effective teamwork plays in improving the quality and safety of healthcare. Shared moral agency, shared ethical decision making, and shared ethical reflection honor the tenets of interprofessional collaborative practice and help build a moral community. The challenge of remaining ethical in peer evaluation situations was discussed, as were serious challenges that arise when a colleague is engaging in unethical or illegal behavior.

Questions for Thought and Discussion

1. You and Uri enjoy a good working relationship as members of an interprofessional care team, although you do not know much about his personal life outside of the work situation. You notice that during the past few days he has become increasingly irritable toward you. You wonder if something you have said or done is making him angry.
   a. What steps, if any, should you take to address this issue?
   b. Do you proceed differently if it appears that his attitude is interfering with the quality of his work? Why?
   c. How do you handle it if another member of the team expresses her worry about his behavior and asks whether you have noted anything disturbing about him in recent weeks?
2. You are a member of the interprofessional care team working in an acute rehabilitation setting. You have been working with Mary Andre, a 63-year-old woman status post coronary artery bypass grafting complicated by a small stroke. Mary is gaining strength and independence in her mobility

and activities of daily living, but she lives alone and continues to have some memory impairments and lapses in safety that impact her level of functioning in home management tasks such as cooking and medication management. At the team meeting, the agreement was that Mary would remain at rehabilitation for 5 more days to advance her independence and safety with instrumental activities of daily living before transitioning back home. You arrive at work and find out at morning rounds that Mary will be going home today. The case manager who is running morning rounds says, "We (the rehabilitation facility) need the bed, and Mary is close enough to meeting her goals. We can get her home care services and just tell her not to cook until the home care agency clears her." Articulate your next steps in discussing this decision with the interprofessional care team. What principles of interprofessional collaborative care are being challenged by this case? What are some possible alternatives to ensure the outcome of a caring response for Mary and the restoration of your (and her) faith in team decision making?

3. You are told by a young patient, whose complications from child-birth required her to remain hospitalized on the obstetrics ward, that Dr. Redmarck, a medical resident assigned to her case, is acting "inappropriately" toward her. She says she is scared, and she looks it. When you ask what she means, she says, "Twice this week he has stopped in during the late evening and has asked to examine my breasts. At first I didn't think anything about it, but then I started thinking that it didn't have anything to do with my condition…He pulls the covers way back and lifts up my gown. The way he looks at me and touches me down there—there's something strange. I dread seeing him." What steps would you take in response to this information?

References

1. World Health Organization (WHO): *Framework for action on interprofessional education & collaborative practice*, Geneva, 2010, World Health Organization.
2. Interprofessional Education Collaborative. Core competencies for interprofessional collaborative practice; 2016 update. Retrieved from www.ipecollabora-tive.org/resources.html.
3. Institute of Medicine (IOM): *Measuring the impact of inter-professional education on collaborative practice and patient outcomes*, Washington, DC, 2015, The National Academies Press.
4. Frenk J, Chen L, Bhutta Z, et al: Health professionals for a new century: transforming education to strengthen health systems in an interdependent world, *Lancet* 376:1923–1956, 2010.
5. National Academies of Sciences, Engineering, and Medicine: *Strengthening the connection between health professions education and practice: proceedings of a joint workshop*, Washington, DC, 2019, The National Academies Press.

6. National Academies of Practice: *State of the science: a synthesis of interprofessional collaborative research*, National Academies of Practice, Washington, DC, 2019.

7. Weiss D, Tilin F, Morgan M: *The interprofessional health care team: leadership and development*, Burlington, MA, 2014, Jones and Bartlett Learning.

8. Doherty RF: Building effective teams. In Jacobs K, editor: *Occupational therapy manager*, ed 6, Bethesda, MD, 2019, AOTA Press.

9. Frost JS, Hammer DP, Nunex LM, et al: The intersection of professionalism and interprofessional care: development and initial testing of the interprofessional professionalism assessment (IPA), *J Interprof Care* 33(1):102–115, 2019 Jan-Feb. doi: 10.1080/13561820.2018.1515733.

10. Stern DT: *Measuring medical professionalism*, New York, 2006, Oxford University Press, as cited in the Interprofessional Professionalism Collaborative Glossary. Available at http://www.interprofessionalprofessionalism.org/resources.html.

11. Haddad A, Doherty R, Purtilo R: Respect for self in the professional role. *Health professional and patient interaction*, ed 9, St. Louis, 2019, Elsevier, pp 42–59.

12. Purtilo R: Thirty-first Mary McMillan lecture: a time to harvest, a time to sow: ethics for a shifting landscape, *Phys Ther* 80:1112–1119, 2000.

13. Clark PG, Cott C, Drinka TJ: Theory and practice in interprofessional ethics: a framework for understanding ethical issues in healthcare teams, *J Interprofessional Care* 21(6):591–603, 2007.

14. Crocker A, Trede F, Higg J: Collaboration: what is it like? Phenomenological interpretation of the experience collaborating within rehabilitation teams, *J Interprofessional Care* 26:13–20, 2012.

15. Blackmer J: Ethical issues in rehabilitation medicine, *Scand J Rehab Med* 32: 51–55, 2000.

16. Edmondson AC: *Teaming: how organizations learn, innovate, and complete in the knowledge economy*, San Francisco, 2012, Jossey-Bass.

17. Haddad A, Doherty R, Purtilo R: Professional boundaries guided by respect. *Health professional and patient interaction*, ed 9, St. Louis, 2019, Elsevier, pp 28–40.

18. Hsiao T: The case for marijuana prohibition, *Ethics Medicine* 35(1):17–26, 2019.

19. Wong SS, Wilens TE: Medical cannabinoids in children and adolescents: a systematic review, *Pediatrics* 140(5):e20171818, 2017.

20. Aggarwal S, Blinderman CD: Cannabis for symptom control #279: fast facts and concepts, *J Palliative Med* 17(5):612–614, 2014.

21. Health Resources and Services Administration (HRSA) the Josiah Macy Jr. Foundation, the Robert Wood Johnson Foundation (RWJF), and the ABIM Foundation in collaboration with the Interprofessional Education Collaborative (IPEC): *Team-based competencies: building a shared foundation for education and clinical practice*, Conference Proceedings, Washington, DC, February 16-17, 2011.

22. Child Welfare Information Gateway: *Definitions of child abuse and neglect*, Washington, DC, 2019, U.S. Department of Health and Human Services,

Children's Bureau. Available at https://www.childwelfare.gov/pubPDFs/define.pdf#page=5&view=Summaries%20of%20State%20laws.

23. Deutsch SA: A struggle for certainty: protecting the vulnerable, *N Engl J Med* 372(36):506–507, 2015.

24. James JT: A new, evidence-based estimate of patient harms associated with hospital care, *J Patient Safety* 9(3):122–128, 2013.

25. Mackery MA, Daniel M: Medical error—the third leading cause of death in the US, *BMJ* 353. doi: https://doi.org/10.1136/bmj.i2139, May 2016.

26. Purtilo R: Teams, healthcare, ed 3. In Post S, editor: *Encyclopedia of bioethics*, vol 5, New York, 2014, McMillan and Company, pp 2495–2497, Revised from original, 1995, and ed 2, 2004.

27. Ugaddan, RG, Park SM: *Do trustful leadership, organizational justice, and motivation influence whistle-blowing intention?* Evidence From Federal Employees." Public Personnel Management, vol. 48, no. 1, Mar. 2019, pp. 56–81.

28. Purtilo R: Interdisciplinary health care teams and health care reform, *J Law Med Ethics* 22(2):121–126, 1994.

29. Jamison K: *Night falls fast: understanding suicide*, New York, 1999, Knopf, p 255.

30. Brigham TC, Barden AL, Dopp A et al: A journey to constuct an all-encompassing conceptual model of factors affecting clinician well-being and resilience. *NAM Perspectives*. Discussion Paper, 2018, National Academy of Medicine, Washington, DC. Available at https://nam.edu/journey-construct-encompassing-conceptual-model-factors-affecting-clinician-well-resilience/.

31. Oreskovich M, Kaups K, Balch C, et al: The prevalence of alcohol use disorders among American surgeons, *Arch Surg* 147:168–174, 2011.

32. Shanafelt TD, Balch CM, Dyrbye LN, et al: Suicidal ideation among American surgeons, *Arch Surg* 146:54–62, 2011.

8

Living Ethically Within Healthcare Organizations

Objectives

The reader should be able to:

- Identify several areas of healthcare addressed by organizational ethics.
- Define the term mission statement and the role of a mission statement in an organization.
- Describe what policies are and what they are designed to accomplish within healthcare and other organizations.
- Explain how the utilitarian approach to policies and practices serves everyone well and the conditions under which serious shortcomings may arise from relying solely on this approach.
- Apply several ethical principles in the analysis of organizational ethics problems.
- Identify and discuss the rights of professional employees in healthcare organizations.
- Name some virtues of organizations and why they are important in today's evolving healthcare delivery system.
- Identify strategies organizational systems can use to support moral resilience and well-being in health professionals.
- Compare basic values of health professionals with those of healthcare organizations and strategies for bringing the two into agreement around their common goals.

New terms and ideas you will encounter in this chapter

organizational ethics	conflict of loyalty	Patient Protection and
mission statement	stakeholder	Affordable Care Act
policy	cost-effectiveness	principle of participation
conflict of interest		principle of efficiency

Topics in this chapter introduced in earlier chapters

Topic	Introduced in chapter
Values and duties	1
Moral agent	3
Moral distress	3
Ethical dilemma	3
Locus of authority considerations	3
Virtue	4
Prima facie and absolute duties	4
Utilitarian theory	4
Principles approach	4
Beneficence	4
Nonmaleficence	4
Justice	4
The six-step process of ethical decision making	5
Moral courage	6
Moral resilience	6
Well-being	6
Interprofessional collaborative practice	7

Introduction

So far, the ethical challenges that individuals and interprofessional care teams face in their professional roles and work environments have been a focus in this text. In this chapter, you will explore the organizational dimensions of healthcare. The suggestions in the previous chapter regarding your ethical survival are not complete without including your placement within the larger organization of healthcare and the challenges it presents. Thus another critical area of ethical reflection in healthcare is *organizational ethics*. Organizational ethics pays attention to the values, needs, traits, rights, and duties expressed in mission statements, business practices, policies, and other administrative arrangements.

Organizational ethics cuts a wide swath across your professional life. The field addresses ethical issues in the institutional structures that deliver healthcare or are involved in remuneration for professional services, agencies that regulate health professionals or healthcare practices, professional associations, businesses that provide healthcare equipment or material for procedures, and pharmaceutical companies. Subsets of organizational ethics are business ethics, management ethics, administrative ethics, and legislative ethics, to name a few. Each addresses the conditions under which an organization's and society's moral expectations can be reconciled. They focus on the larger societal and bureaucratic organization of modern healthcare; therefore goals are not limited solely to the ethical goals of individual health professionals and teams.[1] At the same time, often in the cases we have already presented, we note that in addition to what is accomplished at the point of decision making, institutional policies and actions affect patient care, so the outcome in part is determined by the relationship between healthcare organizations and its professionals. For instance, a business goal of increasing the profit margin each year is legitimate for a business enterprise. Business ethics addresses the conditions necessary for that profit margin to be gained, with adherence to high ethical standards set by the consumers of the business' products or services, society, and the organizations themselves. Healthcare organizations have ethical problems that in many ways are similar to good business management anywhere, but because of the special place the professions have in society, these organizational structures must be styled to fit the type of role their employees and clients play. The "product" of the professionals' skilled efforts is high-quality patient care outcomes. As a participant in various healthcare organizations, your challenge is to assess whether their values, rights, and duties affect your ability to achieve this end with patients when measured against the standard of your professional values, rights, and duties. To illustrate one version of how the ethical challenges of working within an organization affect health professionals, consider the following story, which serves the purpose of showing how professionals' tasks sometimes may appear to be removed from an individual patients' well-being but always are informed by that purpose.

 ### The Story of Simon Kapinsky and the Interprofessional Ethics Subcommittee to Implement a Green Health Plan

The chief executive officer (CEO) of StarServices, Inc., a for-profit major health plan, has asked Simon Kapinsky, a senior member of the professional staff in one of the plan's units, to chair an interprofessional ethics subcommittee of the health plan's greening advisory council. The advisory council recently was formed to set new policy and practices for StarServices, Inc. to operate as a "green health plan." The CEO explains that the council decided that an interprofessional care team made up of several leaders of the unit's clinical departments should be in charge of assessing the clinical implications of this change in regard to the health services it offers. On review of the material from the CEO, Simon learns that the board of trustees of the health plan signed a contract 2 years ago to build or remodel all of its treatment (not research) units according to principles of ecological architectural design. Simon is aware that the flagship hospital in the health plan (where he is employed) already has undergone major renovation, but he was not fully aware of the scope of the project. In the proposal, the greening of the health plan is being financed one-fourth by StarServices, Inc.; one-half by municipal bonds in the city in which the major institutions of the health plan are located; and one-fourth by Green International, a private architectural firm whose purpose is to showcase ecological architecture in public buildings. Green International claims that the new health plan structures will become the showcase for eco-friendly medical facilities over the next 50 years. The estimated overall cost is $46 million, but Green International emphasizes that much of that cost will be recovered by offsetting operating costs and by the amount of business this ecofriendly model project will generate. When Simon returns the material to the CEO, the latter emphasizes, "With our flagship hospital in the health plan already partially renovated, StarServices, Inc. is positioned to move ahead substantially toward its strategic goal of becoming the greenest health plan in the world. Now the next step is to rescale our clinical services according to the overall ecological impact of the range of clinical services we offer. We can do well financially by doing what is right for the environment! As you are the chair of the subcommittee, we look forward to you becoming a member of the advisory council; you will meet with us to keep us up-to-date on your subcommittee's findings and recommendations. Of course, all members of your team will receive release time from their clinical duties during this period as we at the top are aware of the immensity of the task we are asking of you."

Simon is not exactly thrilled at the prospect of chairing this subcommittee, but with his CEO appointing him to the post, he also feels that he does not have any good alternative but to accept. That night, he goes home and discusses it with his partner, who is also a health professional. Over dinner, they come up with some questions that Simon will urge the subcommittee to raise about the project. They agree that, as concerned and ethically informed professional leaders, they have more to take into account than to jump on the bandwagon of excitement about being the "greenest health plan in the world," as laudable as that goal is.

Some of their questions include:

- Should a healthcare plan alter or select its range of patient services on the basis of environmental ecological impact?
- Assuming that the decision has been made to take this approach:
  - Has the organization already developed its own set of criteria for selecting the current clinical services that will be discontinued, and, if so, what are they?
  - Which specific services or categories of patients that could be excluded would raise the most concern for the administration (if any), and is the administration willing to consider keeping these groups in the plan at the price of ecological efficiency if the subcommittee recommends it?

- If the subcommittee can come up with a plan, is the administration willing to consider ways to honor the goal to be "green"—or even "the greenest"—without tinkering with the types of patients or range of services currently offered?

At the first meeting of the interprofessional ethics subcommittee, Simon is gratified to learn that everyone has the same questions as well as some other concerns. They wonder whether or not every stone has been turned to look for cost-saving and ecologically responsible changes in the way things are done at the various institutions of the health plan to warrant this jump to a cut or cutback in direct patient care services.

By the end of the meeting, the subcommittee is confident that their questions raise serious enough concerns that they should be submitted to the CEO and chairperson of the advisory council for further discussion. Simon agrees to carry their request to the chair of the advisory council and sends a copy to the CEO. He is surprised when, at the next meeting of the full council, he notes that the subcommittee's questions are not on the agenda and the chairperson does not mention it.

Finally, Simon calls the chairperson. She says, "I have just been writing a letter to you and the subcommittee thanking you for your thought-provoking questions, and, of course, the administration shares your concerns or we would not have chosen the best clinical leaders we could identify to carry this aspect of the project forward. We recommend that you not delay in the larger task of assessment and recommendations, rather to be informed in your own thinking with respect to the important issues you raise." Simon responds with a stunned silence. The chairperson, noting this, continues, "I think in time any ethical problems your subcommittee thought may be barriers will iron themselves out."

Simon thinks it over, discusses it with his partner, and calls the subcommittee together. They agree to take the advice of the chairperson but not to let go of their own questions, which they believe are extremely relevant to the basic purpose of the organization and their ability to keep optimal patient care at the center of their discussions.

Reflection

Before reading on, write down all of the values and priorities implied or expressed by the members of the administration. Then do the same for the interprofessional ethics subcommittee.

Administration:

_____

_____

_____

_____

Interprofessional ethics subcommittee:

_____

_____

_____

_____

The Goal: A Caring Response

Simon and the health professionals on the subcommittee are moral agents whose "voice" must reflect values, needs, duties, and rights guided by the goal of a caring response in the health professional and patient encounter. For the interprofessional care team to be effective, patient-centered analysis and strategy must govern their recommendations. The "voice" of the organization is expressed through the administrators and others who look out for the administrative interests of the organization (i.e., the chief executive officer [CEO] and chief financial officer [CFO], trustees, and in privately owned institutions, the stockholders). You can correctly think of them as the moral agents charged with protecting the values, needs, duties, and rights of the organization as a whole. Thus you can expect their analysis and strategy priorities to reflect their position and responsibilities. In Chapter 2, you also learned that to live by the goal of a professional caring response requires acknowledging that care cannot be "bottled"; it must be tailored for each situation. Right off, the subcommittee recognizes that in this situation their care for patients includes accepting it as a sign of good faith on the part of StarServices, Inc. that administration included direct care providers in the project, giving the members an opportunity to help shape the plan. Of course, as one member of the subcommittee added, "The proof is in the pudding!" as to how seriously their recommendations will be taken. A third added, "So, let's put the right ingredients in the pudding!" Having generated this amount of energy for what is possible, Simon reminded them of the assumptions of a relationship-centered approach that you read about in Chapter 2: What may seem conflicting purposes may be brought together and finally reflected in a changed organization overall. Simon concluded the meeting with encouraging them to identify strategies to engage effectively with the administration, reassuring them that the priorities they were representing would be recognized and their recommendations implemented. What follows is the process this meeting initiated.

The Six-Step Process in Organizational Matters

Given that several moral agents are found in this situation, you will gain some important insights by walking with Simon and the subcommittee through their experience with the use of the six-step process of ethical decision making as a framework.

Step 1: Gather Relevant Information

Simon and the subcommittee need to gather data in different places than if the issue pertained solely to their search for an optimal plan of care between themselves and their patients. As noted at the outset of this chapter, the values and priorities of organizations can be found in their mission statements, policies and administrative practices, and business approaches. The subcommittee would be wise to turn to these documents to gain support for the professional values they are trying to protect.

Mission Statements as Relevant Information

A *mission statement* is an organization's brief description of its ideals and aspirations. The mission statement drives an organization's strategic priorities, and it is from these values and ideals that goals, behavioral objectives, and expectations of all users (e.g., patients and all employees) are derived. Sometimes, the values of the organization are reflective of religious assumptions. In the United States, many hospitals and schools are owned and operated by religious groups, a situation visitors to other parts of the world may not see. Such an organization makes reference in its mission statement to its understanding of the relationship of humans to a higher being and each other and to the way in which the organization views itself as participating in the larger spiritual and social scheme of things. In contrast, the U.S. Veterans Administration healthcare plan is an example of a government-owned and government-operated healthcare system, which now partners with various private companies for goods and services. One expects its mission statement to read quite differently from that of a religiously based nonprofit healthcare organization. Box 8.1 contains an example of a hospital mission statement.

Box 8.1   Mission Statement—Massachusetts General Hospital

> Guided by the needs of our patients and their families, we aim to deliver the very best healthcare in a safe, compassionate environment; to advance that care through innovative research and education; and to improve the health and well-being of the diverse communities we serve.

From Massachusetts General Hospital, Boston. Available at http://www.massgeneral.org/about/overview.aspx. Courtesy Massachusetts General Hospital.

● ◣ *Reflection*
What does this mission statement tell you about the nature of this institution?

_____

_____

_____

Suppose this is the mission statement of StarServices, Inc. Does this statement say some things that would support the ethics subcommittee regarding arrangements they can recommend based on the organization's mission? If so, what are they?

_____

_____

_____

● Go back to the subcommittee's questions. Do any specific phrases in the mission statement help provide a basis for taking the question(s) seriously? Which questions are they?

_____

_____

_____

Because mission statements are public documents that become the basis for more specific policies and expectations, it is prudent and responsible to check the mission statement with as much care as possible before becoming part of an organization. This checkpoint should enable you to avoid moral distress or ethical dilemmas further into your affiliation with this body and its policies and practices if you find you do not subscribe to the overall nature of the organization's mission.

Summary

Like codes and oaths for health professionals, a mission statement is an organization's public statement designed to declare the type of organization it is, including its core ethical purpose, values, and ideals.

Policies and Administrative Practices as Information

A *policy* is a statement designed to establish formal and informal guidelines for practice within an organization. Obviously, policies should be consistent with the values of the organization. They also should be specific expressions of how the ideals in the mission statement can be performed by the people in the organization and how the organization hopes to attract or serve. If policies are to be followed, they must also be clear, practical, flexible, and consistent with the values of the people or groups to whom they apply.

Currently, policies in healthcare reflect both traditional healthcare ethics and business ethics. The hospital administrator of a religious group whose mission clearly was to deliver high-quality patient care once commented, "No money, no mission." The goals of an organization are not fully met simply by focusing on the model of a single patient and the health professional or interprofessional care team. In fact, it is often at the level of policy that goals for an individual patient's well-being come into direct conflict with business interests. This concern was high in the minds of the ethics subcommittee members, and they wanted to hear from the administration that they could trust that patient-centered values and practices would not be unduly compromised.

The subcommittee will have to spend considerable time accessing policies that pertain to patient care in StarServices, Inc. Some of them will include statements of patient rights introduced in Chapter 2 and include protections for and responsibilities of professionals administering care. Statements in these key documents also can provide substance to the approach they take.

 Summary

Few health professionals today are in situations in which they can ignore organization policies. Still, professional values must guide their own decisions.

As you recall from Chapter 5, step 1 of the six-step process of ethical decision making includes identifying the facts, including the relevant stakeholders and contextual factors in the problem you face. The organization is a stakeholder, and a policy in that organization is a contextual factor. The Realm-Individual Process-Situation (RIPS) model of ethical decision making developed by three physical therapists maintains that partially because

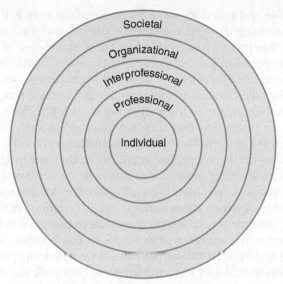

Fig. 8.1. Framing ethical decision making across realms.

of the changes in the healthcare system, almost all ethical issues that involve patient care now also have business or administrative and larger societal dimensions.[2] Similar to the work of Glaser,[3] their three realms of ethics (individual, institutional [i.e., organizational], and societal) must be identified for their relevance.[3] Reflecting on these realms as a schema can be helpful in framing the ethical decision-making process for individual health professionals and members of the interprofessional care team (Fig. 8.1). This type of template also is useful to the subcommittee as they gather information.

Step 2: Identify the Type of Ethical Problem

Simon and his colleagues on the ethics subcommittee of the greening advisory council are experiencing moral distress. Their guts tell them that something may be wrong in the entire approach StarServices, Inc. is taking in its pursuit of an otherwise laudable goal of becoming "the greenest [healthcare] plan in the world."

They also feel the pinch of an ethical dilemma. On the one hand, they recognize that they have a duty of loyalty to the goals of their employing healthcare organization, StarServices, Inc. Honoring its organizational goals is an expression of these employees' willingness to acknowledge that being an employee provides the context for them to make a living while honoring their professional commitments. They are brought face to face with the reality that the values, needs, duties, and rights of the organization must be taken deeply into the equation as a part of their overall analysis. At the same time, they know that they have a responsibility to how that loyalty is expressed in light of the current challenge they face. They were placed in a consultative role and asked to make recommendations to help ensure that the health plan succeeds in its worthwhile project, but their dilemma is in knowing that this project's success could come at the cost of compromising a caring response to patient groups that use the facility. At this point, they are on the horns of a dilemma with two right courses of action facing them—one being their loyalty to the organization, and the other, more compelling course, their loyalty to the well-being of patients. The subcommittee is also facing the possibility that they are involved in a conflict of interest situation. A *conflict of interest*—or as it is sometimes correctly identified, a *conflict of loyalty*—occurs for professionals when they are in situations that significantly threaten their professional duties and commitments.[4]

Simon and the subcommittee must consider the differences in decision-making authority between them and the administration. Although aware that their role ultimately is advisory, they believe that they bring an essential ethical perspective and area of expertise to this business enterprise. In fact, they were appointed to do so. Their positions as leading professionals in this organization should give them the say-so to have their recommendations taken seriously by the administrators and advisory council. In fact, their concerns are based on thoughtful ethical reasoning, which causes them to take their moral agency as guardians of patients' well-being seriously. They believe they are on solid ground regarding their assumption that this healthcare organization should protect quality care for patients above all other priorities.

One important lesson the subcommittee members are learning is that there are many stakeholders in the type of project they have been pulled into, with different and sometimes conflicting values and priorities. A *stakeholder* is a person, group, or other entity that has a deep and compelling interest in a situation that it wants to protect. Because ethical issues are involved, the stakeholders all are moral agents with their part to play in arriving at ethically acceptable courses of action. Two major stakeholders are the professionals and the administration or management. In order of priority, some common loyalties that cause ethical conflict between health professionals and the top-level administration of a healthcare organization are listed subsequently.

Where Do Health Professional and Organization Priorities Lie?

Health Professional	Organization
• Individual patient care	• Fiscal viability
• Other professionals, teammates	• Employee protection
• Patient satisfaction	• Competitiveness in the marketplace
• Workplace effectiveness and efficiency	• Patient/consumer safety and satisfaction
• Societal expectations/laws upheld	• Laws, regulations upheld
• Professional values	• Community support
• Self-fulfillment	• Institutional efficiency/effectiveness

● ▰ *Reflection*
In examining these two sets of loyalties, where, if any place, do you see complementary interests in which the administration of StarServices, Inc. and the ethics subcommittee of professionals are likely to find common ground for discussion and eventual agreement? List them here.

_____

_____

_____

Why have you chosen these? Describe in a sentence or two before going on.

_____

_____

_____

_____

● ## Step 3: Use Ethics Theories or Approaches to Analyze the Problem

Several ethical approaches can be considered when a policy or procedure proposal is being assessed, and the interprofessional ethics subcommittee goes to work on this part of their task.

Utilitarian Reasoning in Organizational Ethics

Utilitarian reasoning is the usual approach to a potential structural change in an organization. Understandably, from the administrative and business standpoint, an ethically supportable policy or procedure is one that brings about the best outcomes overall based on a utilitarian value system designed to provide the greatest good for the greatest number. It follows that from an organizational standpoint, considerations of individual autonomy may be submerged in favor of such utilitarian considerations as efficiency of operations and economic stability. Simply stated, the organization that fulfills its function of providing a worthwhile service efficiently usually is believed to justify the means used to attain that end as long as the net result is a greater balance of benefits to humanity than would be realized if the organization did not exist.

The idea of *cost-effectiveness* often is cited as the appropriate goal of health plans. A definition of cost-effectiveness is that the highest quality of care possible is provided at the lowest price. No one can argue with that underlying utilitarian ideal. As you know, however, the ethics subcommittee wants to be sure that the administrative arrangements, however laudable, do not succumb to the serious criticism that such efficiency can best be achieved through cutting costs by means that unnecessarily compromise high-quality care. They know that successful institutions today are influenced by the idea of being "fit for purpose," meaning that the organization itself is responsive to particular needs and priorities of the public it services, and this, in turn, requires that all institutional arrangements are geared ultimately to that end.[5]

Taking these general considerations into account, the combined group can profitably discuss the question of whether StarServices, Inc's proposed course of action to cut back or cut out some services appears to encourage practices that will do more good than harm overall. No one will argue against the idea that a green organization is a benefit to the environment and to the community and, from a market competition and community support standpoint, benefits the organization greatly. The ethics subcommittee is convinced that the burden of proof on the organization is to show that the goal of high-quality patient care is protected and encouraged.

The criticism often leveled at pure utilitarian thinking generally applies to the current situation under discussion. The policy or procedure that works as a general touchstone cannot provide the optimal solution to every situation. It may be inappropriate or inadequate to handle specific problems faced by the organization and its constituents. Therefore the utilitarian equation merely provides boundaries. We all find ourselves breaking general guidelines when overriding them is ethically justified—for example, parking in a no-parking zone to assist at the scene of an accident. That is, of course, why there is a prima facie, but not an absolute duty, to honor organizational arrangements based solely on utilitarian reasoning. What may be best for most people most of the time may not be best in a specific situation. It is from this level of concern about whether a caring response to individual or groups of patients will be compromised that the addition of several ethical principles helps enrich and fill out the ethics subcommittee's ethical analysis.

Principles Approach in Organizational Ethics
From a principles approach, several ethical principles can further delineate values and duties to which this particular organization must answer.

The principle of beneficence is one key. Although utilitarianism emphasizes overall good consequences that are brought about by a course of action, beneficence requires the moral agents to delineate what type of good is the act itself. For instance, consider specific benefits that may be a part of the combined group's discernment about the next step. If a proposed course of action allows some members of the organization to be exemplars in terms of improving patient satisfaction while increasing employee morale and demonstrating good stewardship of environmental or other resources, these specific benefits can be heralded apart from the overall good consequences.

The principle of nonmaleficence also is an essential corrective to utilitarian theory used alone. The administration that creates moral distress by ignoring the voice of concern brought by thoughtful professionals such as the ethics subcommittee is harming its employees and risking a decrease in professional staff morale more widely. Moreover, as StarServices, Inc. looks toward implementing its ideal of a green healthcare organization, the combined group of administrators and subcommittee members must work together to minimize undue harm that would ensue through new policies and procedures, practices, or resource priorities. In this case, part of the harm would be a compromise of the professionals' ability to bring about optimal patient care policies and practices because of inappropriate cuts in goods or services.

The philosopher John Rawls, to whom you were introduced in a previous chapter, holds that the principle of justice is a fundamental virtue of institutions. His position is that if an organization is fair in its assignment of rights and duties and makes provision for a fair distribution of its resources, then all individuals in those institutions will be able to live more moral lives.[6] If the administration of StarServices, Inc. can show that its proposed course of action will continue to honor the distribution of patient care resources based on patient-centered considerations of need (rather than on market and other business benefits alone), a major concern of the ethics subcommittee can be laid to rest.

The principle of respect also is relevant. All stakeholders in this situation deserve respect. The interests of administrators and trustees counsel toward a green organization because it shows respect to the larger community through saving and protecting natural resources and by being accountable regarding health-related environmental pollution and other harms. They are aware that healthcare institutions are among the highest waste-producing and toxin-producing entities and are committed to demonstrating a viable alternative.[7] The professionals' goal of showing respect for patients can factor in benefits to the latter that a greener workplace will provide. At the same time, this ethics subcommittee comprises an interprofessional team that is well positioned to keep the patients' well-being tantamount, creating a reasonable expectation that their recommendations always will keep professional values and duties at the center of their work. This is a strong argument in the subcommittee's favor that whatever change is made in patient care services, it does not compromise the professionals' duties of a care-centered workplace.

Summary

Utilitarian reasoning is almost always used to determine the best possible balance of benefits over burdens when organizational policies and procedures are being implemented. At the same time, principle-based approaches that involve the dictates of beneficence, nonmaleficence, justice, and respect considerations refine the ethical analysis in a specific situation to guide decision makers.

Step 4: Explore the Practical Alternatives

The subcommittee already has done considerable work on its task. It has examined organizational documents and policies that support its position, identified needs, duties, and relevant ethical principles that it believes should govern future action from the standpoint of its professional role as a moral agent. It has taken into account that "the bottom line" of money does matter in organizations and that administrative decisions always must keep "the big picture" in focus, weighing the costs of one priority against another and honoring the importance of efficiency within the organization as a whole. Although the subcommittee has concluded that a utilitarian approach by itself is not a sufficient basis for ethical analysis, it agrees that this approach is one critical aspect of ethical concern when it comes to an organization's general positions, policies, and practices. It also has reckoned with the moral rights and reasonable expectations with which it undertook the responsibility of trying to help address a major change in the character, public image, and internal practices of StarServices, Inc. In all of this, the subcommittee has moved forward believing that through diligence the top administration and trustees will have an opportunity to foster an environment consistent with the high moral and service standards of patient-centered healthcare. Note, too, that the subcommittee did not refuse to participate in this important planning, even though it did not feel completely supported at the outset. It showed up and worked diligently to create a context in which everyone involved has a chance to bring their best thinking and core priorities to the table of negotiation. Now the subcommittee has convened again to hone in on the alternatives it sees in framing its recommendations.

Reflection
List some practical alternatives that you think Simon and the ethics subcommittee have open to them.

_____

_____

Consider the following alternatives:

- Surely one course of action is to do nothing more than submit its recommendations at the level of the framework for ethical decision making the subcommittee has deployed and turn the strategic next steps over to the administration.
- Simon may continue to attend the meetings of the greening advisory council and communicate privately with the CEO and chairperson of the council to become the point person for the ethical reasoning that will inform future decisions about how to address clinical services within the new "greened" system. He can also seek guidance from an ethics committee in his place of employment for further insight into how to proceed.[8]
- The entire subcommittee may now move vigorously to the task with which they were originally charged by choosing to focus on research findings from other green healthcare institutions about how they reckoned with their mission of maintaining or improving quality care; by appealing to government and other agencies for information regarding environmental issues related to healthcare procedures; and by a more service-by-service assessment, asking the CEO and council for the appropriate documents, experts, and staff support to engage in a thorough study of possible areas of waste or administrative "fat" that could be eliminated without altering quality care.
- A version of the previous alternative is to recommend that the current subcommittee be refocused, with some members remaining and others being added to discuss their understanding of how quality care can best be maintained or enhanced across the organization while educating them to the larger goals of the greening project.

Steps 5 and 6: Complete the Action and Evaluate the Process and Outcome

In considering which alternative to pursue, you will note that each one involves a willingness to move ahead in the face of some unanswered concerns, to honor professional loyalties while respecting key organizational concerns, and to develop an ethical framework that can be applied to many specific decisions. Notably, the subcommittee has also interpreted its task in such a way that its moral agency has not been compromised, courageously rising to the challenge of patient advocacy in a changing environment in which policies and practices seem at odds with the demands of their moral roles. Importantly, by all of these means, it has avoided experiencing a feeling of loss of control, stress, discontent, and disheartenment.[9]

The ethics subcommittee's goal to help set direction that upholds the organization's high ethical standards of patient care is on its way to being realized.

As with all important ethical challenges, the subcommittee's willingness eventually to reconvene as a "reflection group" (see Chapter 6) to evaluate the process and outcome of its experience will strengthen it for future leadership efforts within its organizations. Moreover, the subcommittee can find ways to share its successes with other staff and interprofessional colleagues attempting to deal with similar challenges regarding the increasingly rich mix of priorities that health plans are facing.

Educating for Moral Agency Within Organizations

As an educational opportunity, at least two areas of the StarServices, Inc. ethics subcommittee experience may make good professional development activities in their workplace or at meetings in professional organizations. These opportunities are introduced here.

Living With the Business Aspects of Healthcare

Healthcare organizations are businesses, but not only businesses. Bodenheimer and Grumbach[10] maintained that the following three major forces drive the organization of healthcare in the United States and, to some degree, in all economically developed nations: (1) the biomedical model, (2) financial incentives, and (3) professionalism. The service of healthcare is expressed through the biomedical and clinical skills of the professionals, the financial grounding through financial incentives, and the particular ethical standards through professionalism. Still, the financial incentives often are targeted in the literature as creating the biggest challenge to the professionals. In other words, the challenge for health professionals is the requirement of living with the "business" of healthcare but not letting it govern all the values and priorities of practice.

Business language often conjures up negative images of greedy healthcare institutions driven by profit at all costs. Such organizations do exist and, of course, create ethical dilemmas for any health professional who works in them because they fail to meet reasonable expectations of patients and society. Not all healthcare institutions, however, are driven solely by a monetary bottom line. Many healthcare organizations are distinguished by their vision, mission, and sensitivity to the implications of each when making decisions about the business. The business functions of any organization are designed to help meet the appropriate goals of that organization, whatever those goals may be. An examination of the priorities of an organization in chart form earlier in this chapter highlights why some major themes in business ethics are honesty in advertising, transparency in dealings with partners and clients, fairness in the treatment of employees and others, criteria for quality control of the product or service, the meaning of fiscal accountability from the standpoint of taking everyone's legitimate interests into account, and the duty of respect for others in all the organization's interactions.

Workplace Wellness

As discussed in Chapter 6, burnout in the health professions is an urgent problem in the United States, and one that healthcare organizations have begun to take seriously.

A major area of attention in today's healthcare organizations is building moral capacity to ensure provider wellness and resiliency. Health professionals who experience burnout are more likely to take short cuts, make diagnostic errors, communicate poorly with their patients and colleagues, suffer from emotional exhaustion, and experience mental health conditions.[11] Evidence also shows that dissatisfaction and wanting to leave one's job and the professional altogether often follow morally distressing encounters.[12] Organizations that foster a culture of compassionate care and support recognize that clinician well-being is a sign of a healthy, healthcare organization. Organizations can commit to resilience by learning and growing from ethical tensions experienced by the patients, families, interprofessional care teams, and the communities they serve. Activities such as ethics education, peer counseling, critical incident debriefing, and ethics rounds all contribute to organizational wellness. When organizations attend to the resilience of the workforce, mindful, caring responses are achieved.

Healthcare Reform

The healthcare delivery system is continuously evolving. The passage of the *Patient Protection and Affordable Care Act* of 2010 marked a major shift in the United States from treating healthcare as a commodity to a right. This landmark legislation had three main goals: to expand access to health insurance, to protect patients from arbitrary actions by insurance companies (such as refusing to cover individuals with preexisting conditions), and to reduce costs. Healthcare regulations are changing at a rapid pace. The Affordable Care Act (ACA) and other health reform initiatives incentivized integrated and coordinated care delivery, changing the way care is delivered across multiple settings and organizations.[13] Alternative payment models and value-based payments have been implemented, and payment is now linked to quality outcomes under Medicare, private payers, and health systems. Although a full discussion of the ACA, value-based payment, and reimbursement models is beyond the scope of this book, note that the emphasis on measurement of quality and patient experience will hold organizations (and the leadership of these organizations) accountable to navigate change and ensure that ethics and data-driven decision making are central in care redesign and delivery.[14]

Reflection

Specify some ways a healthcare organization such as a health plan, hospital, nursing home, or home health agency has to gear its business goals, policies, and practices to meet high ethical standards of patient care.

_____

_____

_____

_____

To thrive ethically within the organization in which you work, you need to identify the business realities and critique them. Although it goes beyond the parameters of this book to fully address the business dimensions of your practice setting, the next generation of health professionals, to which you will belong, will be forced to be more cognizant of them. One of the most interesting challenges for you is that the organizational structures in which you may find yourself are much more diverse than even a few years ago. For example, in addition to the more familiar settings of a hospital, clinic, rehabilitation center, school system, home health agency, or hospice, you may be working aboard a cruise ship, in the military, at a children's camp, with a sports team, or for a retail corporation. In each instance, your professional values must be honored and the business aspects of the workplace understood for how well they match up with the demands of the health professions.

---

⑥ Summary

A firm grounding in professional ethics and astute awareness of the business dimensions of healthcare are necessary for a full picture of ethical problems in today's healthcare organizations.

Rights of Professionals in Organizations

The ultimate administrative decisions in most organizations are made by those in leadership positions, although multilevel input is often invited. The greening advisory council and its ethics subcommittee are examples of StarServices, Inc.'s mechanisms to invite multilevel input. In other words, more and more people from all echelons of an organization hierarchy are currently being recruited to provide input and share governance in administrative decisions. The sections that follow discuss the rights of professional employees in healthcare organizations.

The Right to Participate

This stance is consistent with the idea that everyone in an organization has a basic moral right to become involved in appropriate ways. The moral *principle of participation* is seldom included in lists of ethical principles applicable to healthcare ethics but is often cited in social ethics and political treatises on democratic societies. It arises partly from the more familiar principle of autonomy because it supports the idea that you, in your role as a professional, have a right to help determine aspects of your workplace that directly affect your well-being. Your involvement in organizational arrangements and the review of practices or policies are the only ways you can ensure that you will not be forced to sacrifice important personal and professional values to overriding organization values such as efficiency. Workplace efficiency can be applauded when it is brought in line with the professional values of faithfulness to patients' and professionals' rights and prevention of harm to anyone. But only with participation of concerned professionals is that outcome assured. Simon and his colleagues were offered—and took—the opportunity to participate in ensuring that patient-centered care was not compromised.

A good place for you to start exercising your right of participation at the organizational level is in your own place of employment or your professional association. Part of the ability to be involved in policy is to be able to ascertain where organizational arrangements are being made and revised. Pertinent questions include:

1. What are the names of groups responsible for making organizational arrangements and setting policies and practices? To whom, exactly, does each report?
2. Who sits on the organization's various committees, and what are their qualifications? Are there frontline providers on the committees to inform discussion?
3. What must you do to be nominated for or appointed to a group?
4. To whom must you speak to learn more about a group and express your interest?

The Right to Employment Protections and Guidance

It is your right to assume that your organization will have a range of policies and other administrative arrangements that give clear direction for you to practice ethically. Depending on the nature of your patient population and the services offered through the organization, you should be able to find the following types of policies or guidelines related to patient care:

- Informed consent policy
- Advance directive policy
- Surrogate decision making, healthcare agents, durable power of attorney for healthcare, and guardianship process policies
- Withholding and withdrawing life-sustaining treatment policy
- Assisted suicide and abortion policies

- Do not resuscitate (DNR) policy
- Confidentiality and privacy policy
- Organ donation and procurement policy
- Human experimentation regulations (policies and procedures)
- Conflicts of interest policy (including patient care and research policies)
- Patient admission, discharge, and transfer policy
- Impaired providers policy (including reporting procedures for impaired professional colleagues or preventable adverse events)
- Conscientious objection policy and procedures
- Reproductive technology policies
- Grievance procedures

Reflection
Can you think of other policies, procedures, or guidelines that pertain to your professional responsibilities?

_____

_____

_____

_____

The Right to a Virtuous Organization

As you recall, virtue theory provides tools to examine the type of person one ought to be. Philosophers, economists, and others acknowledge the power of organizational structures to affect the lives of individuals in our highly bureaucratized society. You have a right to be assured that your workplace administration shows sincere and intense commitment to creating a humane or "virtuous" organization. Because most organizations are governed by a small number of leaders who have the final say over what happens to everyone, this commitment must begin with the individuals who have the most power and authority. When leaders demonstrate, mentor, and endorse ethical decision making, their staff are more likely to focus on their own moral reasoning.[15] The interprofessional ethics subcommittee in this chapter recognized the difference in decisional authority between the top administration and themselves. The traits of healthcare organizations are one important focus of serious reflection today, and we invite you to participate in this exciting dimension of your professional career.

You already have learned that efficiency is one virtue of organizations because they are designed to meet multiple needs and render multiple services. The *principle of efficiency* can provide a moral basis for conduct that benefits all. From a social standpoint, many say that a "good" or "well-run" organization is an efficient one. From the standpoint of your tasks within a healthcare organization, however, you benefit from institutions and systems that reflect other virtues too.

For example, you have also already learned in this chapter that a commitment to justice in the organization's assignment of benefits and burdens is a virtue that organizations can strive to meet.

Can you imagine what a courageous organization is like and what type of policies and administrative guidelines you can find there? What about a compassionate institution? Consider the following findings from the Schwartz Center for Compassionate Care[16]:

- Organizations that place a high priority on delivering compassionate care benefit from lower staff turnover, higher retention, recruitment of more highly qualified staff, greater patient loyalty, reduced costs from shorter lengths of stay, lower rates of rehospitalization, better health outcomes, and fewer costly procedures.
- Caregivers who express compassion for patients, families, and each other experience higher job satisfaction, less stress, and a greater sense of teamwork.
- Patients who are treated compassionately benefit from improved quality of care, better health, fewer medical errors, and a deeper human connection with their caregivers.

These data help support your role in constructing policies, practices, and other arrangements that allow your workplace to exhibit a commitment to organizational virtue. Institutions that create and sustain times, places, and processes for moral dialogue support this commitment.[17]

Summary

Organizations have a moral obligation to help prevent destructive conditions from occurring to their employees and others who make up the organization. Because so many people spend more time each week in the organizations of work than they do in their own homes, all organizations must assume an influential role in helping to foster high moral standards.

This chapter takes you, the moral agent out of the one on one or team clinic environment and into the committee room and administrator's offices in which a new interprofessional care team is called on to help meet an organizational goal. As the complexity of the health professions and healthcare environment continues to grow, so do the necessity and opportunity for becoming involved in the development of mission statements, policies, and administrative and business practices. Such involvement should enable you to maintain professional standards and a high level of ethical practice. The six-step process of ethical decision making can guide you in your role in this situation. Despite the help that the organization's policies, practices, and environment can provide, they are not an automatic guarantee of high-quality patient care or fair practices toward employees, patients, or others. You still must apply skillful ethical reasoning about ethical dimensions of care delivery as they present themselves.

Questions for Thought and Discussion

1. Can you describe an employment situation in which you can imagine quitting in protest over an ethically unacceptable policy of the organization? What is it? List the pros and cons of quitting. Now list some changes that would allow you, in good faith, to continue in the organization.

2. You are part of the interprofessional care team that works with the autistic population in a charter school setting. Your program has been highly sought out by parents of children with autism and other developmental disorders, so much so that currently 10 students are on the wait list. The team receives a referral for a new child to be transferred into the program. The child is placed on the wait list, but the administration communicates a request to the team to see whether there is "anyway they can accept the child now since he is the grandson of one of the school's employees." The team is split on what recommendation they should give. They deeply regard and respect the child's grandmother but also know that several students are ahead of this child on the wait list and are likely just as deserving. Should the team approve the acceptance? Defend why or why not, drawing on the duties, rights, and role issues discussed in your study of ethics so far.

3. Eudora Cathay has been a unit clerk at the same for-profit privately owned hospital in an affluent, largely white suburb for 2 years. The position of unit clerk is a demanding one that involves answering the phone, relaying messages, coordinating laboratory personnel in their rounds, responding to physicians' and nurses' requests, and making sure that patients are in the right places at the right times. Eudora's professional dress style is informed by her African heritage. Some members of the staff, particularly physicians and administrators, are displeased by her style of dress. Others find it attractive and an interesting change from the wall-to-wall white uniforms worn by the professional staff everywhere in the hospital. The dress policy does not require unit clerks to wear a uniform and stipulates only that they be neat and well groomed (which she is) and dressed appropriately. Someone in an administrative position asks Eudora to dress more conservatively. She refuses on the grounds that she is neat and well groomed and any further demands are an invasion of her personal rights. She is fired for her refusal to comply amidst rampant rumors of racism. Discuss her situation in light of good organizational policy. Should there be a dress code? Is there anything ethically relevant about how employees dress? Why or why not?

References

1. Johnson C: *Organizational ethics: a practical approach*, ed 3, Thousand Oaks, CA, 2015, Sage Publications.
2. Swisher LL, Arslanian LE, Davis CM: The realm-individual process-situation (RIPS) model of ethical decision making, *HPA Resource* 5(3):1, 3, 8, 2005.
4. Gabard D, Martin WW: *Honesty and conflicts of interest: physical therapy ethics*, Philadelphia, 2003, FA Davis, pp 142–158, definition 143.
3. Glaser JW: Three realms of ethics: an integrative map of ethics for the future. In Purtilo RB, Jensen GM, Royeen CB, editors: *Educating for moral action: a sourcebook in health and rehabilitation ethics*, Philadelphia, 2005, FA Davis, pp 169–184.
5. Kanter RM: How great companies think differently. *Harvard Business Review*, 2011. Available at https://hbr.org/2011/11/how-great-companies-think-differently.
6. Rawls J: *A theory of justice*, ed 2, Cambridge, MA, 1991, Harvard University Press.
7. Pierce J, Jameton A: *The ethics of environmentally responsible health care*, New York, 2004, Oxford University Press, pp 43–60.
8. American Society of Bioethics and Humanities: *Core competencies for health care ethics consultation*, ed 2, Chicago, 2011, American Society of Bioethics and Humanities.
9. Blau R, Bolus S, Carolan T, et al: The experience of providing physical therapy in a changing health care environment, *Physical Ther* 82(7):648–657, 2002.
10. Bodenheimer TS, Grumbach K: How health care is organized—I: primary, secondary, and tertiary care. *Understanding health policy: a clinical approach*, ed 6, New York, 2016, McGraw-Hill, pp 45–60 (Lange paperback ed).
11. Epstien R: *Attending: medicine, mindfulness, and humanity*, New York, 2017, Simon and Schuster.
12. Whitehead PB, Herbertson RK, Hamric AB, et al: Moral distress among healthcare professionals: report of an institution-wide survey, *J Nurs Scholarsh* 47:117–125, 2014.
13. Burwell SM: Setting value-based payment goals—HHS efforts to improve U.S. health care, *N Engl J Med* 372(10):897–899, 2015.
14. Counte MA, Howard SW, Chang L, et al: *Global advances in value-based payment and their implications for global health management education, development, and practice.* Front Public Health. 2019; 6;379 Published 2019 Jan 18. doi:10.3389/tpubh.2018.00379.
15. Newton L: Ethical leadership means empowering your followers, *Alberta RN* 69(1):30–31, 2015.
16. The Schwartz Center for Compassionate Care: *Building compassion into the bottom line: the role of compassionate care and patient experience in 35 U.S. hospitals and health systems*, Boston, 2015, The Schwartz Center for Compassionate Care.
17. Hamric AB, Wocial LD: *Institutional ethics resources: creating moral spaces, nurses at the table: nursing, ethics, and health policy, special report.* Hastings Center Report, 2016, 46, 5, S22-S27. doi: 10.1002/hast.627.

Ethical Dimensions of the Professional–Patient Relationship

9

Honoring Confidentiality

Objectives

The reader should be able to:
- Define the terms confidentiality and confidential information.
- Identify the relationship of a patient's legal right to privacy with his or her reasonable expectations regarding confidential information.
- Recognize the three different forms of privacy related to health professional–patient interaction.
- Describe the concept of need to know as it relates to maintaining confidentiality.
- Discuss the ethical norms involved in keeping and breaking professional confidences.
- Name the general legal exceptions to the professional standard of practice that maintains that confidences should not be broken.
- Consider practical options that a health professional or interprofessional care team can take when faced with the possibility of breaking a confidence.
- Discuss some important aspects of documentation that affect confidentiality.
- Compare ethical issues of confidentiality traditionally conceived with those that have arisen because of electronic medical records and patient care information systems.
- Describe the key privacy considerations related to the use of social media in healthcare.

New terms and ideas you will encounter in this chapter

trust
confidentiality
confidential information
right to privacy
need to know
patient care information systems (PCIS)
health information managers

the medical record
Health Insurance Portability and Accountability Act (HIPAA)
protected health information
covered entity

Health Information Technology for Economic and Clinical Health (HITECH) Act
electronic health record (EHR)
social media
panel of laboratory tests

Topics in this chapter introduced in earlier chapters	
Topic	Introduced in chapter
Hippocratic Oath	1
Character traits or virtues	2
Codes of ethics	2
Ethical dilemma	3
Beneficence	4
Nonmaleficence	4
Fidelity	4
Autonomy	4
Policy	7

Introduction

In this chapter and the next several chapters, you have an opportunity to think about specific ways in which patients learn to put their *trust* in you as a health professional and your colleagues who are part of their interprofessional care team. You already have met some patients through the stories that have been presented to help focus your thinking. The idea of *confidentiality* in healthcare has ancient roots as a basic building block of trust between health professionals and patients. For instance, the Hippocratic Oath, written in the 4th century BC, says,

> And whatsoever I shall see or hear in the course of my profession, as well as outside my profession… if it be what should not be published abroad, I will never divulge, holding such things to be holy secrets.[1]

And so confidentiality is a splendid place to begin this focus on basic components of trust building. The story of Twyla Roberts, a physical therapist, and Mary Louis, a patient, helps set the stage for reflection on confidentiality.

💝 The Story of Twyla Roberts and Mary Louis

Twyla Roberts works as a physical therapist for Marion Home Care Agency. Her patients are primarily elders, but she also occasionally treats children. All of Twyla's visits are performed in the home setting. She evaluates and treats throughout the community, and the agency is interconnected with two of the area hospitals and several outpatient clinics. The organizations are well connected electronically in one patient care information system. This arrangement allows Twyla to enter her patient information into the hospital's database and also to receive instant, thorough information on any activity her patients may have in the larger healthcare system. This electronic record also contains the patient health history and treatment activity. She refers to it many times each day and enters her own data each evening.

Thus the clinical record of her patient, Mary Louis, is in "the system," and her progress after a fall is documented. Mary has just been discharged from the hospital after a fall at home. She was seen by a surgeon, several nurses, a physical therapist, an occupational therapist, and, when she was preparing for discharge, a social worker. She is now referred to the home care agency for a home safety evaluation and for ongoing therapy to regain function of her right knee, which was injured in the fall.

Twyla has been taught to document all relevant information about a patient; therefore she is surprised by her own reluctance to record a conversation that occurred with Mary today. During their treatment session, Mary blurts out that the reason for her injury was not a fall. She has fallen in the past; however, this time her injury was the result of a domestic dispute. Mary's husband, who has middle-stage Alzheimer's disease, has been showing more signs of agitation. He became confused one evening, and a struggle ensued. Mary tried her best, but she was neither able to effectively reorient her husband nor manage his aggressive behavior. The incident ended abruptly when Mary's husband pushed her down the stairs. Despite her disorientation at the time, no one asked specifics regarding how she fell, and so in the ambulance she told them she tripped rather than revealing the truth.

She says to Twyla, "I probably shouldn't have told you about this either. Now my secret is out. Please don't tell anyone. I am actually ashamed for my husband, you know. I don't want anybody to know about this. I am really afraid it might affect his ability to stay home. If my daughter finds out, she will surely have him sent to a nursing home. I know he is getting worse, but I would just die if we could not be together. Promise me you won't say anything!" Twyla does not promise, but neither does she tell Mary that her secret is not safe. Instead, she tries to talk with her about the importance of seeking respite care and of getting more assistance for her husband. But Mary says once again, "Please don't tell anyone."

Twyla completes her treatment and logs in to her laptop computer to begin her clinical documentation. She opens Mary's electronic health record and notes that the social worker, Michael White, was concerned about the home situation. He found Mary's husband to be quite irritable during hospital visits; he interviewed Mary several times without her husband but did not elicit any evidence that would classify him as an overt safety risk. Twyla realizes that if she documents this conversation, Mary's secret will be out for everyone on the patient information system to read. She realizes that Mary has shared information with her that she really wishes she had not. Now Twyla wishes, too, that when Mary started talking about it she would have stopped her and said she could not promise to keep it confidential. But she did not. Still, she fears that if she does not document their conversation, she could regret it later.

⚖ Reflection

What should Twyla do next? Why? What should she ultimately do in regard to this situation? Why?

_____

_____

_____

_____

Many dimensions of Twyla's ethical quandary are identical to questions that have made confidentiality a compelling issue over the centuries. At the same time, because she lives in an era of computerized data entry, storage, and retrieval of patient information, her situation also is highly contemporary.

The Goal: A Caring Response

In light of all you have learned about Twyla and Mary, you know that her ethical goal of finding a caring response requires her to address both traditional and contemporary dimensions of confidentiality and the specific type of confidential information that this patient has shared. She needs to be clear about what confidentiality is and its appropriate use and limits. She needs to understand the related concept of privacy and be savvy about new challenges regarding the use of computerized networks designed to manage information about patients.

Identifying Confidential Information

The most commonly accepted idea of *confidential information* in the professions is that it is information about a patient or client that is harmful, shameful, or embarrassing. Does it necessarily have to come directly from that person? No. Information that is furnished by the patient directly or comes to you in writing or through electronic data, or even from a third party, might count as confidential.

Who should be the judge of whether information is harmful, shameful, or embarrassing? The person himself or herself is the best judge, but any time you think a patient has a reasonable expectation that sensitive information will not be spread, it is best to err on the side of treating it as confidential. Of course, as Fig. 9.1 illustrates, it is possible to go to extremes so that the best interests of the patient are lost in the process. A good general rule regarding potentially confidential information is to treat caution as a virtue.

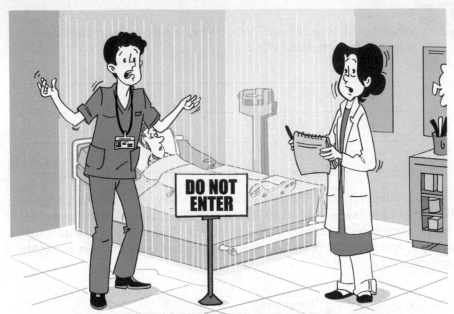

"I'D LIKE TO TELL YOU WHAT THE PATIENT'S CONDITION IS, DOCTOR.
BUT IT'S TOO CONFIDENTIAL!"

Fig. 9.1.

Confidentiality and Privacy

Sometimes the notion of confidential information is discussed within the framework of the U.S. constitutional *right to privacy*.[2] In this framework the right to privacy means that there are aspects of a person's being into which no one else should intrude. We return to this idea of privacy later. At the same time, confidential information creates a situation a little differently than privacy, taken alone.

There are three different forms of privacy: physical, informational, and decisional. Patients who share private information have chosen to relinquish some aspects of their privacy because they have a reasonable expectation that sensitive information shared with certain people will further their own welfare.[3] The patient thinks, "I may have to tell/show you something very private, perhaps something I'm ashamed of, because I think you need to know it to plan what is best for me. But I do not want or expect you to spread the word around." There is an implicit understanding in the relationship that you, the professional, can perform your professional responsibilities only with accurate information from and about the patient. Patients and family caregivers trust that health professionals have the competency

● to maintain professionalism in communicating information necessary for healthcare delivery.

When you have confidential information from patients, they have a right to expect that you will honor your professional promise of confidentiality.

> ⑤ **Summary**
>
> Confidentiality is one of the most basic principles in healthcare practice, and it is the most long-standing ethical dictum in healthcare codes of ethics. Confidentiality is the practice of keeping harmful, shameful, or embarrassing patient information within proper bounds. The right to privacy gives legal standing to this ethical principle.

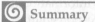 *Reflection*

Go to the code of ethics or other guidelines of your profession and write down what it says about confidentiality.

_____

_____

_____

_____

● **Confidentiality, Secrets, and the Need to Know**

Developmental theory informs us that concern about confidentiality begins when a child first experiences a desire to keep or tell secrets. Secrets manifest a developing sense of self as separate from others, and the desire to share secrets is an expression of reaching out for intimate relationships with others. How secrets are handled in those early stages of development can have long-lasting effects on an individual's sense of security, self-esteem, and success at developing intimacy.[4] The power of a secret, or of being in a position to tell a secret, is nowhere conveyed more clearly than when a 2-year-old child has a secret pertaining to someone's birthday present! When was the last time that you had a secret that was so potent it was difficult, maybe impossible, to keep?

Sharing of clinical information must occur so that the healthcare system can effectively care for a patient. The sharing of "secret" information with members of the interprofessional care teams or others involved in the patient's care is not considered a breach of confidentiality as long as the information has relevance to their role in the case. In fact, sharing is deemed essential for arriving at a caring response because up-to-date, thorough information is the structure on which high-quality healthcare delivery to a patient depends.[5] Some information comes from your clinical evaluation of the patient's condition; the rest has to come from the patient.

A reliable general test for which team members should be given certain types of information is the *need to know* test. Need to know information is necessary for one to adequately perform one's specific job responsibilities. Does the person need this information to help provide the most caring response to the patient? Information that passes the need to know test must be distinguished from that which a teammate might be interested to know and especially from information that has no bearing on the teammate's ability to offer optimal care.

Ⓢ Summary

Together, the immediate aims of confidentiality are to:
1. Facilitate the sharing of sensitive information with the goal of helping the patient.
2. Exclude unauthorized people from such information.
3. Discern need to know information from mere interest when deciding what to share.

 Reflection

Susan is a nurse who works in the orthopedic department of a large urban hospital. Her son's girlfriend was admitted to the medical department of the same hospital for treatment of a staphylococcus infection in her right ankle. Susan's son asks his mom to "look in the computer and find out what is going on with his girlfriend." What should Susan do?

_____

_____

_____

_____

If you answered that Susan should not access her son's girlfriend's record, you are correct. Susan is not a health professional on the team caring for this woman, so she does not have a need to know the details. She could go to visit the girlfriend in the hospital and offer her support; however, accessing her medical record is a breach of confidentiality. Any information about a patient should never be passed along to someone not involved in the care of a patient. All patients have a right to privacy.

What if Susan worked in that department and was the nurse assigned to take care of her son's girlfriend? In this case, Susan would have a need to know. If she was assigned to care for the girlfriend, she would need to access the medical record for relevant clinical details. Susan may choose to recuse herself from the case and seek an alternative patient assignment given that she knows the girlfriend; however, this decision would depend on other factors such as the needs of other patients on the unit and staffing. Her need to know still would not warrant her sharing the information with her son.

Keeping Confidences

In Chapters 2 and 4, you were introduced to the ideas of caring and the character traits that a health professional should cultivate. Keeping secret information that flows from patient to health professional is not valued as an end in itself but rather as an instrument that serves trust, and the ultimate value that both the keeping of confidences and the subsequent building of trust points to is human dignity.

 Summary

Keep confidences
to
Build trust into the relationship
to
Maintain patient dignity

Health professionals are motivated to keep the confidences entrusted to them because it has long been understood that a trusting health profession-al–patient relationship must be built. Confidentiality serves as one corner-stone for that solid foundation. However, conflicts often arise in regard to keeping patient confidences, and health professionals must decide how to best balance these competing interests. This is reflected in a number of codes of ethics. Many contain statements similar to this one from the American Medical Association (AMA) Principles of Medical Ethics:

> *A physician shall respect the rights of patients, colleagues, and other health profes-sionals, and shall safeguard patient confidences and privacy.*[6]

In such statements, the conflict is presented as one in which the health professional's duty to benefit and refrain from harming patients by keeping their secret is pitted against a duty to prevent harm to the patients them-selves, to someone else, or to society.

Breaking Confidences

As you have seen previously, the importance of confidentiality is recognized in both law and professional practice; however, in certain cases, the most caring response requires breaching the patient's confidence.[7] Historically, such cases involved preventing harm to others, such as with carriers of contagious diseases who wished to keep the condition a secret. The person does not have the prerogative of keeping the secret by requiring the professional to keep silent about the condition.

Legal exceptions to the standard of practice that confidences must be kept, except with the patient's consent or at the patient's request to break it, include the following[8]:

- An emergency in which keeping the confidence will harm the patient.
- The patient is a danger to, or threatens to harm, themself (e.g., is suicidal).
- The patient is incompetent or incapacitated, and a third party needs to be informed to be a surrogate decision maker for the patient.
- Identified third parties are at serious risk for harm (e.g., sexually transmitted diseases, child or elder abuse).
- Request for commitment or hospitalization of a psychiatrically ill patient.
- A serious risk that many others may be harmed (e.g., a terrorist threat).
- A court order.

A general rule of thumb is that you must not share confidential information unless it is required by the conditions of the law such as those listed or authorized by the patient personally. The presumption is that health professionals try to minimize the number of exceptions. Most patients do not know about the limits of confidentiality. As you learned in the story of Twyla and Mary, Twyla wishes she had exercised the good judgment of advising Mary of this before rather than after the patient divulged sensitive information.

The Six-Step Process in Confidentiality Situations

With the previous description of what confidentiality is and when it may legally or ethically be breached, let us return to the story of Twyla Roberts and Mary Louis to see how confidentiality works in everyday practice.

Step 1: Gather Relevant Information

One aspect of Twyla's concern arises from the nature of Mary's comments. She always assumes that patients are telling the truth (until she has had it proven to the contrary). If so, she may want to talk to Mary more about her knowledge of the event to help understand the situation better. Was this the first time such an event occurred? Does Mary feel unsafe in her home? Is Mary's daughter involved in the care of her parents? How well is the spouse's dementia condition being managed? Increasingly, adults with dementia receive care in the community sector. What resources are available to Mary and to her spouse? How will Mary's role as a caregiver be impacted by her new injuries? Who are the other stakeholders in this case?

Another avenue of discussion Twyla may wish to pursue is why Mary does not want "anyone" to know. She has blurted out some reasons. Often spouses of patients with Alzheimer's disease withhold information on the basis of detailed moral, social, and psychological considerations that involve deep emotional investment. Family dynamics are often complex, and dissenting opinions regarding care plans can negatively impact the quality of life for couples.[9]

Steps 2 and 3: Identify the Type of Ethical Problem and the Ethics Approach to Analyze It

Twyla knows that, despite these caring responses, in the end her dilemma boils down to whether she should document their conversation in Mary's medical record, knowing that by doing so she is opening this information to others.

 Reflection

What kind of ethical problem does Twyla have? Is it moral distress? An ethical dilemma? Take a minute to jot down your response before proceeding.

_____

_____

_____

_____

In some instances of confidentiality, the moral agent faces moral distress. However, Twyla has not been prohibited from documenting the conversation. She is experiencing such distress from her belief that she should document the conversation with the knowledge that it may cause harm to Mary. At the very least, she is justifiably concerned that it may shake Mary's trust in her. She cannot achieve both the outcome of keeping the confidence and the one of doing her duty to document relevant information. She is facing a classical version of an ethical dilemma.

 Reflection

From the standpoint of a health professional's goal of arriving at a caring response, name three ethical principles that will help guide your thinking about your conduct in regard to keeping or reluctantly breaking confidences.

Principles

1. _____

2. _____

3. _____

Name some character traits that will help you in these challenging situations.

Character traits

1. _____

2. _____

3. _____

If you answered with the principles of beneficence, nonmaleficence, or fidelity and the right to autonomy, you are grasping the ethical principles or elements that support confidentiality. A key character trait is trustworthiness (i.e., your part of the bargain when you ask the patient to trust you). Other traits include kindness, compassion, and moral courage to break confidences when it is ethically or legally necessary to do so.

In conclusion, breaking of confidences always entails at least one harm. Two questions we always ask when faced with such a decision are:

1. When is the harm of threatening the fragile trust in the relationship outweighed by the benefit?
2. How can the amount of harm be kept to a minimum when it becomes ethically appropriate to break a confidence?

The burden of proof is always on the health professional to minimize the harm.

Step 4: Explore the Practical Alternatives

What options does Twyla have in trying to discern what to do?

One way that Twyla can handle this situation is to keep the confidence by sharing it with the other members of Mary's interprofessional care team who have a good reason to learn about this information. Often a health professional's inability to assess whether a person outside the immediate care team should be given information leads the professional to discuss it with a trusted colleague first. For Twyla, one person seems to be the obvious choice: the social worker who treated Mary at the hospital. Part of the motive of this discussion among professionals is to clarify whether Mary has spoken to anyone else and to confirm how she should proceed.

Often, an additional outcome of this type of in-house discussion is to determine whether further action on behalf of the patient should be taken. Social workers are well trained in the policies and procedures that relate to elder abuse and neglect. By collaborating with the social worker, Twyla expands her knowledge and maximizes resources. If Mary remains unwilling

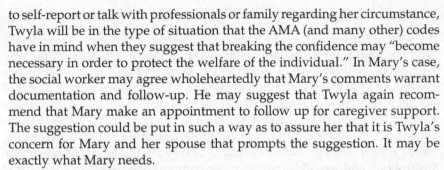

to self-report or talk with professionals or family regarding her circumstance, Twyla will be in the type of situation that the AMA (and many other) codes have in mind when they suggest that breaking the confidence may "become necessary in order to protect the welfare of the individual." In Mary's case, the social worker may agree wholeheartedly that Mary's comments warrant documentation and follow-up. He may suggest that Twyla again recommend that Mary make an appointment to follow up for caregiver support. The suggestion could be put in such a way as to assure her that it is Twyla's concern for Mary and her spouse that prompts the suggestion. It may be exactly what Mary needs.

Another option for Twyla is to say nothing but still make note of the conversation on the patient's record.

This option is not recommended as it breaks the confidence of the patient without taking any further direct action to let her know what has been done and why. Although the health professional's anxiety would be relieved, at least momentarily, in this case, the action would serve little useful moral purpose in regard to helping Mary. In some cases, Twyla may see this as her only alternative, but she has not yet tried to go back to Mary to advise and discuss with her what she has determined she must do.

If Twyla goes directly back to Mary and reveals to her in a supportive way that the conversation was deeply troubling, Mary quite possibly could gain better insight into the seriousness of her comments. Mary may be suffering from mental stress and caregiver fatigue, two common outcomes of spousal caregiving in long-term, serious conditions.[10,11] Twyla can be a help in referring Mary to someone who can assist her and her husband. At least she will know that in choosing to proceed as she did (in telling her about his serious condition), Twyla did not take this plight lightly. She used her ethical reasoning to honor her own goal of providing optimal care for this patient.

Step 5: Complete the Action

This case, like many discussed in this text, does not have simple answers. However, given all the aspects of her role as a moral agent, Twyla should go back to Mary immediately to discuss her concern. She also should let her know that she is compelled to at least document the conversation because the information is highly relevant to Mary's care and it is a part of her moral duty to document such exchanges.

Step 6: Evaluate the Process and Outcome

Obviously, any caring professional would be concerned about the consequences of overriding a patient's wishes in a situation in which the latter thought she could count on the professional to keep a "deep, dark secret." Whatever Twyla decides to do, she will benefit by taking time to review her actions and motives each step of the way.

Confidentiality, Records, and Patient Care Information Systems

Another important aspect of confidentiality raised in this story is the process of information sharing and record keeping that goes on within today's healthcare (and other institutional) systems. For example, Mary's report of abuse, if documented, will remain in her *electronic health record (EHR)*. The issue of how far this information should and can go takes on greater importance when one considers modern, computerized systems of record keeping called *patient care information systems (PCIS)*. Virtually all major healthcare institutions and agencies currently use computerized systems that enable easy entry, storage, and retrieval of almost any information. This aspect of the patient's care has become so sophisticated that a group of professionals called *health information managers* are key members of the healthcare team. Their primary role is to be "responsible for designing and maintaining the system that facilitates the collection, use and dissemination of health and medical information."[12] Depending on what is requested and the policies of the healthcare plan at her institution, the information regarding Mary's self-report may be released to insurance agencies, other care providers, people conducting research, or state agencies. In short, Mary's and her husband's living situation is in danger of changing because of information documented in her record. Twyla must be aware that if she records their discussion, Mary's husband may receive a stigmatizing profile, even though her intent may be to act in accordance with what her professional ethics guides her to do in relation to her patients.

Although ethics as expressed in the codes of ethics of most health professions requires that information about patients be kept confidential unless some strongly overriding argument for disclosure exists, the realities of modern healthcare make this difficult. As noted previously, these EHRs are accessible to many different people and agencies, for many different reasons, and computerized data systems compound the problem. Thus any information that may impair the patient's ability to function freely and confidently in society must be more carefully weighed than ever before it is recorded in the medical record. Challenges to confidentiality as traditionally understood arise in several ways, some of which are highlighted in the following pages.

The Medical Record

The medical record is an extremely useful document for health professionals. Medical records can be found in both paper and electronic form. Records are systematic accounts of a patient's encounter with a health provider. They serve as a repository of information. They are generated by and contributed to by many providers in and across a various health delivery settings. An EHR is an electronic record of patient health information. Similar to the paper medical record, EHRs include patient demographics, progress notes, problems, medications, relevant social history, medical history, vital signs, laboratory data, and diagnostic reports. Most readers, thinking back to a recent healthcare encounter, can recall a provider who was either entering data or retrieving it from a computer in the examination room. The EHR has now been officially inserted into the patient–provider interaction. The key is to ensure that the caring relationship does not suffer as a result. Research shows physicians in ambulatory practices spend at least as much time looking into their computer screens as they do into their patient's eyes.[13,14] Many healthcare organizations have begun to integrate the use of voice recordings and medical scribes to decrease the amount of time providers spend **computing**, and increase the amount of time they spend **relating**. As discussed in Chapter 9, these efforts support work place well-being and provider wellness as they restore compassionate care at the center of the interaction.

Regardless of the type of medical record used, information about a patient that is true and relevant to his or her healthcare ought to be recorded there. At the same time, harm can be done if faulty, erroneous, speculative, or vague information is included because it can be duplicated and spread to several locations in both paper and electronic medical records. The harm that ensues is caused not only by the spread of the information but also may involve the carelessness on the part of professionals. As you return to the story of Twyla and Mary presented at the beginning of this chapter, it is important to recognize the great power of the information about your patients or others. Three guidelines are applicable:

1. Questionable information should be clearly labeled as questionable.
2. True information that is not relevant should not be recorded.
3. All information should be handled among health professionals with regard for the privacy and dignity of patients.

Information recorded in the medical record can be of great help or harm to the patient. For this reason, the medical record needs to be treated with a great deal of respect. Health information managers and others involved with medical record information are usually highly aware of the power of these documents. They function as the gatekeepers for the records and rightfully take great pains to keep the records in order and to make sure that they are available to those professionals who need them and who have a right to see them. Conversely, they also need to be careful that the records are not abused or released to unauthorized persons. Sugarman notes:

> The increasing use of electronic medical records and the creation of computerized databases, while clearly beneficial for many aspects of patient care, raise important questions regarding privacy and confidentiality. The easy retrieval and transmission of such records make them tempting targets for those interested in unauthorized access.[15]

Electronic communications are discussed further in Chapter 10; however, remember that confidentiality applies to all information communicated regarding the patient, whether in verbal conversation, handwritten documentation, or electronic communication.

Reflection

Have you ever seen this disclaimer on the end of an email communication?

> *The information transmitted in this email is intended only for the person or entity to which it is addressed and may contain confidential and/or privileged material. Any review, retransmission, dissemination or other use of or taking of any action in reliance upon this information by persons or entities other than the intended recipient is prohibited. If you receive this email in error, please contact the sender and delete the material from any computer.*

Why do you think that disclaimer is there? How does it relate to confidentiality?

_____

_____

_____

_____

In the end, everyone is responsible for the confidentiality of patient information, whether professional colleagues engaged in a conversation in the corridor, those handling the management of formal records, or the individual health professional properly disposing of worksheets and notes, taking care to log off shared computer stations after use, encrypting electronic devices used to access health information systems, or being vigilant in the use of email, fax, or copy machines. The technology of healthcare information is only as effective as the professionals and others who use the devices allow it to be.

 Summary

Confidentiality comes down to each health professional being vigilant about the flow of patient information, guided by the goal of using information to help the patient.

Patient Privacy: Health Insurance Portability and Accountability Act

Concerns about the collection, storage, and use of sensitive information have led to much discussion by patients and the public in recent years, so that the notion of private information increasingly has been mentioned as relevant to considerations of confidentiality. In 1996, the United States passed regulations under the *Health Insurance Portability and Accountability Act (HIPAA)* that imposed considerable new constraints on the use and disclosure of a patient's personal and clinical information. These regulations went into effect in April 2003 and continue to govern patient privacy as related to healthcare communications. A major goal of HIPAA is to ensure that an individual's health information is properly protected while allowing the flow of information needed to promote high-quality care.

This set of regulations, called the New Federal Medical-Privacy Rule,[16] took 5 years to go into effect. The basic intent was to control the use or disclosure of *protected health information*. This rule strongly affects the handling of information for purposes of research. It also has been interpreted to mean that information about patients (including family members) cannot be released. The rule concerns all "individually identifiable" health information created or maintained by covered entity, defined broadly as information about physical or mental health that either identifies an individual person or with respect to which there is a reasonable basis to believe the information can be used to identify the person.[17] A *covered entity* is defined as a health plan, data processing company, healthcare professional, or hospital.

The Health Information Technology for Economic and Clinical Health Act

The *Health Information Technology for Economic and Clinical Health (HITECH) Act*, which was Title XIII of the American Recovery and Reinvestment Act of 2009, was signed into law in February 2009. Parts of this act expanded and strengthened the privacy laws that protect patient health information originally outlined in HIPAA. The 2013 HITECH Act Final Rules went into effect in March of 2013 and stipulated new obligations on covered entities, business associates, and subcontractors. These additional provisions regarding privacy and security breaches, reporting of breaches, accounting of disclosures, and restrictions of disclosures for sales and marketing purposes, are in response to developments in health technology and the increased use, storage, and transmittal of electronic health information.[18,19] The act also designated funding to expand the federal government's effort to establish a national electronic patient records system along with comprehensive records privacy and security standards. One of the challenges in the national adoption of EHRs in the United States was ensuring the privacy of electronically accessed information. Although one of the primary goals of HITECH Act was to foster the transition to EHR and improve quality care and patient communication, the results have been mixed. For many health professionals, the EHR has led to decreased face-to-face interaction with patients. As you learned in Chapter 6, it also has been correlated with burnout caused by the cognitive demand and workload required as a result of the quantity of documentation and imposed entry fields to meet payer/organizational requirements. As one colleague reported at a recent ethics rounds: "I am exhausted. I spend my whole day on my laptop during patient visits and then return home to spend my evening responding to all the patient inquiries that have come in through the electronic patient health portal. It is too much!"

Century Cures Act

Although implemented in most every care delivery setting, many EHRs remain unintegrated with little unification across systems. In 2016 the 21st Century Cures Act was signed into law to improve EHR usability. The Century Cures Act mandates the use of open healthcare Application Programming Interfaces (APIs). This law has led to the customization of interfaces (third-party apps) and workflows to better meet the needs of health professionals and organizations. Although some feel these tools are overdue, others raise concerns regarding the vulnerability and security of so many electronic interfaces.

No matter the technology, tool, or legislation, what is essential is that health professionals and patients participate in technology and policy discussions. Only then can important ethical issues be contemplated and decisions regarding health record databases and their approved collection, storage, and usage can be articulated nationally and globally.[20] You will learn more about professional citizenship and moral advocacy in Section V of this text, which looks at ethical dimensions of the social context of healthcare.

As you can see, you are entering the health professions at a time when new and evolving legal parameters about what can and cannot be shared, and by what means, will continue to be a source of discussion, revision, and refinement. Hopefully the intent of preventing undue invasion of a patient's privacy can be balanced against the legitimate incursions into privacy that have served patients' interests well over the centuries. The details of how this will be best accomplished continue to unfold.[21]

Confidentiality and Digital Technologies

The evolution of new media and technology has changed how we access, communicate, and protect health information. Communication is discussed in more detail in Chapter 10; however, we pause here to reflect on confidentiality as it relates to the digital age. Consider the following scenario. Dijiana is an occupational therapist working full-time at Turner Heights Preschool, a private preschool for children with autism and other developmental disabilities. Her mother calls her at work one day to say that she just left her book club where one of her friends asked, "Doesn't your daughter work at Turner Heights?" Dijiana's mom answers, "Yes" to which her friend replies, "Well that place is in big trouble. My grandson's photo showed up on their Instagram page yesterday with the caption 'look at this cutie—focus on ability—not disability.' My daughter is very upset and is going in today to speak to the owner. She wants the post taken down immediately and is going to demand that whoever posted it gets fired." Dijiana quickly opens the site, reads the post, and sighs.

As this scenario highlights, more and more patients and professionals are using web-based platforms and social media for communication, patient engagement, professional development, health education, and advocacy. According to the PEW Research Center, as of 2019, 96% of Americans have a cell phone, 90% of U.S. adults use the Internet, and 72% of the public uses some type of social media.[22] In addition, it is estimated that 80% of Americans look up health information online. The online conversation about health is being driven forward by two forces: the availability of social tools and the motivation, especially among people living with chronic conditions, to connect with each other.[23] Ressler and Glazer define *social media* as "the constellation of Internet-based tools that help a user to connect, collaborate, and communicate with others in real time."[24]

Social media has become a part of everyday life, but once you become a health professional, restrictions and additional guidelines must be considered. The most popular forms of social media are social networking sites, such as Facebook, Snapchat, and Twitter, and media-sharing sites, such as Instagram and YouTube. Social media is changing the communication paradigm, but the unregulated nature of the Internet allows for the possibility of unintended self-disclosure and possible violation of confidentiality.[25,26] Health professionals are obligated to both understand these technologies and ensure their safe use in healthcare and education.

The most significant confidentiality concerns associated with social media use are the inappropriate sharing of information and professional–personal boundary issues. However, social media engagement does not create ethical distress if best practices are observed and online communication adheres to terms of service, professional standards, and organizational policies.[27] Most organizations have codes of conduct and specific policies on the use of social media. We suggest that you read these documents carefully to inform your professional practice. Given the fact that social media platforms create digital footprints that cannot be erased, many of these policies are zero tolerance should a health professional violate patient confidentiality in a post.[26] In addition to your organizational policies, many professional organizations have white papers or professional guidelines regarding social media use. Consensus is building around principles that help guide social media use in the health professions. Several authors have summarized these well, including offering competencies for online professionalism. The following are key considerations to guide social media use for health professionals.[27–33]

- Have clear objectives. Why are you using social media? Is it to learn, share, or network? The objective should drive the choice of technology. For example, an organizational Facebook page may be a good place to post educational material for patients and families, whereas a private, members-only blog may be where you network with colleagues.

Separating private and professional social media platforms allows for a clearer boundary.

- Acknowledge sources of information and control information sharing. Think thoughtfully about who may be viewing your posts, share good health information, and refute the bad. Correct misinformation, be respectful, and uphold good netiquette.
- Clearly delineate personal opinion from organizational positions. Refrain from posting anonymously and state any conflicts of interest.
- Ensure security of self and other users. *Never share patient-specific information.* Follow the elevator rule: If you shouldn't say it in a public elevator, do not post it online.
- Appropriately use mobile devices and applications. Use dual password authentication and enable encryption on your devices. This includes understanding intellectual property as it relates to downloading and sharing content and researching mobile applications before downloading.
- 80% of social media is accessed via mobile devices. For this reason, these platforms can be effective tools for research recruitment and scholarly dissemination, however, user beware. Social media and smartphone sensors generate vast amounts of data, so additional protections are required to ensure proper data protection and patient privacy.

The growth of social media and other forms of electronic communication presents both opportunities and challenges for the health professional. Upholding one's duty to maintain and protect patient confidentiality is an expression of the care for both the individual client and society as a whole.

Summary

Keeping confidences is an ethical guideline that health professionals can rely on to maintain trust and to foster dignity in the health professional–patient relationship. Sometimes, however, the interests of another person or society or even the best interests of the patient advise against keeping the confidence.

The digital age of EHRs and social media raise attention to difficult ethical questions related to confidentiality. As a health professional, you must rely on sound clinical reasoning regarding the various moral obligations of professional practice, the rights of all involved, and the character traits that enable you to maintain a relationship of trust to arrive at a decision that is the most consistent with the goal of a caring response.

Questions for Thought and Discussion

1. Sonia is a nurse practitioner student who is completing her final clinical in an ambulatory internal medicine/primary care setting. She is caring for Lea, a 42-year-old woman who visited the office last week for ongoing

fatigue and generalized malaise and weakness. Sonia conducted several blood tests on Lea (called a *panel of laboratory tests*) and told her she would get back to her with the results. Sonia's supervisor concurred with the laboratory tests Sonia requested but also added a human chorionic gonadotropin (hCG) test to the panel to rule out pregnancy as the cause of Lea's symptoms. Sonia accessed the laboratory work via the computerized system and found all of Lea's laboratory test results were within normal limits with the exception of the hCG levels, which were elevated, indicating pregnancy. This afternoon Sonia picked up the phone to dial Lea's number and inform her of the results. The call went to Lea's voice mail, and, as Sonia prepared to leave a message, she hesitated.

Why do you think Sonia hesitated?

What should Sonia say? Defend your response with ethical principles that support confidentiality.

2. The following story of Mr. Shaw provides a good basis for thinking about some of the things you have just learned.

Ann von Essen is a health professional, and David Shaw is a patient in the hospital where she works. He has been referred to her for discharge planning. Mr. Shaw is a pleasant man, 42 years old, whose family often is at his side during visiting hours. He was admitted to the hospital with numerous fractures and a contusion after an automobile accident in which his car "skidded out of control and hit a tree." He has no memory of the accident, but the person traveling behind him reported the scene. The arrangement for his discharge is going smoothly. During one of Ann von Essen's visits, however, Mr. Shaw's mother, a wiry woman of about 80 years, follows her down the corridor. At the elevator, Mrs. Shaw says, "I wish you'd tell Sonny not to drive. It's those epileptic fits he has, you know. He's had 'em since he was a kid. Lordy, I'm scared to death he's going to kill himself and someone else, too." Ann is at a loss about what to say. She thanks Mrs. Shaw and jumps on the elevator. She goes down the elevator for one flight, gets off, and runs back up the stairs to the nurses' desk. She logs on to the computer to review Mr. Shaw's EHR and finds nothing about any type of seizures. Put yourself in the place of Ann von Essen. Do you have confidential information? What should you do? Why?

Let us assume that in the state in which you work the law requires that people with epileptic seizures be reported to the Department of Public Health, which in turn reports them to the Department of Motor Vehicles.

a. What do you think is the morally "right" action to take regarding Mr. Shaw once you have become the recipient of the information about his possible problem?

b. What duties and rights inform your decision about what to do?

c. Suppose you believe that it is morally right for the Department of Motor Vehicles to be advised of this situation. The obvious course of action is for you to inform the physician, the physician to report to the Department of Public Health, and the Department of Public Health to report to the Department of Motor Vehicles. If any of the usual links in this process are broken by failure to communicate the information, do you have a responsibility to make sure the Department of Motor Vehicles has actually received this information? Defend your position regarding how far you believe you and anyone else in your profession should go in pursuing this matter.

3. Cassandra Egan is a social worker who practices in a community health center. She treats clients across the life span but specializes in care of adolescents and young adults. Cassandra often posts public health research and other educational materials to the health center's Facebook page. Recently, when visiting the page, she notes that her patient Emily Ingemi has posted information regarding her life with celiac disease, including some rather personal health information. Cassandra is surprised to see this level of detail up on the site because its acceptable use policy states that information is not protected from public view and cautions patients regarding posting such details. Emily is coming to Cassandra's support group later this week. What do you think Cassandra should do? What is her obligation as a health professional? As an employee of the community health center?

References

1. Hippocrates: The oath. In Jones WHS, editor: *Hippocrates I*, Cambridge, MA, 1923, The Loeb Classic Library, Harvard University Press, pp 299–301.
2. *Griswold v. Connecticut*, 1965, 381 U.S. 479. 85 S Ct. 1678.
3. Purtilo R: Professional-patient relationship III: ethical issues. In Jennings B, editor: *Encyclopedia of bioethics*, ed 4, vol 3, Farmington Hills, MI, 2014, MacMillan Reference USA, pp 2150–2158.
4. Allen A: *Privacy and medicine*. In Zalta EN, editor: *The Stanford encyclopedia of philosophy*, 2011, spring ed. Available at http://plato.stanford.edu/archives/spr2011/entries/privacy-medicine/.
5. Klapman S, Sher E, Adler-Milstein J: A snapshot of health information exchange across five nations: an investigation of frontline clinician experiences in emergency care, *J Am Med Inform Assoc* 25(6):686–693, 2018.
6. American Medical Association: Principles of medical ethics, adopted June 1957; revised June 1980; revised June 2001, 2016. Available at https://www.ama-assn.org/sites/ama-assn.org/files/corp/media-browser/principles-of-medical-ethics.pdf.
7. Reamer FG: Ethical issues in integrated health care: implications for social workers, *Health Soc Work* 43(2):118–124, 2018.
8. Gutheil TG, Appelbaum PS: Confidentiality and privilege. *Clinical handbook of psychiatry and the law*, ed 5, Philadelphia, 2020, Wolters Kluwer, pp 1–33.

9. Tracy CS, Drummond N, Ferris LE, et al: To tell or not to tell? Professional and lay perspectives on the disclosure of personal health information in community-based dementia care, *Can J Aging* 23(3):203–215, 2004.

10. Khalaila R, Cohen M: Emotional suppression, caregiving burden, mastery, coping strategies and mental health in spousal caregivers, *Aging Ment Health* 20(9):908–917, 2016.

11. Ornstein KA, Wolff JL, Bollens-Lund E, et al: Spousal caregivers are caregiving alone in the last years of life, *Health Affairs* 38(6):964–972, 2019.

12. American Health Information Management Association: The 10 security domains (updated), *J Am Health Inform Manage Assoc* 83(5):50, 2012.

13. Ming T-S, Olson CW, Li J, et al: Electronic health record logs indicate that physicians split time evenly between seeing patients and desktop medicine, *Health Affairs* 36(4):655–662, 2017.

14. Maki SE, Bonnie Petterson B: *Using the electronic health record in the health care provider practice*, Clifton Park, NJ, 2014, Delmar.

15. Sugarman J: *20 Common problems: ethics in primary care*, New York, 2000, McGraw-Hill, pp 158–159.

16. U.S. Department of Health and Human Services: *Federal Register* 67:53182-53273, 2002. Available at the Federal Register Online via the Government Printing Office, www.gpo.gov; FR Doc No: 02-20554.

17. Kulynych J, Korn D: The new federal medical privacy rule, *N Engl J Med* 347(15):1133–1134, 2002.

18. American Recovery and Reinvestment Act of 2009, One Hundred and Eleventh Congress of the United States, First Session, January 6, 2009. Available at http://frwebgate.access.gpo.gov/cgi-bin/getdoc.cgi?dbname=111_cong_bills&docid=f:h1enr.pdf.

19. Salz T: HIPAA: training critical to protect patient practice, *Med Econ* 25(Sep):43–47, 2013.

20. Milton CL: Information sharing: transparency, nursing ethics, and practice implications with electronic medical records, *Nurs Sci Q* 22(3):214–219, 2009.

21. Terry N: Health privacy is difficult but not impossible in a post-HIPPA data-driven world, *Chest* 143(6):835–840, 2014.

22. Pew Research Center: *Internet and tech fact sheets*, 2019. Available at https://www.pewinternet.org/fact-sheet/.

23. Fox S: *The social life of health information*, Washington, DC, 2011, Pew Research Center's Internet & American Life Project. Available at http://www.pewinternet.org/2011/05/12/the-social-life-of-health-information-2011/.

24. Ressler PK, Glazer G: Legislative: nursing's engagement in health policy and healthcare through social media, *Online J Issues Nurs* 16(1):2011. Available at http://www.nursingworld.org/MainMenuCategories/ANAMarketplace/ANAPeriodicals/OJIN/TableofContents/Vol-16-2011/No1-Jan-2011/Health-Policy-and-Healthcare-Through-Social-Media.html.

25. Wang Z, Wang S, Zhang Y, Xiaolian J: Social media usage and online professionalism among registered nurses: a cross-sectional survey, *Int J Nurs Stud* 98:19–26, 2019.

26. Westrick SJ. Nursing students' use of electronic and social media: law, ethics, and e-professionalism. *Nurs Educ Perspect*. 2016 Jan 1;37(1):16-22.
27. Gagnon K, Sabus C: Professionalism in a digital age: opportunities and considerations for using social media in health care, *Phys Ther* 95(3):406–414, 2015.
28. Eysenbach G: Social media use in the United States: implications for health communication, *J Med Internet Res* 11(4):e48, 2009. Available at http://dx.doi.org/10.2196/jmir.1249.
29. Ramage C, Moorley C: A narrative synthesis on healthcare students use and understanding of social media: Implications for practice, *Nurse Educ Today* 77:40–52, 2019.
30. Anuja Jain A, Petty EM, Jaber RM, et al: What is appropriate to post on social media? Ratings from students, faculty members and the public, *Med Educ* 48:157–169, 2014.
31. Lacham V: Social media: managing the ethical issues, *Medsurg Nurs* 22(5): 326–329, 2013.
32. Kouri P, Rissanen M-L, Weber P, Park H: Competences in social media use in the area of health and healthcare: studies in health technology and informatics. In, Murphy J, et al, editor: *Forecasting informtics competencies for nurses in the future of connected health*, 232, Washington, DC, 2017, IMIA and IOS Press, pp 183–193.
33. Torous J, Ungar L, Barnett I: Expanding, augmenting, and operationalizing ethical and regulatory considerations for using social media platforms in research and health care, *Am J Bioethics* 19(6):4–6, 2019.

● 10

Communication and Shared Decision Making

New terms and ideas you will encounter in this chapter

communication	hope	affective
active listening	disclosure and	value-based transfer
shared decision	nondisclosure	health literacy
making	patient rights and	handoffs
do not resuscitate	responsibilities	shared mental models
dignity	duty to share	sentinel event

Topics in this chapter introduced in earlier chapters

Topic	Introduced in chapter
Interprofessional care team	1
A caring response	2
Honesty and integrity	2
Cultural humility	2
Moral distress	3
Deontology	4
Ethics of care	4
Narrative reasoning	4
Autonomy, beneficence, nonmaleficence, veracity	4
Six-step process	5
Responsibility	5
Moral courage	6
Competencies for interprofessional collaborative practice	7
Administrative policies	8
Confidentiality	9
Trust	9

Introduction

Communication is an essential part of healthcare delivery. You read in the previous chapter about the importance of confidentiality. Confidence in another is a foundational aspect of the patient–health professional relationship. Confidentiality is about holding sensitive but relevant information. *Communication* is about sharing information. How information is shared in healthcare is vitally important. In this chapter, the ethical dimensions of sharing information to actualize a caring response are discussed.

Consider the following scenario. Mary Beth is riding the train on her morning commute into work. She works as a recreational therapist in an inpatient mental health clinic. Sitting across from her is a young woman having a conversation on her cellular phone. The young woman disregards her public surroundings and talks loudly throughout the call. Others on the train cannot help but overhear her as she talks openly in this shared space. Her conversation details a discussion she had last night with her mother about her sister's new husband. She elaborates how they suspect that the new husband has a serious problem with alcohol. She talks in detail about his drinking patterns and behaviors. She shares her concern regarding potential depression and abuse. Many individuals try to distance themselves from this young woman, but the train is full. They look away, reading their papers and listening to music. Mary Beth has neither with her. She closes her eyes and secretly hopes the young woman's cellular phone will run out of battery life.

Reflection
Have you ever experienced such a situation? If so, what has been your reaction?

_____

_____

_____

Is anything happening in this conversation that seems unethical? Why or why not?

_____

_____

_____

This scenario highlights a social communication shared between two individuals through the long-accepted mode of telephone technology. The communication was not unethical, per se, but clearly showed poor judgment and etiquette. The cellular phone user may have seen the conversation as normal social discourse; however, it violated the privacy of both the people in the conversation and the commuters.

Reflection
What if the young woman talking on her cellular phone was a healthcare provider sharing the story of a patient she treated? Would that be different? If so, how?

_____

_____

_____

Communication

Communication is a key foundational aspect of therapeutic relationships and a core competency for interprofessional collaborative care delivery.[1-4] Multiple research studies have shown that effective communication is an essential tool for the development of a successful treatment plan, improved patient knowledge, adherence to treatment regimes, and improved psychosocial and behavioral outcomes. Communication happens on many levels and in many ways. We do it so often that we often neglect to think of it or actualize its importance. Levetown helps highlight this well when she states, "communication is the most common 'procedure' in medicine."[5] Health professionals communicate through spoken and written words and languages and nonverbally through body language, gestures, and mannerisms. They also communicate through a variety of technological means. Some of these are well established, such as phone and email. Some are newer technologies, such as text messaging, video conferencing, social networking sites, and mobile applications (apps). Health professionals communicate directly with patients themselves and are also responsible for communicating effectively with other providers, family members, schools, interpreters, payers, and other stakeholders to achieve the best care delivery. To do so, skilled communication is necessary.

The goal of this chapter is not to provide a comprehensive overview of communication in healthcare settings but rather to highlight how ethical problems may present surrounding such communications. Miscommunications and poor communications often precipitate ethical problems. In the pages that follow, you will gain a broader understanding of the role of skilled communication in achieving a caring response.

The Purpose of Communication

A primary goal of healthcare communication is to achieve successful information transfer and exchange. It is a means of informing and advising our patients. But it is also about much more. It includes *active listening*. Active listening is used when a health professional listens and attends to cues in the patient's verbal and nonverbal communication. It includes responding and validating to convey understanding. Communication also includes educating, collaborating, coordinating, decision making, and partnering. Through communication, healthcare professionals develop a relational dynamic with the patient, which when successful, serves to facilitate shared decision making. *Shared decision making* is a communication process in which information is exchanged not *from* professional to patient but *between* professional and patient.

Shared Decision Making

Shared decision making is the concept that decisions are made based on an underlying assumption of mutual respect and joint interest. Shared decision making values patient autonomy and recognizes the need to support self-determination. Through shared decision making, health professionals inform and educate patients regarding their health options and the best available evidence supporting those options, *and* patients share with health professionals their values, goals, and preferences.[6] In this way, decisions are informed, and the professionals and patient work together to arrive at the best decision. In this model, because information is shared, health professionals and patients can effectively partner to consider options, negotiate, and commit to making care decisions aligned with what matters most to the patient.[7-9]

---

⑨ Summary

Shared decision making is a tool for a caring response that requires attention to the type and content of communication.

To recognize the ethical relevance of communication in achieving a caring response, we turn to the story of Beth Tottle and the Uwilla family.

🍃 The Story of Beth Tottle, Mrs. Uwilla, and the Uwilla Family

Mrs. Uwilla is a 67-year-old woman from Haiti. She came to the United States to visit and assist her daughter's family with the birth of their second child. She is a widow and the mother of six children: two deceased, three in Haiti, and one in the United States. Mrs. Uwilla is non-English speaking; her native language is a dialect of French Creole. Of modest means, Mrs. Uwilla supported herself caring for her grandchildren and other children in her rural Haitian village. A short while after arriving in the United States, Mrs. Uwilla collapsed on the sidewalk while walking with her daughter. She was taken to Mercy Trauma Center, where she was determined to have sustained a severe subarachnoid hemorrhage from a ruptured cerebral aneurysm. She was admitted to the hospital and underwent a lifesaving, emergent hemicraniectomy, a procedure in which the neurosurgeon removes a portion of the skull bone to allow for brain swelling. While in the intensive care unit, she underwent placement of a tracheostomy and a gastrostomy tube. She was successfully taken off of mechanical ventilation but was unable to eat and continued to need artificial nutrition and hydration. Mrs. Uwilla was nonverbal (i.e., unable to express herself through words) and maintained a very low level of consciousness. She was immobile, minimally interactive, and dependent in all activities of daily living.

Beth Tottle, the case manager assigned to care for Mrs. Uwilla, kept up-to-date with the interprofessional care team regarding Mrs. Uwilla's clinical condition. Her job was to help coordinate a safe discharge plan for all patients on the neurosurgery unit. Mrs. Uwilla's daughter, Mica, delivered her new child and was able to visit her mother only sporadically as she was recovering from childbirth and had no other help at home. Beth was helping to coordinate Mrs. Uwilla's care and asked Mica if anyone else could help. Mica told Beth that Mica's older brother, Rene, might be able to come to the United States to help. Rene had called the unit several times and kept up-to-date via phone conversations with the nursing staff. He was a religious man and showed consistent care and concern for his mother. The doctors had told him a few months would be needed for them to replace Mrs. Uwilla's skull bone and for the swelling to resolve. They also had told him that she may be able to receive rehabilitative care in the United States but that they would not know her options for sure until the case management team was able to research additional options.

After several phone conversations, Beth Tottle was able to convince Rene Uwilla to travel to the United States. He obtained a visitor's visa and arrived 1 month into her hospitalization to assist the family in decision making regarding the next steps. He cried when seeing his mother for the first time. The day after he arrived, a family team meeting was scheduled, during which Mrs. Uwilla's slow but steady progress to date was outlined. The resident physician told Mr. Uwilla that they needed to make some decisions regarding her future care, most significantly her "code status." He stated, "We are recommending your mom be made *do not resuscitate* (DNR). This means if her heart stops, we won't restart it." The case manager and other members of the interprofessional care team also begin to educate Mr. Uwilla regarding the discharge planning process. Because Mrs. Uwilla was not a U.S. citizen and lacked health insurance, her options for continued rehabilitative services were limited. They asked Mr. Uwilla to consider taking his mother back home to Haiti, although they realized that the care there would be suboptimal.

Mr. Uwilla, was overwhelmed, responded angrily saying, "Now I see why it was so urgent to come here. You told me she would be rehabilitated here but now say that option is 'very limited.' Not only do you want me to get my mother out of here, you also want me to kill her. You see her as work—she is a human being! This is the woman who taught me to love. I cannot be expected to immediately manage all of this. I am only one person." The team was caught off guard by his response, and many of them looked to each other for assistance.

Reflection

What factors do you think led to Mr. Uwilla's response?

_____

_____

_____

_____

What are the communication needs of this family?

_____

_____

_____

The Six-Step Process in Communication

Step 1: Gather Relevant Information

Beth Tottle's and the interprofessional care team's duties of beneficence and veracity dictate that they must attempt to assess Mr. Uwilla's statement accurately. Mr. Uwilla may be asking the team this question because he wants them to reassure him that he does not have to face the uncertainty of his mother's recovery alone. He also may want reassurance that he is part of the decision-making process for his mother's care. Differences in power are quite prevalent in communication. These differences should be lessened in the shared decision-making model; however, research shows that they continue to be prevalent in how professionals communicate with patients and families.[10]

It is important to be as sensitive as possible to the implicit, unspoken messages that are contained in language. This is true of all verbal communications between individuals. Here, Mr. Uwilla is expressing a nameless fear with the statement that the team wants him "to kill his mom." We know that he is a religious man and that religious or spiritual beliefs may be associated with what he hears. He may have heard that in the United States individuals of an older age are not valued, and he may perceive that the staff would like her to die. He is in a vulnerable situation at the moment. Often times, when a do not resuscitate (DNR) status is raised, it can be perceived as abandonment of the patient or family.

The health professionals must also acknowledge the fact that Mr. Uwilla and his family are from a Haitian culture. This is a different culture from that of the Western, predominantly white care providers. Currently, no one on the care team shares this cultural background. Beth herself knows very little about Haitian culture and traditions. As you recall from Chapter 2, cultural humility is needed to help ensure that the Uwilla's feel respected, understood, and cared for. Beth cannot help but wonder what illness or disability even means in the Uwilla family's culture. The team must understand the meaning of the illness for Mr. Uwilla and his family. What are the Uwilla family's cultural expectations? What is the role of the healer? The caretaker? The interprofessional care team needs to use narrative and contextual reasoning to think about who Mrs. Uwilla was, who she is now, and who she may become. They must reason about the patient's prospective story and how her son fits into that story. Narrative can give meaningful structure to life throughout time, and tapping into Mrs. Uwilla's narrative will give her son and the care team a better way to make compassionate and collaborative decisions with her best interests as a guide.[11]

Mr. Uwilla's anxiety is likely heightened by the feelings of helplessness and insecurity that arise when a loved one has an uncertain prognosis. Patients and family members are not the only ones who do not like uncertainty; health professionals often have difficulty with it as well. Uncertainty is a concept that implies limitations to knowledge of a particular outcome.[12] Often there are no adequate predictors of functional outcome for patients with conditions as seriously compromised as Mrs. Uwilla's condition. In neurosurgery, outcome after hemicraniectomy has been traditionally measured according to survival and level of disability; however, researchers and clinicians are now looking at measures of quality of life as well. Mr. Uwilla's real question may concern the extent of his mother's anticipated recovery. How will he know how much and when she will get better? Everyone has told him her recovery will be a long road. What does that mean? He may be asking beyond "What if her heart stops beating" to "Will you still care for her?" or "What is at the end of this tunnel?"

Beth and the interprofessional care team must also consider the organizational and societal resources available (or the lack thereof) and how they impact Mrs. Uwilla's care. As you recall from Chapter 8, considerations of the organization as a stakeholder, along with the administrative and societal dimensions of the case, are part and parcel to the ethical decision-making process.

In summary, the first important step in Beth Tottle's assessment of this situation is to gather the relevant information by gaining a better understanding of what Mr. Uwilla heard, what he is asking, and what the sources of his discomfort are.

● ⬛ *Reflection*
   We have listed some types of information about the communication
   (or lack of it) we think are relevant. What other types of information
   would you want to have before proceeding in this situation?

   _____

   _____

   _____

   _____

Step 2: Identify the Type of Ethical Problem

This case provides an example of suboptimal communication that precipi
tates moral distress. Indeed, a central problem for Beth, and the interprofessional care team, has to do with professional relationships and care planning. Nurses, therapists, chaplains, technologists, dieticians, pharmacists,
social workers, case managers, clinical administrators, and others may find
themselves in the difficult position of being caught in the middle between
the medical need for timely decision making and their own assessment of
how a caring response consistent with the best interests of the patient can
be realized. As you recall from Chapter 7, a well-coordinated team effort
on behalf of the patient makes the most efficient use of resources, time, and
energy and supports the patient's attitude of trust toward those entrusted
with his or her care. Working together to communicate information in a responsible, responsive, and respectful manner is a skill and competency all
teams must develop.

This story also highlights the impact of the context on ethical decision
making. The role of the family caregiver (Mr. Uwilla) in this case is to protect
hope. The role of the interprofessional care team is to predict hope. These
roles are currently challenged by the clinical ambiguity, sociocultural barriers, health systems regulations, and other factors.

Dignity as a Foundational Concept

As you recall from previous chapters, respect for self and respect for persons are important character traits of health professionals. Haddock defined
dignity as "the ability to feel important and valuable in relation to others,
communicate this to others, and be treated as such by others."[13] This definition highlights the necessary regard for dignity in health professional and
patient communications as it has shared meaning in the relational dynamic.
Because communication is a relational dynamic, dignity can be considered
as two values: other-regarding by respecting the dignity of others, and
self-regarding by respecting one's own dignity.[14] You should recognize this

concept from previous chapters in which the concept of self-care was introduced.

Dignity and respect are also the foundations of cultural competence. Inclusion is achieved when individuals feel heard, valued, and appreciated. When health professionals demonstrate dignity and respect in their behaviors and communications, they uphold the moral obligation to inclusive excellence and culturally informed care.

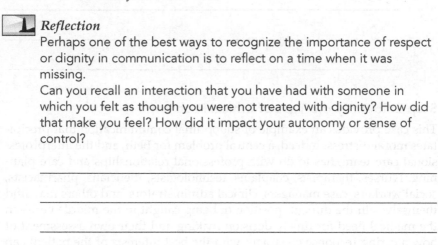

Reflection

Perhaps one of the best ways to recognize the importance of respect or dignity in communication is to reflect on a time when it was missing.

Can you recall an interaction that you have had with someone in which you felt as though you were not treated with dignity? How did that make you feel? How did it impact your autonomy or sense of control?

_____

_____

_____

_____

Communication: Hope and Disclosure

Hope. It has long been debated how to honor *hope* through discussion of *disclosure and nondisclosure*. Health professionals must balance how to best communicate clinical information as it relates to hope. Hope engenders the possibility of a future good.[15] Hope is related to coping and quality of life; however, it has multiple meanings to multiple people, at various times of their lives. In their study of hope in patients dying of cancer, Eliott and Olver[16] found that patients rated hope as essentially human. It was essential to and for life. It was not static but rather dynamic and life affirming. They summarized this well from a narrative perspective when stating, "Hope works to connect the individual to the past, present and future. The patient's value is made tangible through the expression and engagement of hope, with and for others."[16] Whether patients present to a health professional with a chronic condition or a new diagnosis, they look to the clinical information for hope. They listen to what their health professional says with an ear to the future. Sometimes this information carries bad news in it. The idea of bad news or uncertainty has led to a long debate for disclosure versus nondisclosure in healthcare communications. The paragraphs that follow outline key ethical arguments in that debate.

● *Arguments against disclosure.* The main argument advanced against disclosure of "bad news" is that the health professional's role is to predict the clinical basis for a patient's hope and hope may be shattered by bad news. Bad news is often thought of as information related to a diagnosis, prognosis, or functional outcome. That may be what Mrs. Uwilla's son was concerned about, and often health professionals have the same thoughts.

Throughout most of the history of Western healthcare, the patient has been understood as the one who needs to be cared for, who has little knowledge of medical science, who suffers passively from a disease, and who comes to the healthcare system much in the same way that a car is brought to an automobile mechanic. This image has changed. Most 21st-century patients are more informed regarding their own health and the health of their loved ones. In Western society, patient responsibility has evolved into that of an informed consumer, and in general, an informed patient is a healthier patient. We cannot assume that the Uwillas share this mainstream understanding, but we can assume that hope matters. Mr. Uwilla's religious background is a hint in this direction because in many religions, faith and hope have an established connection.

Patients come to us with knowledge obtained from various sources, including communications with friends and exposure to all types of media. Research by the Pew Internet Project and California Health Care Foundation found that 80% of Internet users look online for healthcare information.[17] Most people trust web-based social media and find information posted useful, but all media and Internet information is not quality information. Some websites are peer reviewed and primary source websites; others are opinion based. This impacts health communications in both positive and negative ways. Quality information can help broaden a patient's ● understanding of a condition, but it can also serve to challenge the information exchange process. Health professions must embrace these challenges and acknowledge that they serve as a starting point for improved patient education experiences.

Both character traits and duties are involved in professional-patient communications. A professional's benevolent disposition has been regarded as more important than an honest one, although both are extremely important. Duties involved in communicating uncertainty include beneficence, nonmaleficence, and veracity. All of these may counsel against disclosure.

Arguments against disclosure of difficult information are traditionally based on paternalistic thinking. The health professional is privy to the awful truth of the inexorable progress of many diseases and decides what patients ought to be told based on an assessment of their welfare. Of course, such perceptions are heavily influenced by the professional's own concept of his or her role in the situation and attitudes about illness and disability or death.

Arguments for disclosure. In the 1960s, the physician Elisabeth Kübler-Ross[18] spearheaded a then revolutionary movement in healthcare. She was convinced that patients with fatal illnesses could handle the truth about that awesome knowledge and therefore that information ought not be swept under the rug delicately but rather dealt with honestly, carefully, and realistically. She cited many cases of people having come to terms with the meaning of death and dying for themselves and their loved ones because they knew the truth about their own condition and its prognosis. In her view, the truth is a power that is most likely to allow shared decision making and maintain informed or realistic hope.

Currently, thanks to Kübler-Ross and others since her, the topics of dying and death are not as taboo as they were several years ago; there also is a new openness in communication about many kinds of sensitive information. The idea that patients can handle difficult news, and may even benefit from knowing, has taken health professionals down a new line of reasoning: The truth, rather than being a barrier to hope, may set the patient free. In the 1990s, the acquired immunodeficiency syndrome (AIDS) epidemic raised truth-telling questions and concerns to the forefront of health professionals' consciousness because if the patient does not know, then he or she cannot be responsible for preventing the spread of the disease. The advancement of gene identification and preclinical genetic diagnosis in this century will continue to drive discussions in the ethical dimensions of disclosure versus nondisclosure of clinical information.

In this interpretation, an honest disposition is at least as important as, and not necessarily in conflict with, a benevolent one. Acting truthfully is consistent with acting beneficently. You cannot discern what is "best" for a patient by making decisions independently on his or her behalf. Caring entails sharing pertinent information. The best way to maintain trust is to share relevant information with patients but to do so in ways that will be supportive of them.

Successful disclosure communications are both sensitive and concise. Underlying this bias toward greater disclosure of information is the conviction that if you convey the message that you still care and have the intention and ability to comfort, then it is possible to both tell the truth and maintain the patient's trust and hope. Benevolence is expressed through honesty rather than played off against it.

Patient rights and responsibilities. An additional factor that supports direct disclosure of information to patients is the understanding of patient rights. Patients have a right to information about their conditions if they want this information. As introduced in Chapter 2, *patient rights and responsibilities* documents outline these patient (or consumer) protections. The goal of a patient's rights and responsibilities statement (Box 10.1) is to strengthen consumer confidence that the healthcare system is fair and responsive to consumer needs, to affirm the importance of a strong relationship between patients and their providers, and to highlight the critical role that patients play in safeguarding their own health.[19] In such documents, patients are assumed to have a right to the truth about their condition, and it is reasonable

Box 10.1 Patient's Rights and Responsibilities

As a patient at Tingsboro Hospital, we want you to know your rights and responsibilities. We encourage you to communicate openly with your healthcare team and to advance your own health by being well informed regarding your care. Listed below are your rights and responsibilities.

Your Rights

- You have the right to receive accurate and understandable information to assist you in making an informed decision regarding your healthcare.
- You have the right to considerate and compassionate care that respects your culture, values, and beliefs. You have the right to this care regardless of your age, race, ethnicity, religion, sex, sexual orientation, gender identity and expression, socioeconomic background, or disability.
- You have the right to know the names of the healthcare providers involved in your care.
- You have the right to communicate with your providers in confidence and to have the confidentiality of your health information protected. You have a right to review and request copies of your medical records.
- You have the right to access emergency health services when and where the need arrives.
- You have the right to fully participate in all decisions regarding your healthcare, including the decision to refuse or discontinue treatment to the extent permitted by the law.
- You have the right to voice your concerns about the care you receive. This includes the right to a fair and efficient process for resolving differences with health plans, healthcare providers, and the institutions that serve them.

Your Responsibilities

- You are expected to provide to the best of your ability accurate and complete information regarding your identity, condition, past illnesses, medicines, and any other information that relates to your health.
- You are expected to ask questions when you do not understand or believe that you cannot follow through with your treatment plan. You are responsible for your health outcomes if you do not follow the mutually agreed-on care plan.
- You are expected to treat all hospital staff, other patients, and visitors (and their property) with courtesy and respect.
- You are expected to keep appointments, be on time for appointments, or call your healthcare provider if you cannot keep your appointment. If financial needs arise, you are expected to be honest with us so we may connect you to the appropriate resources.

to believe that you, the health professional, do not have the prerogative of withholding it.

There is a *duty to share* the information with the patient and withholding it can be viewed as a type of injury to the patient's trust. If information is withheld, it must be on the basis of other moral considerations deemed more compelling than the patient's right and your corresponding duty to disclose in a given situation.

Summary

It is the ethical duty of the health professional to balance hope and disclosure while respecting the dignity and rights of each individual patient. You cannot discern what is "best" for patients by making decisions independently on their behalf. Caring entails sharing all pertinent information.

Reflection

Give an example of when you think it is benevolent to share difficult information with a friend. What principles or dispositions guide your thinking?

_____

_____

_____

_____

Let us return to the story of Beth Tottle and Mrs. Uwilla. Now that Beth has gathered the facts and identified the type of ethical problem, she must continue in her ethical decision-making process.

Step 3: Use Ethics Theories or Approaches to Analyze the Problem

Step 3 is designed to encourage conscious reflection on your basic ethical approach to complex problems, such as moral distress, illustrated by the story of Beth Tottle and Mrs. Uwilla and her family.

Drawing on an ethics of care approach for analyzing this issue is ethically appropriate. As the relationship between Beth Tottle and the Uwilla family further develops, we come to understand how this relationship, the context surrounding the Uwilla family's complex situation, and the overriding cultural significance drive the decision making. Communication is relational.

The ethics of care is a need-centered and individualized relational approach. It involves analyzing the Uwilla family's situation with care, empathy, involvement, and the maintenance of harmonious relationships.[20] Beth reflects on how the team's communications have impacted the relationship with Rene Uwilla and sees the moral significance of a more patient-centered approach.

You probably have also recognized that a heavy reliance on the duties and rights that come into conflict in this story places the analysis within the deontological framework or approach to this issue. Much of the traditional healthcare approach to ethical problems relies on an understanding of our various duties, commitments, rights, or loyalties. Do you also find yourself thinking as a deontologist about this problem?

If you depend solely on neither duties nor rights, your approach may look more to the consequences that will be brought about by this unsuccessful communication. In this case, you are reasoning as a utilitarian.

Reflection

Which consequences are relevant for your consideration in the story of Beth Tottle and Mrs. Uwilla? Which ones weigh the most heavily? Why?

_____

_____

_____

_____

Once you have identified relevant duties, rights, and consequences and have determined the approach you will use, you are in a position to determine an ideal course of action for Beth and the team. This ideal course also should be guided by character traits of compassion and integrity. Compassion requires a balance in healthcare communications between providing guidance and allowing autonomy to achieve shared consensus in complex situations.[21]

Because we live in a less than perfect world, however, Beth must now begin the arduous task of identifying the several practical alternatives.

Step 4: Explore the Practical Alternatives

Seemingly good rapport exists between the members of the interprofessional care team; however, this rapport has not yet been developed with Mr. Uwilla. Building a trusting relationship and truly sharing decisions is a process that happens over time.[22] Still, Mrs. Uwilla's son has now directly asked the team what their intentions are in treating his mother. Beth Tottle and the team now need to come up with some alternatives. Consider the following alternatives.

Alternative A. The team could consider the information exchange complete with the clinical information as shared. This alternative is one based on diagnostic reasoning alone, and, as you know from your reading in previous chapters, rarely is one mode of clinical reasoning used in isolation. This leads to alternative B.

Alternative B. The team could offer support to Mr. Uwilla. Mr. Uwilla's anger and anxiety illustrate well that fears of abandonment can reflect a lack of respect toward the patient and family. At such times, the therapeutic encounters in which the health professionals are involved must become the vehicle for such comfort. Active gestures of caring, and just simply being there, can assure patients that the health professional, and by implication, all the powers of the healing professions, will not abandon them. Beth may also decide to engage Mr. Uwilla at a deeper level in ongoing communications. The door is still open for Beth and other members of the team to clarify their intentions. Little was done before this meeting to legitimize the reality and complexity of Mrs. Uwilla's care. This led to a focus on the scientific and economic issues, but not the moral or emotional ones, which led to an obstacle in their relationship with the son. Mr. Uwilla shows resistance to the team because of these poor initial communications, and trust must be re-established. Thus the fourth step in Beth Tottle's process of moral judgment and action may well be to offer support to Mr. Uwilla right away and tell him that these decisions do not need to be made today; rather they are ones that her colleagues would like him to begin to think about. She may take a lead in the meeting and redirect the conversation to Mr. Uwilla. She will need to use her interprofessional collaboration and communication skills to balance duty to the client and duty to her teammates.

Alternative C. Beth and the team can address the emotional, in addition to the cognitive, communication needs of the Uwilla family. Beth knows from her health professional training in effective communication that two types of patient needs must be addressed: the cognitive and the affective. *Affective* refers to the deep emotional need. The healthcare team has attempted to meet Mr. Uwilla's cognitive need by giving him diagnostic information and asking questions. They have not met his affective need. Beth may choose to alter the direction of the meeting to one that ensures he feels understood by reflecting his feelings and showing respect through validation, concern, and compassion. She may use a reflective response, such as "When you say 'I can't be expected to immediately manage this; I am only one person,' I think this must be so overwhelming. What is the hardest thing about your mom's illness for you and your family?" By using her interpersonal skills, Beth will show Mr. Uwilla that she values his thoughts; this may start to close the information gap between him and the team. Beth is fulfilling her professional loyalty to the team in a way that is likely to benefit the patient as well.

Alternative D. Beth can more fully explore with the hospital administration a value-based transfer option. Because Mrs. Uwilla is not a U.S. citizen, she does not qualify for the typical rehabilitative care that others in her clinical condition would. The Emergency Medical Treatment and Labor Act (EMTALA), enacted in 1986, requires that hospitals provide stabilizing treatment for patients with emergency medical conditions regardless of their ability to pay. It is through this law, and the hospital's mission to provide care to all regardless of ability to pay, that Mrs. Uwilla has been cared for to date; however, secondary care facilities such as rehabilitation hospitals and skilled nursing facilities are not under the same obligation. Many provide free care, but at a limited capacity. Beth and the interprofessional care team will need to explore with the administration and outside agencies whether any "free care" beds are available inside or outside of the hospital network. At times, networked healthcare organizations implement a *value-based transfer*, which means that the organization allows a patient to be cared for in a less expensive, more appropriate treatment environment regardless of ability to pay. This is often a more compassionate, and ethically supported, option than medical repatriation, which is the process of returning a person to their place of origin or citizenship.[23]

Reflection
Now that you have read some ideas about the practical options open to Beth, add some more of your own if you have them.

_____

_____

_____

_____

Step 5: Complete the Action

Whatever Beth decides to do, she now needs the courage to do what she reasons is a caring response in this situation. The most difficult part of her action will be if she decides to redirect the communication with the family and that results in her breaking faith with the team. Beth will need moral courage to identify the good and change the context of care for the Uwilla family. Addressing this moral distress allows for health professionals to move forward with integrity.

Step 6: Evaluate the Process and Outcome

When Beth has completed the action, has she performed her professional responsibility? If on reviewing her action, she realizes it followed the most thorough and careful ethical analysis that she was able to exercise in this situation, she can rest assured that she has given everyone involved her best effort. Review of your thinking with colleagues can further help you make an accurate assessment.

Beth may also ask an institutional resource to come and meet with the caregivers on the unit to help them learn methods to improve their cross-cultural and value-based communications. Communication is often learned during professional training, but it is a skill that must be practiced. This story highlights, as many do, that how we communicate has an impact on the quality of the relationship with an individual patient, family, and other team members. It follows that healthcare professionals have an ethical duty to develop their skills in communication. Many professional organizations rank communication high among the needed practice skills and continuing competencies. Knowledge of how to best communicate can give health professionals a strong footing when interacting for a caring response. This reinforces that on a professional level, the "good outcome" is upheld when professionals possess technical *and* interpersonal abilities to supplement their professional reasoning.

Communication Standards, Technologies, and Tools

National Standards

Communication is so vital to healthcare delivery that many national accreditation standards are in place to ensure that communication is both safe and effective. The Joint Commission, a not-for-profit independent organization that accredits healthcare facilities in the United States, includes communication among its top elements necessary for providing safe, quality care. Standards are currently in place that support effective communication in a variety of areas, including, but not limited to, the environment of care, provision of care, treatment and services, human resources, record of care, national patient safety goals, medication management, information management, and leadership. Two examples of such standards relate to patient education and caregiver-to-caregiver communication in patient handoffs.

Patient Education

Standards are currently in place and resources available to ensure that patients receive information about their care that they can understand, both verbally and in writing.[24] Health professionals are responsible for evaluating a patient's readiness to learn and preferred learning styles. As you recall, responsibility as a moral agent includes both accountability and responsiveness. These basic distinctions support effective communications. Patient education must also take into consideration health literacy as it relates to education material. *Health literacy* is defined by the Agency for Health Care Research and Quality as "the degree to which individuals have the capacity to obtain, process and understand basic health information and services needed to make appropriate health decisions."[25] Health literacy is not just the ability to read. It is a complex set of reading, listening, analytical, and decision-making skills *and* the ability to apply these skills to health situations. Health literacy is a function of an individual's skills and social demands. It varies by context and setting and greatly impacts health professional and patient communications. Many health-related communications are limited in that the patient or family does not understand the information being presented (Fig. 10.1). Health professionals must attend to and accommodate for health literacy in their professiomunications. Doing so upholds one's duty to ensuring the moral good in communicating for a caring response

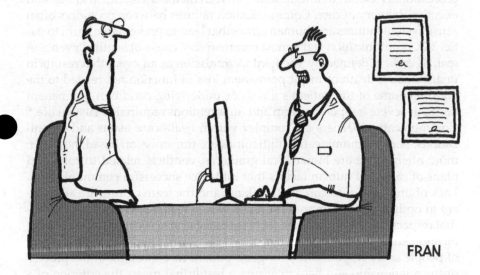

FRAN

So the epithelial cells recovered by the fiberoptic branschoscopy suggests that your phosphotyrosine levels are higher than expected, which questions the appropriateness of your current asthma treatment ...what do YOU think?

Fig. 10.1. The complexity of health literacy. (*Copyright www.cartoonstock.com.*)

Handoffs

No one provider can care for a patient 24 hours a day. *Handoffs*, by definition, involve the transfer of rights, duties, and responsibilities from one provider or team to another.[26] Since 2006, The Joint Commission has required hospitals to establish standards for handoff communications. Most organizations and agencies use both verbal and written handoff procedures, as well as *shared mental models* for effective and efficient team communication. Shared mental models are a common technique for ensuring accurate and succinct communication about patients within and across teams. Two examples that have shown positive effects on team functioning include SBAR (situation, background, assessment, recommendation) and IPASS (introduction, patient, assessment, situation, safety concerns).[27,28] Handoffs and shared mental models are excellent opportunities to ask questions and participate in shared decision making so the patient's high quality of care remains seamless.[29]

Team Communication

As you learned in Chapter 7, care is almost always provided by teams of professionals. Good communication between members is critical to safe and effective delivery of care. Communication failures between providers often cause system failures and human errors that lead to preventable harm to patients. Communication is the most common root cause of sentinel events. A *sentinel event* is defined by The Joint Commission as an event that results in unanticipated death or major permanent loss of function not related to the natural course of the patient's illness or underlying condition, permanent harm, or severe temporary harm and interventions required to sustain life.[30] Communication barriers are complex within healthcare teams and organizations. Some communication difficulties are transmission based; however, more often, there are hierarchical gradients, conflicts related to roles and plans of care, and human factors that influence successful communication. Lack of time, use of jargon, multitasking, and the team culture are all barriers to optimal team communication. Effective teams have leadership, mutual respect, cohesion, and high levels of collaboration with reliable communication among the team.[31] The story of Mrs. Uwilla highlights how a team of people share responsibility for good patient care throughout the process of the relationship and help to ensure a result that meets the criterion of a caring response.

Communicating With and Through Technology

In Chapter 9, you learned about privacy of health information in a digital world. Communication technologies such as blogs and social networking sites are alternative points of connection for user-generated content. These connections create new communication cultures, demands, professional considerations, and opportunities.[32,33] Social networking sites allow individuals to engage with users of similar interests, build and maintain relationships, share information, and feel more connected. They have an impact on communication from a privacy, safety, and professional reputation standpoint. Given the evolving nature of these technologies, we encourage you to consider the relevant ethical dimensions each time a new technology is introduced. Ask questions such as:

- How does this technology ensure patient privacy?
- How does this technology enhance team communication or patient care?
- How will oversight and accountability for the technology be ensured?
- What are the potential benefits and burdens that may be realized from this new communication technology?
- How can this technology engage relevant communities to improve health?
- Are there related governmental or organizational policies that dictate the use of the technology for patient care delivery or research?

Asking such questions can help the interprofessional care team and the organization uphold their shared moral agency to ensure best practice in communications.

Reflection

Vanessa is a 25-year-old social worker who practices in an outpatient pediatric mental health setting. Recently, the clinic implemented a "no cellular phones in the treatment rooms" policy. They have posted the policy in the waiting area. What do you think of this proposal? Use your clinical reasoning and ethics knowledge to help Vanessa support or reject the proposal.

_____

_____

_____

_____

Tools for Communication

Research studies have found that effective patient–health professional communication is associated with better health outcomes and greater patient satisfaction and follow-through with care.[34] It can also prevent ethical dilemmas.[35] In an ideal world, all communications would go well, but we know that in reality that does not happen. We all lose our cool. We all encounter conflicts and differences of opinion. Conflict creeps in and, when not addressed, interferes with a caring response. Several tools can assist the health professional in achieving more effective communication.

Numerous tools have been shared throughout the chapter; add the items in this list to help fill up your toolbox.

- Value and appreciate what the patient or family member communicates.
- Practice presence. Presence is the quality of listening without interrupting, interpreting, judging, or minimizing.[36]
- Acknowledge the patient's emotions through the use of reflective summary statements.
- Slow down, talk less, and listen more. Listen for content, meaning, and emotion.
- Watch nonverbal messages.
- Seek to understand the other person's position.
- Be honest, clear, and direct.
- Simplify communication and confirm comprehension.
- Encourage questions. Instead of saying do you have any questions, reframe to say what questions do you have.
- Understand the patient's story. Understanding the patient as a person can help you reason narratively and give you insight into the patient's illness experience.
- Encourage other members of the interprofessional care team to give communications the time they deserve and give timely, instructive feedback to colleagues regarding their performance in this realm.
- Practice and reinforce new communication skills interprofessionally as part of routine continuing professional development.

Summary

Effective healthcare communication is vital to a caring response. You have learned about various components of communication throughout this chapter. It is a complex topic that is often at the root of many ethical issues in healthcare. As you learn more about essential elements of communication, you will be better prepared to actualize your role as a moral agent. Communicating as a health professional is about being and doing. Skilled communication will help you uphold your ethical duty to treat patients in a dignified, respectful, and caring manner.

Questions for Thought and Discussion

1. Anjali works as a nurse in the pediatric oncology unit. She has just finished working a 12-hour shift. She is tired because it has been a busy and stressful day. Two of the children she was caring for needed intense interventions, and she had a family meeting for a client with a recent diagnosis of terminal cancer. On top of it all, Anjali is worried that she will be late to relieve her mother-in-law, who is caring for her daughter while she

is at work. She must now communicate with Dacy, the incoming nurse, to hand off her patients at change of shift. The unit is noisy, and the secretary has just paged Anjali. Dacy is ready for report but is socializing with the unit secretary.

What are the potential interferences with Anjali's ability to communicate? If handoff of her patients is ineffective, what are some of the potential results?

Are there any strategies that Anjali or Dacy can use to help improve the quality of the handoff process?

2. Pooja is an occupational therapist who works in an outpatient hand clinic. She has just met her new client Darren, who has arrived at the clinic for evaluation and treatment of a radial nerve injury after an open reduction and internal fixation of an elbow fracture. Darren is concerned by his lack of hand motion and sensation as a result of the nerve injury. He talks with Pooja about his injury and operative course. He had full hand use before the surgery. He reports having minimal conversations with his surgeon to date. He was sedated after the procedure, and his follow-up visit was quite brief. He asks Pooja what her opinion is, saying, "I get the feeling something went wrong during my surgery. I asked why my hand is like this now, and they gave me some technical jargon. Do you think the surgeon made a mistake?"

If you were Pooja, how would you handle this communication? What would be your first step? Why?

Role-play your response with a student colleague or out loud. How did you do? Was it easy or hard to respond to?

What duties must be considered in this situation?

References

1. Taylor R: *The intentional relationship: occupational therapy and the use of self,* Philadelphia, 2008, FA Davis.
2. Interprofessional Education Collaborative: *Core competencies for interprofessional collaborative practice: 2016 update,* Washington, DC, 2016, Interprofessional Education Collaborative.
3. IOM (Institute of Medicine): *Interprofessional education for collaboration: learning how to improve health from interprofessional models across the continuum of education to practice: workshop summary,* Washington, DC, 2013, The National Academies Press.
4. Haddad A, Doherty R, Purtilo R: *Health professional and patient interaction,* ed 9, Philadelphia, 2019, Elsevier.
5. Levetown M: American Academy of Pediatrics Committee on Bioethics: communicating with children and families: from everyday interactions to skill in conveying distressing information, *Pediatrics* 121(5):1441–1460, 2008.

6. Scheunemann LP, Ernecoff NC, Buddadhumaruk P, et al: Clinician-family communication about patients' values and preferences in intensive care units, *JAMA Intern Med* 179(5):676–684, 2019.
7. MGH: Available at https://mghdecisionsciences.org/about-us/shared-decision-making/.
8. Barry MJ, Edgman-Levitan S, Sepucha KR: Shared decision-making: staying focused on the ultimate goal *N Engl J Med Catalyst*, September 6, 2018.
9. Elwyn G, Frosch D, Thomson R, et al: Shared decision making: a model for clinical practice, *J Gen Intern Med* 27(10):1361–1367, 2012.
10. Karnieli-Miller O, Eisikovits Z: Physician as partner or salesman? Shared decision making in real time encounters, *Soc Sci Med* 69:1–8, 2009.
11. Mattingly C, Fleming MH: *Clinical reasoning: forms of inquiry in a therapeutic practice*, Philadelphia, 1994, FA Davis.
12. Purtilo RB, Robinson EM, Doherty RF, et al: *Maintaining compassionate care: a companion guide for families experiencing the uncertainty of a serious and prolonged illness*, Boston, 2008, MGH Institute of Health Professions and Kenneth B. Schwartz Center. Available at https://www.mghihp.edu/sites/default/files/publications/compassionate-care-booklet.pdf.
13. Haddock J: Towards further clarification of the concept "dignity," *J Adv Nurs* 24:924–931, 1996.
14. Gallagher A: Dignity and respect for dignity: two key health professional values: implications for nursing practice, *Nurs Ethics* 11(6):587–599, 2004.
15. DePalo R: The role of hope and spirituality on the road to recovery, *Exceptional Parent* 39(2):74–77, 2009.
16. Eliott JA, Olver IN: Hope, life and death: a qualitative analysis of dying cancer patients' talk about hope, *Death Stud* 33:609–638, 2009.
17. Fox S: *The social life of health information*, Washington, DC, 2011, Pew Research Center's Internet & American Life Project. Available at http://www.pewinternet.org/2011/05/12/the-social-life-of-health-information-2011/.
18. Kübler-Ross E: *On death and dying*, New York, 1969, Macmillan.
19. U.S. Department of Health and Human Services: *Patient rights and responsibilities*. Available at https://www.hhs.gov/answers/health-care/what-are-my-health-care-rights/index.html.
20. O'Sullivan E: Withholding truth from patients, *Nurs Stand* 23(48):35–40, 2009.
21. Sanghavi DM: What makes for a compassionate patient-caregiver relationship? *Jt Comm J Qual Patient Saf* 32(5):283–292, 2006.
22. Karnieli-Miller O, Eisikovits Z: Physician as partner or salesman? Shared decision making in real-time encounters, *Soc Sci Med* 69(1):1–8, 2009.
23. Kuczewski M: Clinical ethicists awakened: addressing two generations of clinical ethics issues involving undocumented patients, *Am J Bioethics* 19(4):51–57, 2019.
24. Angela G, Brega AG, Barnard J, et al: *Health literacy universal precautions toolkit*, ed 2, Rockville, MD, 2015, Agency for Healthcare Research and Quality. Available at http://www.ahrq.gov/professionals/quality-patient-safety/quality-resources/tools/literacy-toolkit/healthlittoolkit2.html.

25. Agency for Healthcare Research and Quality: *Health literacy measurement tools (revised): fact sheet*. Available at http://www.ahrq.gov/professionals/quality-patient-safety/quality-resources/tools/literacy/index.html.
26. Denham CR, Digman J, Foley ME, et al: Are you listening... are you really listening? *J Patient Saf* 4(3):148–161, 2008.
27. Agency for Healthcare Research and Quality. (2017). Team-STEPPS® 2.0 leadership briefing. Retrieved from www.ahrq.gov/teamstepps/about-teamstepps/leadershipbriefing.html.
28. Doherty RF: Building effective teams. In Jacobs K, editor: *Occupational therapy manager*, ed 6, Bethesda, MD, 2019, AOTA Press.
29. Haddad AM, Doherty RF, Purtilo RB: *Health professional and patient interaction*, ed 9, St. Louis, 2019, Elsevier.
30. The Joint Commission: *Sentinel event*. Available at http://www.jointcommission.org/sentinel_event.aspx.
31. Mickan SM, Rodger SA: Effective health care teams: a model of six characteristics developed from shared perceptions, *J Interprof Care* 19(4):358–370, 2005.
32. McGill M, Loveless B, McGill M: Social media in healthcare: a 360-degree view, *Am Nurse Today* 14(10):4, 2019.
33. Gagnon K, Sabus C: Professionalism in a digital age: opportunities and considerations for using social media in health care, *Phys Ther* 95(3):406–414, 2015.
34. Silverman J, Kurtz S, Draper J: *Skills for communicating with patients*, ed 3, New York, 2013, Radcliffe Publishing.
35. Mueller PS, Hook CC, Fleming KC: Ethical issues in geriatrics: a guide for clinicians, *Mayo Clinic Proc* 79:554–562, 2004.
36. Epstein R: *Attending: medicine, mindfulness, and humanity*, New York, 2017, Simon & Schuster.

11

Informed Consent in Care Delivery and Research

Objectives

The reader should be able to:

- Evaluate how informed consent, as both a procedure and a process, helps one express care and respect patient dignity.
- Describe three basic legal concepts that led to the doctrine of informed consent.
- Name three approaches to determining the disclosure standard for judging that a patient has been informed.
- Discuss three major aspects of the process of obtaining informed consent.
- Differentiate between patients who were never competent and those who were once competent, and identify the challenges posed by each in regard to informed consent.
- Compare informed consent used in healthcare delivery with that used in human studies research.
- Understand the role of institutional review boards in supporting ethical research.
- Define the terms placebo and placebo effect, and explain why placebo use is a challenge to the general idea of informed consent.
- Discuss the possible benefits and harms of placebo use and the ethical principles that are important in analyzing placebo use.
- Identify three general guidelines for information disclosure of genetic information and the challenges to informed consent that genetic testing raises.
- Recognize considerations that must be taken into account to ensure that sociocultural differences are honored in informed consent.
- Describe the function of the ethical idea that patients have a right not to know.

New terms and ideas you will encounter in this chapter

informed consent
battery
disclosure
fiduciary relationship
contract
disclosure standards
general consent
special consent
voluntariness
mental competence or
  mental capacitation
informed refusal

limited English
  proficiency (LEP)
capacity
competence
never competent
once competent
surrogate or proxy
  consent
legal guardian
best interests standard
substituted judgment
  standard

advance directives
assent
vulnerable populations
therapeutic research
institutional review
  board (IRB)
placebo
sham treatment
placebo effect
genetic information
right not to know
genomics

Topics in this chapter introduced in earlier chapters

Topic	Introduced in chapter
A caring response	2
Interprofessional care team	2
Character traits	4
Virtue	4
Principles approach	4
Autonomy	4
Beneficence, nonmaleficence	4
Patient-centered care	6
Shared decision making	10
Health literacy	10
Rights and responsibilities	10

Introduction

One important avenue to your success as a professional who has learned how to arrive at a caring response is proficiency in the communication, listening, and interpretive skills necessary to honor *informed consent*. Informed consent is one of the cornerstones of the U.S. and Canadian healthcare systems. Although the doctrine is the most formalized in these countries, it is an important concept in many healthcare systems worldwide. With both patients and research participants, basic principles of respect for the person undergird informed consent. Step-by-step through the ethical decision-making process, the importance of several aspects of informed consent in achieving your goals as a moral agent should become apparent. To inform your thinking, consider the story of Jack Burns and Cecelia Langer.

❤ The Story of Jack Burns and Cecelia Langer

Jack Burns, a 74-year-old retired cross-country truck driver, came to the emergency department of his hometown hospital because of "kidney problems" and dehydration. The healthcare team in the emergency department quickly decided that he should be admitted for further tests. Jack balked, saying he was "allergic" to hospitals; however, after talking to the doctor in the emergency department, he agreed to "stay overnight—that's all." Cecelia Langer, a nurse practitioner from the renal unit, accompanied him to the admissions area because he seemed weak and a little disoriented. When the intake clerk presented him with the general hospital admissions informed consent form, he retorted, "I know I got to sign this thing to get some help, but I don't have to like it." Cecelia encouraged him to read it and went over the main points with him.

Jack was admitted to the renal unit. The next day, he was presented with another consent form by the hospitalist, this one for the tests themselves, and he became belligerent. He asked for "that nurse that helped me last night." Cecelia, who was about to begin her afternoon shift, went directly to his room. Jack said he could not understand what they were trying to get him to do. She patiently explained the procedure he would undergo and referred to the informed consent form each step of the way. Although she herself thought it seemed quite well written, she needed almost 20 minutes of talking with him before he decided to sign it. However, when he was taken to the area where the professionals would prepare him with contrast dye for the test, he again became agitated and claimed he had never been told that they were going to "inject poison" into him. The team leader showed him where it had been discussed on the form. He shrugged his shoulders and said, "Okay, but I hope that woman who explained it to me knows she did a terrible job because I would have never signed it if I knew I was going to get injected with chemicals."

The team gave some consideration to postponing Jack's test, but when they asked him whether this was what he wanted, he grunted, "Go ahead. Do the test." The team also wondered whether to tell Cecelia about his comment and decided to do so. At first, she was annoyed, but later, she found herself thinking about what to do to avoid this from happening to a patient again. Maybe he really did not understand.

Reflection

Before you continue, take a minute to jot down your own response to this situation in regard to Cecelia's and the other health professionals'

● roles in explaining the procedure. Can you think of anything else they could have done to help Jack?

_____

_____

_____

_____

You will have an opportunity to revisit their situation as you study this chapter. You can begin to assess it by comparing it with any experience you may have had in which you were asked to give your informed consent for a treatment or diagnostic intervention or for participation as a research subject.

Reflection
If you have ever been asked to sign an informed consent form, could you understand it easily? Did you have to sign your name? Was someone on hand to answer questions you may have had at the time, or was a telephone number provided to reach someone later? Did reading and signing the form make you feel more reassured about what you were about to experience? Why or why not?

_____

_____

● _____

_____

Now that you have a story to refer to and have considered your own experience, if any, you are ready to read on about informed consent.

The Goal: A Caring Response

Informed consent is founded on basic legal and ethical principles. It entails a process of decision making and is both a process and a procedure. Informed consent happens when a patient authorizes a procedure or intervention based on an understanding of the risks, benefits, and alternatives.[1] In short, it is another tool to assist you in your skillful search for enacting a caring response through shared decision making.

An example of a procedure consent document is provided for you in Fig. 11.1. An informed consent document spells out how health professionals intend to use specific diagnostic or treatment interventions for the purpose

Tingsboro Hospital
Procedure Consent Form

Patient Label

Name

Medical Record #

DOB

Procedure: _____

I,_____, consent to the above treatment procedure as deemed medically necessary by my medical provider. My care provider,_____, has explained to me the nature of my condition, the procedure, the risks and the expected benefits of the above procedure compared with alternative approaches.

My provider has also explained to me the likelihood, and some possible complications of this procedure including, but not limited to, bleeding, infection, loss of limb or organ function, drug reactions or possibly death. I also understand that I may need a blood transfusion during or after this procedure.

I understand that Tingsboro Hospital is a teaching hospital and that students and other trainees may participate in this procedure as permitted by law and hospital policy. I also understand that tissues, blood, body parts or fluid may be removed from the body during the procedure. These materials may be used for diagnostic, therapeutic or research reasons.

Any additional comments:

_____

_____

_____

_____

_____   _____
Signature of Patient   Printed Name

_____   _____
Signature of Provider   Printed Name

Date:_____

Fig. 11.1. Informed consent document.

of improving a patient's condition. If designed appropriately, the document enables the person to become well informed before entering the decision-making process. Informed consent, then, becomes a vehicle for protecting a patient's dignity in the healthcare environment, with the fundamental belief that such consent should foster and engender trust between the health professional and the person receiving the services.

Reflection

What strengths and difficulties do you see with use of the informed consent document in Fig. 11.1 to foster the ideal of engendering trust?

Strengths

_____

_____

Difficulties

_____

_____

   To help better understand how informed consent became so central to the health professional–patient relationship, let us engage in the six-step process of ethical decision making with a focus on informed consent.

The Six-Step Process in Informed Consent Situations

As you analyze the specific informed consent–related challenges that face Jack Burns, Cecelia Langer, and the other members of his care team, bear in mind that the informed consent document, process, and procedures were designed to support important ethical dimensions of the relationship.

Step 1: Gather Relevant Information

As you may recall, when the six-step process was introduced in Chapter 5, a long list of types of information you need to ensure optimal patient care was provided. Also noted were other types of information that could help as well, such as information not related to the patient's specific situation. One example is information about the legal principles underlying informed consent; other examples are elements of the process related to disclosure in informed consent. These elements are examined in the pages that follow.

Relevant Legal Concepts That Support Informed Consent

Three important legal concepts have given rise to the thinking about informed consent: battery, disclosure, and the fiduciary relationship. The common-law legal right of self-determination and the constitutional right to privacy also are instrumental in legal thinking. You will consider self-determination for its ethical implications in another section of this chapter.

Battery, based on common law in the United States and other Western countries, is the act of offensive touching done without the consent of the person being touched, however benign the motive or effects of the touching.[2]

Disclosure guarantees the legal right of persons to be informed of what will happen to them. Several landmark legal cases have set precedents for current thinking on the importance of disclosure. Some practical challenges regarding the appropriate standard of disclosure are discussed in the next section.

One of the earliest legal cases in the United States related to disclosure was *Schloendorff v. Society of New York Hospital*; this case emphasized the relationship of disclosure to autonomy. The 1914 ruling stated that all humans of adult years and sound mind have a right to determine what shall be done with their body. For example, a surgeon who performs an operation without the patient's consent is liable on the basis of the harm of nondisclosure.[3] In the 1918 *Hunter v. Burroughs* case, the courts ruled that a physician has a duty to warn a patient of dangers associated with prescribed remedies so the patient is at liberty to decide whether or not the risk is worth it. Both rulings were early attempts by the courts to bring patients' preferences into decisions regarding what would happen to their own body.[4]

A third related legal concept is the idea of a *fiduciary relationship*. You were introduced to this idea in Chapter 2. In such a relationship, a person in whom another person has placed a special trust or confidence is required to watch out for the best interests of the other party. Most health professional–patient relationships are considered to be this type. The physician–patient relationship in the United States was ruled a fiduciary relationship in a 1974 case, *Miller v. Kennedy*, on the basis of the "ignorance and helplessness of the patient regarding his own physical condition."[5] This is, of course, an outdated understanding of the patient as "ignorant and helpless," but that does not negate the basic idea of the need for faithfulness on the part of all health professionals.

The legal case that gave to posterity the term "informed consent" is *Salgo v. Leland Stanford Board of Trustees* (1957). This case stated that physicians violate their legal duty by withholding information necessary for a patient to make a rational decision regarding care. In addition, physicians must disclose "all the facts which materially affect the patient's rights and interests and the risks, hazard and danger, if any."[6] With this ruling, the U.S. courts firmly wedded the notion of a patient's autonomy with that of a health professional's duty to warn of known danger or harm. In other words, the courts recognized that a caring response could not be achieved without those aspects of the interaction.

Relevant Facts Regarding the Process of Obtaining Consent

Let us go on to some practical matters. Currently, the law supports that a patient should gain information about a proposed procedure and should have a voice in the decision. This constitutes a legal contract between patient and health professional. A *contract* is a legal agreement on which

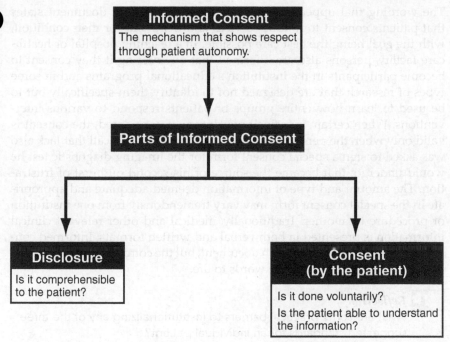

Fig. 11.2. The two dimensions of informed consent.

both parties claim to understand the situation they are agreeing to, including their respective responsibilities and rights.

However, the law also recognizes several challenges in attempting to implement the consent process in a meaningful manner. Some challenges are related to the standard and amount of disclosure, whereas others are related to the person's ability to grasp the situation (Fig. 11.2).

Disclosure standards. Disclosure standards are a key consideration. You have seen that a major legal concern is that a patient be informed. You may wonder what disclosure standard can be used to judge that the level of information is sufficiently clear to be understood? One common suggestion is that "customary medical language" be the standard of disclosure. A second approach, which emphasizes the likelihood that patients misunderstand technical terms used by a health professional, suggests that the standard be determined by what a "reasonable" person needs to understand to make an informed decision. Finding one standard appropriate for everyone continues to perplex many. So, a third common approach is to conclude that the only alternative is to adopt an individualized approach for each patient.

A related aspect of ensuring adequate disclosure focuses on the appropriate amount of information that must be provided. In many healthcare settings, patients are directed to sign a standardized *general consent* form when they are treated. This was the trigger for Jack's first outburst of concern.

The wording that appears on a typical general consent document states that patients consent to routine services and treatment for their condition, with the goal being the best care possible. In a teaching hospital or healthcare facility, persons also are informed that on entering it they consent to become participants in the institution's educational programs and in some types of research that are designed not to identify them specifically but to be used to learn how entire groups of patients respond to various interventions. When certain invasive procedures are considered, the consent is valid only when the person signs a *special consent* form. Recall that Jack also was asked to sign a special consent form for the imaging diagnostic test he would undergo; that became the source of his second outburst of frustration. The amount and type of information deemed adequate and appropriate in the special consent form may vary tremendously from one institution or procedure to another. Traditionally, medical and other relevant clinical information is presented in both verbal and written formats. Informed consent forms constitute the written document, but the communication between the involved parties brings the words to life.

Reflection

What are some practical barriers to institutionalizing any of the three suggested standards for an individual patient?

_____

_____

Do you have any ideas about what an adequate approach to the issue of a disclosure standard fit for all would be?

_____

_____

Anxiety and fear created by the unknown or general distrust of the healthcare system leaves many patients with the sense that unfair advantage is being taken of them. When presenting informed consent documents, you should be found on the side of "taking too much time" with each patient while being attentive to the patient's cues regarding the level of comprehension. The best consent processes always use shared decision making with the patient as the measure of success.

How each patient achieves understanding in the consent process is unique because we all learn, process information, and decision make differently. Studies show that simple verbal and written consent procedures do not always yield adequate patient understanding, but evidence from over 100 randomized trials does show that informed patients have better knowledge of risks and benefits, are more confident in their decisions, and elect more conservative treatment options.[7,8] Many researchers are also studying the effectiveness of alternative consent strategies, such as modified contexts and written materials to combat poor health literacy and assist patients and families in making an authentic, well-informed decision.[9,10] The inclusion of teaching or decision aides, option grids (Table 11.1), and other multimedia formats (e.g., video, interactive computer animation programs) promotes meaningful participation in the consent process and brings attention to the important implications and opportunities of each choice for an informed patient to consider.

Summary

The standard used and the amount of information disclosed combined with the variety of personal factors that influence the patient's decision making must all be taken into account in assessing whether disclosure is consistent with a caring response.

Voluntariness must be ensured. Informed consent assumes that persons voluntarily agree to the procedure or process they are about to undergo. Within informed consent discussions, this is referred to as *voluntariness.* People speak or act voluntarily when no coercion or bias compels them to do so against their own best interests and wishes. For this reason, individuals judged to be in vulnerable situations in which their ability to say "no" or "this is what I want" is compromised should be treated with special regard. As you may recall, Jack told Cecelia, the nurse practitioner, that he felt pressured to sign the consent form. A good informed consent process (in contrast to just an informed consent form) allows him either to increase his comfort level to the point of being willing to sign the form or to go away being clear why he chose to refuse treatment.

Reflection

What steps did Cecelia Langer and the interprofessional care team take to try to meet the criterion of voluntariness? Do you feel confident that they succeeded? Why or why not?

_____

_____

_____

_____

Table 11.1   Sample Option Grid

Spinal Stenosis: Treatment Options

Use this grid to help you and your healthcare professional talk about how best to treat spinal stenosis. It is for people diagnosed with spinal stenosis who have experienced leg weakness, numbness, or pain that worsens with standing and walking and improves with sitting. It is not for people with loss of bowel and urine control due to pinched nerves in their lower back.

Frequently asked questions	Managing without injections or surgery	Injections (epidural steroids)	Surgery
What does the treatment involve?	Being as active as possible to improve blood flow and taking medicine to relieve pain and swelling around the nerves.	Injection of a local anesthetic and steroid where the nerves are under pressure. This takes around 20 minutes.	A small piece of bone is removed to make a larger space for the nerve(s) in your back. This takes about 2 hours and most people spend 1–2 days in the hospital afterward.
How soon will I feel better?	6 weeks after the problem starts, about 20 in every 100 people (20%) say they are better.	Studies have had mixed findings. At best, between 15 and 30 in every 100 people (15%–30%) experience relief. Of those, most feel better in a week or so.	6 weeks after surgery, about 75 in every 100 people (75%) say they feel better.
Which treatment works best in the long-term?	4 years after treatment, about 48 in every 100 people (48%) who manage without surgery say they are better.	It is hard to say. Some studies have shown benefits from steroid injections but others have not.	4 years after surgery, around 59 in every 100 people (59%) say they are better.
What are the main risks/side effects?	The side effects will depend on which pain reliever you use.	Fewer than 1 in every 100 people (<1%) have problems, such as bleeding, headache, and infection.	2 in every 100 people (2%) will get an infection. 1 in every 100 people (1%) will get blood clots. Fewer than 1 in every 100 people (<1%) will get nerve damage.

Table 11.1   Sample Option Grid (*Cont.*)

Frequently asked questions	Managing without injections or surgery	Injections (epidural steroids)	Surgery
How will this treatment impact my ability to care for myself?	You should go about your normal daily activities as much as you are able to.	You will need someone to drive you home after the injection. Most people resume regular activities the day after the injection.	Most people need some help from family and/or friends for 1–2 months following a simple operation. More complex operations require longer healing.
Will I need any other treatment?	No, but you may be asked to see a physical therapist to start an exercise program.	You should take pain relievers as needed and keep active. The injection may be repeated in the future, but usually no more than two or three times in total.	Most people use pain relievers after the operation. Some need physical therapy after their operation, and 15 in every 100 people (15%) need a short stay in a nursing home. Longer term, 6 in every 100 people (6%) need more back operations within 1 year of surgery, 13 in every 100 (13%) within 4 years; and 25 in every 100 (25%) within 10 years.

From Option Grid, May 27, 2015. Editors: Thom Walsh, Benjamin Dropkin, Sohail Mirza, Michael Lewis, Glyn Elwyn. See http://www.optiongrid.org.

One instance that tests the limits of voluntariness as a standard of respect for a person is the psychiatric practice of involuntary commitment for mental illness. This practice has long been condoned by the medical profession and often by society as well. The increasing awareness of the importance of voluntariness, however, has created an environment in which patients are able to maintain control over large parts of their treatment regimen, sometimes including whether to accept or reject medications.

Summary

A conviction that the patient's consent is voluntarily given must be added to the condition of adequate disclosure for the ethical goals of informed consent to be realized.

Patient competence as a consideration. Health professionals have a moral duty to ascertain the level of a patient's ability to grasp the situation so that harm will not ensue because the patient did not understand. This ability is called *mental competence* or *mental capacitation,* two important terms we describe more fully later in this chapter. For the purposes of our discussion here, note that the idea of competence and capacity in the informed consent context allows us to address the assumption that individuals possess certain crucial knowledge without which they are unable to engage meaningfully in a decision. Patients must be knowledgeable about certain crucial aspects of their health and the condition creating the problem to offer true informed consent about proposed procedures to address the clinical problem. However, this formulation of competency, taken alone, is too narrow because it depends almost solely on the professional's clinical evaluation, how much persons are told, and how much they can repeat back to you. This surely is not all you wish to know concerning a patient's decision to give consent. The fundamental concern is whether the patient truly understands the nature of the illness and the basis for consenting or refusing intervention. For example, Jack may be having difficulty comprehending because of cognitive changes often associated with uremic poisoning. This is something that his interprofessional care team must pay close attention to in the process of gathering relevant information about him. They also need to obtain his medical record to determine whether any other conditions in his medical history, such as dementia or mental health disorders, may compromise his mentation.

The widely accepted criteria for ascertaining decision-making capacity in healthcare are:

1. The *ability to communicate choices*. This includes the ability to maintain and communicate these choices consistently over time.
2. The *ability to understand the relevant information* on which the choice is based.
3. The *ability to appreciate the situation and its consequences according to one's own values.*
4. The *ability to reason about treatment options,* which includes weighing the various values and relevant information to arrive at a decision.[11–13]

Ideally, a person should be able to function at all four levels. For instance, nothing the team knows about Jack suggests that previously he was incompetent or incapacitated. At the same time, they have knowledge about the delirium effects of uremic poisoning that may give them pause about his mental acuity and the process in general. Key to assessing Jack's decision is the process by which his decision is reached, not just the outcome or choice itself.

Many patients make decisions that health providers would not necessarily make for themselves. Patients have the right to make an informed refusal of a treatment that the health provider thinks they should accept. An *informed refusal* is when the patient fully understands the information and choices being presented and the consequences of choosing or declining said choices and decides to decline the proposed intervention. Patients have the right to make choices (even ones that health professionals deem unreasonable) for their own healthcare, just as they do in financial and other decisions in their lives. In short, as a part of caring for Jack, Cecelia, as the person on the team he seems to trust most, must take every precaution to ensure he is competent.

Step 2: Identify the Type of Ethical Problem

Cecelia and the interprofessional care team seem to have little doubt about the importance of ensuring that Jack is comfortable in giving his consent for general and special interventions. They recognize themselves as moral agents (A) responsible for a caring response to his concerns. They believe the appropriate outcome (O) is for him to be fully informed and willingly able to give (or refuse) consent. The challenge is *how* to get to that outcome. They are experiencing barriers in the course of action (C) designed by the institution to reach the result of truly informed consent.

In this case, Cecelia Langer (who has become the person Jack seems to trust the most) has a moral distress. She has to overcome the barriers to achieving her intended ethical goal. Because she can speculate what the range of barriers are, her distress falls into moral distress type A. Schematically, her problem looks like this:

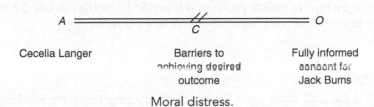

Moral distress.

What possible barriers are there?

First, the wording of the informed consent form may be a problem itself. The readability of informed consent forms has been shown to exceed the average reading levels of most adults in the United States.[14,15] Perhaps the form is so badly worded that no one is really benefited by this mechanism, and Jack is just one of the people to bring it to the attention of the health professionals.

Second, the barrier Cecelia and the other members of the care team might be facing is that Jack may have had life experiences that make him extremely anxious about giving away his autonomy. Has he been a prisoner of war or had other traumatic experiences? Did he see loved ones treated without respect for what he thought were their reasonable requests? We do not know. We certainly can observe that anxiety played a part in his reactions to the requests for him to sign the documents.

Third, he might be afraid of what he, or the health professionals, will find out if they go ahead with the tests. In other words, his reluctance may not be centered on the consent itself but rather on what it represents. His reaction at the time he is about to have the dye injected and the diagnostic test performed may be indicative of his fear of what the tests will reveal.

Fourth, despite the health professionals' good intentions and although Cecelia believes she is doing a good job, the barrier may come from this patient not being able to comprehend what is really happening, even though he appears to. He may be mentally incompetent, lack cognitive insight, have a reading or learning disability, or in some other way be deeply confused about the entire thing.

Reflection
Can you think of other possibilities? If so, jot them down.

_____

_____

_____

Once the type of ethical problem is identified, Cecelia can use the tools of ethics to analyze it (and hopefully move toward resolution).

Step 3: Use Ethical Theories or Approaches to Analyze the Problem

Cecelia, the unit nurse, and the medical imaging team are working well together to address this problem. Cecelia, in particular, has a challenge, as she has other patients to care for in addition to Mr. Burns.

The resolution of her moral distress requires her to call on both virtues and ethical principles to guide her.

Virtues Associated With Caring

In Chapter 4, you were introduced to the idea of virtue, the expression of which is in the form of character traits or dispositions. Character traits help health professionals stand firmly in their commitment to find a "caring response" in a great variety of situations. When we reflect on the challenge facing Cecelia Langer, the common healthcare virtues, such as honesty, compassion, and courage, do not seem entirely fitting for her situation. What dispositions can help her remove the barriers that are keeping her from her desired outcome—that is, confidence that she has supported Jack's right to give (or refuse) informed consent? Character traits that come to mind in observing her at work toward the achievement of this goal include kindness, thoroughness, patience, and empathy. One can assume she knows that if she sloughs off on this task, the self-respect needed for maintaining her own integrity as a professional will receive a blow. Hers is an apt example of how different character traits support moral resilience in different types of ethically challenging situations.

Cecelia will also want to move toward further action, and for that she can find some guidance in the principles approach, applying the principles of autonomy, beneficence, and nonmaleficence.

Principles Approach

Patient autonomy. Beauchamp and Faden noted that, "As the idea of informed consent evolved, discussion of appropriate (ethical) guidelines moved increasingly from a narrow focus on the physician's or researcher's obligation to disclose information to the quality of a patient's or subject's understanding of information and right to authorize or refuse biomedical intervention."[16] The governing ethical principle in informed consent is the right to self-determination or autonomy. It also is reflected in the legal right today.

Health professionals can think of informed consent as a claim to engage in a communication process designed to assist patients in making a healthcare decision in line with their authentic desires, values, and preferences. One could go further and say it is a claim to honor all the conditions, while not interfering with their liberty or autonomy. Anytime you begin communication around informed consent issues with a patient, you are inherently acknowledging an initial imbalance of information between the two of you. Because of this imbalance, the patient's autonomy can be compromised, therefore your goal as a moral agent is to set the conditions for unbiased information exchange and freedom of choice. Only then can both parties enter into dialogue and agreement as equals.

Because Jack Burns still seems upset after he has signed the second consent form, we can conclude that communication (and patient understanding) must have broken down somewhere.

Reflection

Do you think Cecelia Langer met the conditions that would foster good communication between herself and Jack? From what you know, what, if anything, could she have done differently at the outset during their initial exchange to avoid his negative response?

_____

_____

_____

_____

Whatever your suggestion, the key is that the communication should be useful to persons who are making decisions that are fitting for their life situation and within the context of personal values. Therefore you are responsible for informing the person of the conditions under which authentic understanding is achieved. Only then can both parties enter into dialogue and agreement as equals.

Beneficence and nonmaleficence. Two additional principles, beneficence and nonmaleficence, also are basic foundations on which to build your communication with the patient. As you know, these two, together, morally require you to do everything possible to refrain from harming patients and meet your positive obligation of beneficence to help them do what is most beneficial. You as a moral agent can act according to these principles by trying to ensure that patients become equipped with knowledge of what they really want and what it means within the bigger context of their life. Failure to take seriously the process of informed consent constitutes a type of harm. Unfortunately, today, the informed consent form sometimes is treated as a procedural necessity and is handled carelessly, maybe even handed off to a receptionist or aide who is not trained to—and should not be expected to—fulfill this essential component of a caring response. Whatever the process in the institution in which you are employed, failure to take informed consent seriously is tantamount to disregarding the principle of nonmaleficence (do no harm).

> ⑥ Summary
>
> Character traits and ethical principles help informed consent be realized. The patient's autonomy and the health professional's duties of nonmaleficence and beneficence are important markers toward achieving the goal of a caring response.

Step 4: Explore the Practical Alternatives

You are catching Cecelia "downstream" in her moral distress because you know from the story that Jack signed the form and had the diagnostic procedure. You also know that he seemed unhappy at the end and that she, along with the interprofessional care team, are now concerned. However, whether it was at the time Cecelia was first discussing the informed consent form with Jack, or the second time, or even now, after the fact, her concern is that there was or is a barrier to arriving at the outcome the team wanted to achieve to provide optimal care for this patient.

Let us pick up her story at the current time with her pondering what to do because no matter what she did in the past, Jack seemed "dissatisfied."

Cecelia can talk with him again herself, let him know what she heard from the members of the team, and ask him what happened that led him to be so unsatisfied with the outcome of their exchange. Perhaps through that action she will be able to understand better where she let him down (if she did) or if his lingering reluctance had nothing to do with her exchanges with him.

She could go directly to the entire team so that they can have insight into their own future care of him. Perhaps follow-up psychiatric or cognitive evaluations should be pursued should his mentation not clear once his uremia is treated medically.

She also can take the informed consent forms to the appropriate committees within her institution, probably the committees that designed the forms, and ask them to review the documents for clarity, accuracy, and completeness.

Finally, she can let the matter drop. It is over and done.

Steps 5 and 6: Complete the Action and Evaluate the Process and Outcome

Given Cecelia's continued concern and Jack's apparent continued unease, the first through third options combined with further reflection on her experience are warranted. Each may provide insight not only into the possible failures of the informed consent process but also into what the health professionals can do in the future to help ensure a more positive outcome.

One area for reflection will be taken care of by the institution's committees. Cecelia's and the interprofessional care team's experience provides them with an opportunity to review the documents, processes, and procedures of informed consent.

Another area for reflection involves Cecelia and her colleagues trying to better understand the various sources of anxiety and fear that the form, the discussion about the procedures, or other aspects of the informed consent procedure might generate in patients. Are there opportunities for them to learn how to communicate better surrounding these discussions?

A third is that the challenge of arriving at a caring response through the use of informed consent requires diligence regarding how to show respect, taking into account differences among individuals and groups of patients. For instance, the exchange between Jack and Cecelia might evoke for you the picture of two white people. In fact, Jack grew up in a small village in northern Thailand, with a mother of Thai descent and a father who is half Thai and half German. He immigrated to the United States 20 years ago. Language is not much of a barrier for him in his adopted land; however, he was never formally educated in the English language. Cecelia is a fifth-generation "New Englander" who married her high school sweetheart. Nurse and patient come from dramatically different cultural backgrounds and may have different values that guide their communication and decision-making processes.

The well-intentioned but autonomy-dominated principles of informed consent are not universally beneficial to all patients. There are many ways in which language and related sociocultural barriers can diminish its positive effects.[17,18] Although Jack does not have a perceived language barrier, sociocultural ones may make obtaining informed consent more complex. The U.S. federal antidiscrimination laws require that healthcare facilities receiving federal funds provide professional interpretation services for patients with *limited English proficiency (LEP)*. LEP refers to individuals whose primary language is not English and who have limited ability to read, write, speak, and understand English. When examining whether the basic criteria for informed consent were evident in prenatal genetic counseling practices in Texas, Hunt and deVoogd[19] found that patients who needed translation were consistently disadvantaged in the quality and content of their consultations. Some providers feel the burden of additional time and effort to obtain consent when a language barrier is present; however, given how central informed consent is to the practice of safe, legal, and patient-centered care, providers have an ethical obligation to ensure successful information exchange during the consent process. Each case warrants the professional's most vigilant attention if a caring response is to be achieved.

 Reflection

If you can, list some cultural or ethnic groups who would not find the idea of informed consent for each individual member of their group consistent with their moral norms. If you do not know any groups, you have an important task to acquaint yourself with the rich diversity of patients and clients you are bound to see.

_____

_____

_____

_____

Much of informed consent presupposes that patients desire to be independent and in control of their own individual destiny. Your professional goal and privilege of arriving at a caring response goes beyond assuming this. The differences can cause such profound mistakes that a later section of this chapter is devoted entirely to the topic.

---

⑥ Summary

The health professional who provides the patient with pertinent information for informed consent must accurately, and without bias, describe all reasonable treatment options and the risks, benefits, and burdens of each alternative, including no intervention; check for understanding; be clear when framing harms and benefits; and provide patient decision support. Even then, the process of arriving at a caring response has but begun.

In step 6, when Cecelia and the other professionals caring for Jack discuss what happened and why, they may conclude that they "missed the mark" somewhere. If not, they will have at least been diligent in reviewing how their commitment to finding a caring response in this dimension of their professional role depended not only on Cecilia but on all of them working together collaboratively.

We turn now to additional important considerations relevant to your skillful use of informed consent as an ethical tool.

The Special Challenge of Incapacity or Incompetence

Incapacity and incompetence are two terms used to describe the condition of patients for whom the process of truly informed decision making and consent to such decisions are not possible. Capacity and competence mean different things, although they are often used interchangeably. Capacity more commonly refers to clinical judgments and competence to legal ones.[11] *Capacity* is a medical concept that implies that a patient has the ability to understand and weigh medical information to make health decisions.[20] Capacity can fluctuate when patients experience certain medical conditions; for example, fever can temporarily compromise a patient's decision-making capacity. In contrast, certain medical conditions, such as Alzheimer's disease, can progressively worsen a patient's decision-making capacity. *Competence*, introduced briefly previously in this chapter, is a legal term. All persons are presumed competent until legally judged otherwise. Most writing and reflection on the subject urge extreme caution and diligence in discerning how far to proceed with evaluation and treatment if a patient is incapable of making a competent decision. Many patients have decision-making and functional abilities that are task and context dependent. The patient's actual performance along a continuum is key in the determination of capacity. It is not what patients say they will do but rather what they actually do when completing the task. The author recounts many clinical cases in which the patient could verbalize how to do a task, such as using a stove but, when taken to the actual kitchen and asked to prepare a hot beverage, could not safely perform the task. This is why it is so essential that healthcare delivery be a well-coordinated team effort. Whether referred to as capacity or competence, the patient's decision-making abilities are of greatest importance. Wettstein[21] summarized this distinction well as "a person is considered incapacitated when the person is no longer able to perform that specific function and incompetent when a court has ruled so."

Never Competent and Once Competent

The two types of incompetent patients are those who were *never competent* and those who were *once competent*. Some examples of patients who were never competent include newborns, small children, and individuals who have been severely cognitively impaired from birth. In such instances, *surrogate* or *proxy consent* usually is sought, which means that someone is appointed to consent on their behalf. When persons who were never competent become patients, a *legal guardian* is appointed. These patients usually have a guardian for other purposes, and in most instances, the same person is appointed. The next of kin is usually but not always considered the most qualified to be the guardian. The goal here is to determine who can speak for the best interests of this person who has never been in a position to voice her or his informed wishes. (This is called the *best interests standard*.) In contrast, for individuals who were once competent (e.g., those who have organic brain damage that developed in later life, or adult psychoses), a guardian also may be appointed. The guardian must then attempt to make a decision on the basis of what a person would have wanted when competent. (This is called a *substituted judgment standard*.) Sometimes a next of kin or other person makes statements that reflect what the guardian believes the patient said when he or she was competent. Often, this is helpful evidence of what a now incompetent person would want. Other signs are letters, past conversations, comments in the past about other people who became incompetent, or the person's general lifestyle.

In recent years, proxy consent for persons who were once competent has been further formalized by the advent of *advance directives*. The general idea is to allow persons while still competent to make their wishes known regarding decisions that will be made at a time when they become legally incompetent, especially in illnesses that will end in death. Some types of advance directives include living wills, durable power of attorney documents, medical directive documents, and values histories. These are discussed further in Chapter 13. Because these documents vary in focus, you are encouraged to check with your place of employment and with any state laws that may guide the legal use of such documents where you live.

Assent

Assent is a term that arose to cover situations in which persons are not in a position for their consent to be legally honored and so the onus is on the caregivers to try to discern what those persons want in regard to decisions profoundly affecting their life. Assent in children, and in adults with impaired decision-making capacity, honors respect for persons and ensures autonomy (or remaining autonomy in the case of adults). It asserts that the patient is part of the decision-making process by being informed of and included in discussions regarding his or her care. This ensures that patients can, in their own way, communicate a choice and have a say in what happens. Alderson and colleagues[22] highlighted this nicely:

> *The person who is in the body, and is the body, can have unique insights that may be essential for informed decision-making.*

Different countries have established different ages at which children can provide independent consent. In the United States, the legal age of consent is 18 in most states; however, children assent to medical decision making with their families and care providers at much earlier ages. Children often express their deep preferences through their body language, words, and actions. Children need intellectual capacity for true informed and voluntary consent; however, the process is complex because it calls on moral maturity, autonomy, reason, and emotions.[16] Many parents and providers struggle with the balance of asking children to take responsibility for weighty medical decisions given the burden that is often associated with them, knowing that things may not go as expected. That being said, children should be invited to be active participants in the care planning process; through this participation they learn the life skills necessary for successful management of their chronic condition. These experiences essentially help teach self-determination and illness management.

There is reason for serious concern over what happens when adult input capacity is diminished or missing because informed consent is not always taken as seriously as it should be. Patients often are asked to sign such forms with little more than a perfunctory explanation: "You have to sign this, and then we will do the surgery." In all cases, a professional should be present who is able to explain the procedure, its risks, benefits, and burdens; the alternative treatment options (including no intervention) and the evidence supporting these options; and to answer any questions (for the patient or the surrogate, if the patient is incompetent) regarding the fit with the patient goals, values, and informed preferences. Many people have the misconception that if a patient or surrogate signs the form, consent is legally binding no matter what. The form alone is only evidence that they have signed a piece of paper. But in a busy healthcare setting in which patients' lack of willingness to move quickly may be getting in the way of the efficient operation of the institution, there is a great risk that the consent form becomes an empty substitute for truly informed consent.

 Summary

Incompetence and incapacity point to the situations in which patients are judged unable to make informed decisions medically and legally on their own. Respect for autonomy and well-being is attempted through the use of surrogate decision makers, best interests and substituted judgment standards, advance directives, and assent when fully informed consent is not possible.

Informed Consent in Research

Clinical research is essential to advancing the art and science of medicine and improving the quality of care delivery. Clinical trials provide health professionals with new knowledge in how to best prevent and treat illness. As a health professional, you may find that you are a principal investigator or a member of a research team. Obtaining informed consent is a fundamental ethical and legal requirement for conducting human subjects research.[23] To help focus your attention on this important aspect of informed consent, consider an informed consent form used for research, as shown in Fig. 11.3.

Reflection
Would you sign this form? Yes_____ No___
What is clearly stated?

_____

_____

What, if anything, should be written differently?

_____

_____

Almost every experimental procedure within the healthcare setting necessitates some infringement on a person's physical or psychological independence. If the dignity of persons being subjected to an experimental procedure is to be preserved and personal autonomy recognized, they must not be involuntarily submitted to the procedure. Rather, they must freely

RESPONSIBLE INVESTIGATOR:

TITLE OF PROTOCOL:

TITLE OF CONSENT FORM *(if different from protocol):*

I have been asked to participate in a research study that is investigating *(describe purpose of study).* In participating in this study I agree to *(describe briefly and in lay terms procedures to which subject is consenting).*

I understand that

a) The possible risks of this procedure include *(list known risks or side effects; if none, so state).* Alternative treatments include *(list alternative treatments and briefly describe advantages and disadvantages of each; if none, so state).*

b) The possible benefits of this study to me are *(enumerate; if none, so state).*

c) Any questions I have concerning my participation in this study will be answered by *(list names and degrees of people who will be available to answer questions).*

d) I may withdraw from the study at any time without prejudice.

e) The results of this study may be published, but my name or identity will not be revealed and my records will remain confidential unless disclosure of my identity is required by law.

f) My consent is given voluntarily without being coerced or forced.

g) In the event of physical injury resulting from the study, medical care and treatment will be available at this institution.

For eligible veterans, compensation (damages) may be payable under 38USC 351 or, in some circumstances, under the Federal Tort claims Act.

For non-eligible veterans and non-veterans, compensation would be limited to situations where negligence occurred and would be controlled by the provisions of the Federal Tort Claims Act.

For clarification of these laws, contact the District Counsel (213) 824-7379.

_____   _____
DATE   PATIENT OR RESPONSIBLE PARTY

                       _____
                       PATIENT'S MEDICAL RECORD NUMBER

                       _____
                       AUDITOR/WITNESS

                       _____
                       INVESTIGATOR/PHYSICIAN REPRESENTATIVE

Fig. 11.3. Human studies consent form.

Protocol C.A.V.: A pilot study to evaluate short-course irradiation to small cell bronchogenic carcinoma with combination chemotherapy including the drugs Cytoxan, Adriamycin, and vincristine, and prophylactic brain irradiation. The drugs are to be started on Day 1 with the irradiation and repeated on Day 29 and thereafter every 21 days for 6 cycles.

You have been found to have a tumor of the lung which is best treated by drugs because of the extent of disease, metastases, involvement of the lymph glands, or _____ .

Antitumor drugs (chemotherapy) have been found to be effective in slowing tumor growth but are not curative as of now. New drugs and various combinations of new and current antitumor drugs are being tried in the hope of finding better drugs and more effective combinations. The aim of the treatment is to slow or to halt the spread of disease and permit you a longer period of relative well-being.

Radiation therapy is also a proven effective method of killing tumor cells. In this treatment plan for lung cancer, the affected lung will be irradiated for three weeks to maximize the potential reduction of your tumor. Your brain will also be treated with a modest dose of irradiation in order to ward off the spread of disease to this area. A temporary loss of hair may be expected within the field of irradiation.

You will also be given chemotherapy drugs (Cytoxan, Adriamycin, and vincristine) in combination with the irradiation. These drugs will be given to you intravenously on Day 1 and 29 of treatment and thereafter every 21 days for 6 cycles.

Antitumor drugs, such as the ones used in this plan, and radiation therapy may produce some damage to normal cells in the body, even though the treatments are designed to attack primarily the tumor cells. Care will be used to try to minimize the effect of the damage to your normal cells. The particular forms of damage include: nausea, vomiting, diarrhea, lowered white blood cell count, mouth ulcers, and loss of hair. The drug Adriamycin might make worse any cardiac problems you have. During the treatment you will be monitored carefully with blood tests, urine examination, x-ray examination, ECG, chemical tests, and other studies. Should any of these untoward effects occur, your treatment plan will be reevaluated and, if necessary, modified.

If you have any questions, these will be answered prior to starting the treatment program. You are under no obligation to join this study. You will continue to be treated if you refuse. You are free to withdraw your consent to participate in the study at any time without any prejudice to your continued medical care. The confidential nature of your case will be maintained.

I have read the information contained on this page and all my questions have been answered to my satisfaction. I consent to participate in this medical study.

_____
Patient's Signature   Date

_____
Witness (Investigator)   Date

_____
Witness   Date

Fig. 11.3.—cont'd Human studies consent form.

and willingly give their consent to the procedure, considering the relative range of personal risk that may be involved.

Informed Consent Versus Research Consent

There are times in healthcare delivery when standard available treatment options have failed rendering the patient a potential research participant. Patients must understand the difference between being a patient and being a research participant because of a difference in goals. The goal of treatment is to improve or manage the patient's condition with an intended benefit to the individual patient. The goal of research is to answer a clinical question through scientific study and experimentation. It may focus on the development of new treatments or medications, identify causes of illness, study health trends, or evaluate ways in which genetics may be related to an illness.[24] A patient must be provided with safe and effective treatment, whereas a research participant may receive no treatment or one whose likely benefit is unknown.

To ensure informed decision making in the research context, several ethical principles have been implemented into regulations. In 1974, the National Commission for the Protection of Human Subjects of Biomedical and Behavioral Research was charged with identifying the basic ethical principles that should underlie the conduct of biomedical and behavioral research involving human subjects. They developed the now well-known Belmont Report, which serves as guidelines to ensure that research is conducted in accordance with the ethical principles of respect for persons, beneficence, and justice.[25] That report served as foundation for the Common Rule, first published in 1991, and revised in 2017. The Common Rule is a set of federal regulations that govern the protections of human research participation in all federally funded research. The most recent revisions to the Common Rule have been effective since 2018 and place a greater emphasis on the obligation of the researcher to ensure participant understanding, including providing information a "reasonable person" might want to have to make a decision to participate or not participate in research.[26] It also requires explicit disclosure of the role of the researcher, whether that be investigator, entrepreneur, or dual roles as care provider and investigator.[27]

What about people who for some reason cannot give consent for research? Can consent be given on their behalf by someone who is judged to have the person's interests in mind? Because of the possibilities for abuse of such persons, considerable attention has been devoted in recent years to trying to set up reasonable guidelines for ensuring their protection. Disagreement still exists about the morally acceptable way to proceed. Most discussion has taken place within the context of research on children and individuals with disabilities or developmental delays, and on prisoners, pregnant women, neonates, individuals who are economically or educationally disadvantaged, non-English speakers, students, or others who are in a compromised position or in no position to refuse. Sometimes they are referred to collectively as *vulnerable populations*. At one extreme is the position that people in vulnerable populations should not be subjected to research unless it is related to their own illness (i.e., it must be *therapeutic research*). This implies that a parent or other guardian cannot second-guess what the person would do if given the opportunity to consent to a research project that did not also offer possible direct therapeutic benefit to the person, such as a medication or procedure for a fatal condition when no other interventions are available. This topic is among others that require continued debate; on the one hand, vulnerable patients are at risk for abuse, but on the other, when no research takes place in these populations, new clinical discoveries and innovative treatments cannot be actualized for their care. Carlson[28] summarized this well in her work on research ethics and intellectual disability, stating:

> The value of engaging in this dialogue goes beyond research and intellectual disability, as it points to fundamental questions regarding the aims of medicine and science, and the meaning of a good life, and the possibility of solidarity, community, and justice.

 Summary

As in most areas of ethical reflection in the health professions, dilemmas around clinical research require that professionals engage in continual weighing and decision making in their attempt to honor the subject's values. Informed consent has correctly been seen as an essential mechanism to ensure that respect for persons is honored.

Institutional Review Boards

One institutional mechanism that has become a regular means of monitoring the quality of informed consent in research is the *institutional review board (IRB)*. IRBs were implemented in the 1980s to help ensure not only that persons consenting to research understood what they were getting into but also that the research project itself was ethical in its aims and study design. In addition to informed consent considerations, the IRB of an institution assesses whether the risks and benefits of the research is fairly distributed among the individuals or populations that stand to benefit. If you are asked to do a human subjects study as a part of your professional preparation, you will need to complete institutional ethics training. This training provides historic and current information on regulatory and ethical issues important to the conduct of research involving human subjects. The Collaborative Institutional Training Initiative (CITI) Program is one such program. Developed in 2000, this web-based program addresses the educational needs of investigators, staff, and students across a variety of U.S. institutions and in the global research community.[29] The IRB, or research committee governing ethical conduct of research in your institution, will also require that you complete several forms before implementing research.

These forms include a series of questions related to research staff, study population, research aims, study design and methods, data collection, security, and storage, use/security of digital health technologies, specimen collection and storage, conflicts of interest, study communications, recruitment procedures, foreseeable risks and discomforts, expected benefits, equitable selection of subjects, remuneration, study monitoring and quality assurance procedures, confidentiality, privacy, and consent processes. The goal is to protect the rights and welfare of human subjects, ensuring that humane practices in human subject research will be followed. By providing third-party oversight, IRBs ensure that investigators and research staff comply with federal lays and conform to the rigors of review by a panel of concerned professionals and laypeople.

Placebos: A Special Case of Information Disclosure

Informed consent hits a brick wall when placebos are involved because to seek the patient's consent destroys the effect of a placebo. *Placebo* comes from a Latin word that means "I shall please." It consists of any therapeutic procedure (or component of one) that is given for a condition for which it has no known treatment value. A pure pharmacological placebo is a preparation of an inert substance (often a sugar pill) that is not known to have any pharmacological effect. An impure placebo is an active drug given for its psychological effect even though it has no known direct effect on the disorder in question, such as an antibiotic prescribed for a common cold or other viral infection. Administration of the latter type of placebo carries the risk for real side effects, as well as the interpersonal and professional risks we will discuss in regard to pure placebos.

Placebos are often drugs, but they can also be procedures or treatments designed to look like real treatments. This type of placebo is often used in randomized, double-blind control trials when researchers evaluate treatments that are thought to be effective but that have little scientific evidence. A recent example can be found in the controlled trial of arthroscopic surgery for treatment of patients with degenerative tear of the medial meniscus of the knee. The researchers in this multicenter, randomized, participant-blinded and outcome assessor-blinded, placebo-surgery controlled trial found that outcomes after arthroscopic partial meniscectomy were no better than those after placebo surgery. Studies like this often compare traditional treatment over *sham treatment* (a sham treatment is when an investigator goes through the motions but performs no actual treatment; in this case, the sham treatment was simulation to mimic the sensations and sounds of a true meniscectomy (e.g., manipulation of the subject's knee as if the real treatment were being administered; water splashed to mimic the sounds of lavage). The participants were also kept in the operating room for the amount of time required to perform an actual procedure.[30]

The issue of placebo use has received some attention from psychiatrists and ethicists, but most of the literature on this topic has been directed toward physicians. Little research has been done concerning the role of other health professionals and the use of placebo medications and procedures, and yet nurses and pharmacists, in particular, play a direct and essential part in this particular form of deception in healthcare practice. For clear thinking about the ethical problems that may arise in such a situation, it is important to understand the reasons for prescribing a placebo and some of the history and psychology of the placebo response.

Why would any professional give a placebo? It seems to defy the best of clinical discernment and belie the possibility of obtaining consent. One important reason is what is called the *placebo effect*. Virtually all treatments (and some diagnostic studies) have positive effects for some patients over and above the specific effects of their pharmacological mechanisms. In other words, contrary to the immediate response of rejecting the practice, in some cases, the practitioner may judge it to be clinically beneficial for the patient. Beecher[31] in 1955 published the classic study that showed that placebos are effective in treating pain in 35% of patients, regardless of the source of pain or clinical condition of the patient. Over all these years, additional studies have done little to alter these percentages, and the placebo effect is estimated to occur in one of three individuals.[32] Modern neuropharmacology research has discovered that the brain produces its own chemicals, which can act as analgesics and relaxants. These chemicals, called endorphins, seem to work better for some people than for others, which may explain scientifically why some people respond positively to placebos and others do not. A common error made by health professionals has been the assumption that a symptom (e.g., pain) successfully treated with a placebo is therefore not real or is "only psychological."

The placebo effect may be partly responsible for the success of ancient remedies given by shamans, healers, or medicine men. Some of these remedies contained pharmacologically active agents, but others did not, and much of the healer's work consisted of rituals and symbols. That the treatments often were successful is a tribute to the power of the therapeutic partnership.

Modern examples of the placebo effect are the effects of suggestion in decreasing stomach acid in patients with ulcers, alleviating bronchospasm in asthma, and decreasing blood pressure. The phenomenon of the placebo effect is widespread and powerful enough so that no research trials of new medications or even surgical procedures are considered truly rigorous unless the element of suggestion has been effectively eliminated, as in randomized, double-blind, placebo-controlled trials.

Some ethicists and others oppose the use of placebos in healthcare because they see it not only as an end run around informed consent but also as an example of deception or outright lying.

Reflection
Do you think there are times when placebo use justifies the deception? If no, why? If yes, what are they?

_____

_____

_____

_____

A utilitarian approach to the use of placebos supports that their ethical acceptability can be determined by weighing the positive effects against the possible negative ones that could result from placebo therapy. In some specific instances relief of pain has resulted, which by anyone's standard is a positive effect.

Reflection
Thinking as a utilitarian, what do you think are some of the potential harmful consequences of placebo use?

_____

_____

_____

_____

Now that you have listed some consequences, the following are two that often are cited.

Loss of trust in the therapeutic relationship is viewed as one harmful consequence. Deception preempts patients' opportunity to share freely in the responsibility for their health. Allowing deception in our professional and private relationships tends to diminish the overall basis of trust that is so key to the quality of those relationships. For this reason, all health professionals who participate in clinical research must clearly communicate with patients when they are serving in their scientific role versus their clinical role. Best practice standards dictate that when at all possible, the professional treating the patient should be different from the professional researching the patient. In this way, the caring relationship is never compromised by the emotions of randomization.

Inadequate diagnosis is another dangerous consequence.[33] If a health professional is too quick to use a placebo for treatment of a patient's aches and pains, and it seems to be having a positive effect, a potentially serious and treatable medical disorder may be overlooked. Thus a thorough medical and psychological evaluation is important before the use of placebo therapy.

Much of the harm attributed to placebo use comes when it is given without respect for the patient as a person. Health professionals may find it difficult to respect patients who respond to placebos because of our emphasis on mechanistic physiological explanations. Many health professionals believe that a patient's positive response to a placebo indicates that the symptom is not real, even though this has been disproved by many studies, such as Beecher's,[31] and by the recent discovery of endorphins. In fact, cooperative patients who have stable relationships with their caregivers are more likely to respond well to placebos than are the more difficult or less cooperative patients. Thus significant risks ought to be kept in mind, but it seems unwise to rule out the possibility of placebo use completely. We are beginning to learn more about the therapeutic powers (psychological and chemical) of the mind, but we must also remember that we live in a society that has become dependent on pills and potions—symbolically and actually. Compassion allows us to use placebos in situations in which a patient may be respectfully benefited and in which that patient is likely to be unable to produce the desired effect without the symbol of the medication or other medical procedure. However, the health professional must always remember that it is unethical to prescribe placebos when one knows that an effective treatment for the patient's condition is available.

⑥ Summary

Although the administration of a placebo involves scientific deception, which is sometimes held in question from a professional ethics viewpoint, it does not violate the rights of the research subject provided that they have been adequately *informed* that they will receive either a real or placebo intervention.

Disclosure of Genetic Information

Informed consent also arises with interesting challenges in genetic conditions and prediagnostic genetic testing. Because disclosure of *genetic information* almost always is sensitive, it makes sense that each person who comes for testing provide consent for participating in a diagnostic procedure that identifies one's genetic profile or the risk of genetic disease. What to do in regard to others who are affected raises complex questions of disclosure.

♥ The Story of Meg Perkins and Helen Williams

Two years ago, Meg Perkins was diagnosed with ovarian cancer. Recently, she was diagnosed with breast cancer. As she learns more about her condition, she comes to find out from her care team, written material, and her own Internet searches about ovarian-breast cancer syndrome, a genetically linked condition that manifests itself in ovarian and breast cancer. This news is sobering to her because she has two daughters of childbearing age and wants to share any information she can with them about her condition, if she has this syndrome, and what it may mean for them. She learns that some women who have this syndrome undergo prophylactic mastectomy or removal of their ovaries, although this procedure is still somewhat controversial and covered by a limited number of insurers. She tells her daughters about what she has learned from her research and that she plans to be tested. One daughter is anxious to learn everything she can; the other says that she "wants nothing to do with it" and that she prefers to not know the outcome of her mother's genetic testing.

Meg's primary care physician refers her to Helen Williams, the genetic counselor affiliated with the healthcare system in which Meg is treated. Helen shares a multitude of information and options, and ultimately Meg decides to go through with the genetic testing process. On the next visit, Helen is faced with the difficult task of telling Meg that, because her tests reveal the genetic conditions that put her at an 85% risk for having this syndrome, she is correct in thinking about how this involves the entire family. She also tells her that at least one of her two daughters is at a very high risk for development of cancer. The genetic counselor offers to provide Meg's husband and daughters with accurate information elicited from Meg's test findings and to do so in language they can understand so that they will be able to make informed decisions; she needs Meg's and her family members' informed consent to do so. She explains to Meg that this is the job of the genetic counselor and that Meg is not different from many patients who, because of the expansion of genetic information, have found the need to seek professional counsel on this issue.[34]

Meg reveals that she sees a bumpy road ahead and asks Helen what she thinks is best for the family. Helen tells her that this decision varies across families and that it is entirely up to them. She then engages Meg in a discussion about how and what kind of information would be shared if the family members do consent.

As you can see from this scenario, genetic counselors are integral members of the interprofessional care team. They are guided by several best practice standards in informed consent. The first is how the information is conveyed matters. If Helen had said, "You have an 85% risk for a serious defect," it would convey a different story than "You do have an 85% chance of a condition that has the following characteristics, generally speaking, but you also have a 15% chance that you do not have it." This illustrates that the profession of genetic counseling has as one of its ethical tenets to try to convey information in as neutral and encouraging language as possible. The goal is to optimize the autonomy and respect of all family members in their decisions and is a posture that all health professionals guided by the goal of a caring response must exercise.

Second, the extent of information shared also is important. Today, unexpected findings often accompany a genetic screening or laboratory test; therefore health professionals are faced with the challenge of deciding how much of the unexpected information should be included. The desire to determine the appropriate limits of sharing this additional information is not restricted to genetic information. Due regard for the patient and the significance of the additional information for the patient's health are always a consideration. Meg seems to want to know as much as possible, and Helen has been guided by this knowledge.

Third, genetic information sometimes creates a particularly unique situation because the disclosure of this information has ethical, legal, and social implications. A long-standing concern of genetic testing is discrimination. Many patients find that once they are identified as having (or as being at increased risk to have) a medical condition, they are faced with denial of health insurance or employment. The federal Genetic Information Nondiscrimination Act (GINA) was passed in 2008 to prohibit such discrimination.[35] Knowledge can also raise patients' concerns regarding the future of their health and, as scientists gain a better understanding of genetic–environmental interactions, the need to prepare patients for probable life changes.[36] In the case of Meg Perkins, genetic information has a multigenerational dimension with deep relational implications for her offspring.[37] Some individuals with genetic conditions may not want other family members to feel guilty, may have fear about their possible contribution to the syndrome, or may fear that the news will cause psychological harm if the condition will lead to more challenges or suffering for loved ones. Because of the potent nature of genetic information, it also raises the question of whether a patient and family members have a right not to know.

With these weighty considerations in mind, Meg tells Helen that she is going to encourage her family to schedule an appointment to come in to talk with her.

The Right Not to Know

Genetic information has enhanced the questions about the possibilities that individuals have a *right not to know* about information that could be harmful, shameful, or embarrassing about themselves and that they would choose not to know.

Suppose that Meg's daughters are identical twins. If one consents to testing and is found to have the gene composition that gives her a high probability for the development of breast and ovarian cancer, and she decides to undergo a prophylactic radical mastectomy before cancer symptoms appear, her sister (who has the identical genetic makeup as her twin) who did not want to know her genetic profile inevitably will know that she has the gene. What she will not know is the time of onset, severity, duration, or treatability of her own cancer.[38]

Let us assume that the two sisters consent to meet with Helen and discuss their conflict. Twin A says she will consider it abandonment if she is not tested and therefore allowed to make this choice. Twin B says that she will be betrayed if, having been offered the opportunity and refused, Twin A is given the opportunity for testing then takes the steps that will in fact reveal the status to Twin B. Is there any moral claim on the genetic team not to proceed with the genetic testing of Twin A? Most ethicists and clinicians would argue "no", their duty is to provide services to a patient who is in need of it and makes an informed decision about it, but they will do their best to help minimize the amount of hurtful information that trickles to Twin B and to offer their services to her if she wishes to seek it at another time. Unfortunately, the psychological well-being of one twin (A) appears in direct conflict with the other (B), but the resolution between them probably cannot be solved satisfactorily by the health professionals refusing to offer testing, counseling, and treatment to Twin A.

 Reflection
The right not to know in the instance of identical twins might be thought of as a special case because of their identical genetic makeup. Can you think of other instances when patients legitimately may exercise their right not to know?

More generally, the idea of a patient's right not to know supports the idea that the practice of gaining a patient's informed consent to a procedure does not give the professional the prerogative to force the findings on a patient, compromising psychological well-being.

 Summary

Genetic information is especially powerful because of its ability to involve whole kinships. Informed consent for such testing must involve sensitivity to how deeply the resulting information can impact the patient's life. Not only can genetic information disclose essential secrets about individuals, it can challenge familial roles, stigmatize, and lead to social injustices. This has raised the relatively new idea in healthcare ethics that there is a right not to know.

Genomics is a field that has emerged due to the increased use of gene sequencing and the analysis of the human genome in healthcare. Genomics has raised, and will continue to raise, new clinical and ethical debates surrounding questions of informed consent and information sharing regarding genetic tests, gene therapy, and genetic enhancements. Health providers must collaborate as an interprofessional team to balance the client's needs and requests with conflicting demands.[37] Genetic testing and the right to know raise difficult questions, especially when patients may be at high risk for a disease that has no effective treatment or cure. Other questions, such as the storage, sharing, and ownership of genetic information and perhaps even more significantly, how the healthcare community can use genetic information to improve patient care and the health of society, are beyond the scope of this text, but these questions will continue to be considered, particularly with the rise of direct to consumer testing.[39] Use of the six-step process of ethical decision making helps coordinate your ethical reasons with your clinical reasoning in such situations.

Summary

Informed consent in healthcare and human subject research is a standard part of Western healthcare practice and policy. Addressing the shortcomings and adopting varying approaches in different situations are challenges that must be met. Schematically, the idea of informed consent in both healthcare and human subject research has several dimensions that affect the patient's or research subject's effective participation in shared decision making: the information disclosed, the person's understanding of this information, the decision-making capacity, voluntariness, decision support, and deliberate choice. The advent of patient-centered and value-based care is an apt reminder of your responsibility for understanding and abiding by the patient's considered wishes.

Informed consent in healthcare should be yet another means of facilitating effective communication between patient and health professional. Consent-related documents are supposed to be tangible evidence that informed consent was, in fact, given or refused. But healthcare professionals generally place too much emphasis on the form and too little on the informed consent process. Even when the process is emphasized appropriately, the ethical principle of individual autonomy that sometimes dominates must be placed within the larger context of respect for all individuals. At times, respect requires that the participation of the patient or research subject be conducted with respect for sociocultural or other norms that do not place individual autonomy in the prime position. The special challenges of informed consent and information disclosure related to placebo use, vulnerable populations, and genomics will continue to be the topics of lively debate as you enter into professional practice. They will provide you and your interprofessional teammates with an opportunity to help shape ethical principles and guidelines consistent with a caring response.

Questions for Thought and Discussion

1. Scott is a 32-year-old man admitted to an acute psychiatric hospital for suicidal ideation in the setting of noncompliance with his psychotropic medications. Scott voluntarily presented to the hospital, knowing from many years of living with his chronic schizophrenia that he was becoming increasingly psychotic. Scott is refusing to take the recommended psychotropic medications that the weekend staff prescribed. He has begun yelling and throwing medication cups back to the nurses stating, "You guys know you can't make me take this junk! This is what has made me crazy in the first place. Get the hell out of here before I call my lawyer." Scott's mental status has been fluctuating greatly, and you arrive to care for him. The medical team asks you to try to convince him to "be compliant" and take some medications to help get his condition back under control. What do you think about Scott's case? How can the team ensure informed consent in this patient? Can you ethically justify medicating Scott against his will? If so, explain.

2. Suppose you are asked to serve on a national commission to develop guidelines for informed consent for young adults with moderate to severe autism. When do you think these individuals should be viewed as capable of providing full and independent informed consent for treatment? What reasons do you have for your position on the matter? Why are these reasons important from the standpoint of the professional's liability and from the standpoint of the well-being of the adult with autism?

3. Rodger is a 62-year-old male who recently bought his 25-year-old daughter, Elisha, a direct to consumer genetic testing kit for Christmas. Elisha opens the present and gasps, saying "Dad, I can't believe you bought me this for Christmas! I don't really think I want to know if I will get cancer someday." Rodger laughs, saying "What's the big deal? You just spit in an envelope. I already did it, and now I get lots of information from the company about things I can do to live a healthy lifestyle in light of my results." As a health professional, what is your response to Rodger and Elisha in this situation? What do they each need to consider? What ethical principles can guide their decision making?

4. It has been maintained that patients have a right to complete information about their conditions. But what happens when research reveals a genetic disorder that can have known harmful effects on the subject? Should the research subject automatically be told? Who is "the patient" in such situations? What guidelines do you think should guide such information disclosure in research? What if you are serving in a dual role and the research subject is also a patient you are caring for?

References

1. Bester J, Cole CM, Kodish E: The limits of informed consent for an overwhelmed patient: clinicians' role in protecting patients and preventing overwhelm, *AMA Ethics* 18(9):869–886, 2016.
2. Garner BA, editor: *Black's law dictionary*, ed 9, St Paul, MN, 2009, West Group.
3. *Schloendorff v. Society of New York Hospital*, 1914. 211 NY 125, 105 NE 92.
4. *Hunter v. Burroughs*, 1918. 123 Va 113, 96 S.E. 360.
5. *Richard R. Miller, Appellant v. John A. Kennedy, Respondent*, 1974. Court of Appeals of Washington, Division One 11 Wash. App. 27222 P.2d 852.
6. *Salgo v. Leland Stanford Board of Trustees*, 1957. 154 Cal. App 2nd 560, 317 P. 2d 170, 177.
7. Tait AR, Voepl-Lewis T, Moscucci C, et al: Patient comprehension of an interactive, computer-based information program for cardiac catheterization: a comparison with standard information, *Arch Intern Med* 169(20):1907–1914, 2009.
8. Légaré F, Adekpedjou R, Stacey D, et al: Interventions for increasing the use of shared decision making by healthcare professionals, *Cochrane Database Syst Rev* (7), 2018, Art. No.: CD006732.
9. Schuler CL, Dodds C, Hommel KA, et al: Shared decision making in IBD: a novel approach to trial consent and timing, *Contemp Clin Trials Commun* Sept 8: 16, 2019.
10. Berger J: Informed consent is inadequate and shared decision making is ineffective: arguing for the primacy of authenticity in decision making paradigms, *Am J Bioethics* 17(11):45–47, 2017.
11. Grisso T, Appelbaum PS: *Assessing competence to consent to treatment: a guide for physicians and other health professionals*, New York, 1998, Oxford University Press.
12. Applebaum PS: Assessment of patient's competence to consent to treatment, *N Engl J Med* 357(18):1834–1840, 2007.
13. Kolva E, Rosenfeld B, Saracino R: Assessing the decision-making capacity of terminally ill patients with cancer, *Am J Geriatr Psychiatry* 26(5):523–553, 2018.
14. Santel F, Bah I, Kim K, et al: Assessing readability and comprehension of informed consent materials for medical device research: a survey of informed consents from FDA's Center for Devices and Radiological Health, *Contemp Clin Trials* Oct:85, 2019.
15. de la Mora-Molina H, Barajas-Ochoa A, Sandoval-Garcia L, et al: Trends of informted consent forms for industry-sponsored clinical trials in rheumatology over a 17-year period: readability, and assessment of patients' health literacy and perceptions, *Semin Arthritis Rheum* 48(3):547–552, 2018.
16. Beauchamp TL, Faden R: Informed consent: the history of informed consent, ed 3. Post S, editor: *Encyclopedia of bioethics*, vol 3, New York, 2004, Macmillan, pp 1271–1276.
17. Macioce F: Balancing cultural pluralism and universal bioethical standards: a multiple strategy, *Med Health Care Philos* 19(3):393–402, 2016.

18. Deem MJ, Stokes F: Culture and consent in clinical care: a critical review of nursing and nursing ethics literature, *Ann Rev Nurs Res* 37(1):223–259, 2019.

19. Hunt LM, deVoogd KB: Are good intentions good enough? Informed consent without trained interpreters, *J Gen Intern Med* 22:598–605, 2007.

20. Terry PB: Informed consent in clinical medicine, *Chest* 131(2):563–568, 2007.

21. Wettstein RM: Competence, ed 3. In Post S, editor: *Encyclopedia of bioethics*, vol 3, New York, 2005, Macmillan, pp 488–494.

22. Alderson P, Sutcliffe K, Curtis K: Children's competence to consent to medical treatment, *Hastings Cent Rep* 36(6):25–34, 2006, Nov-Dec.

23. Black BS, Brandt J, Rabins PV, et al: Predictors of providing informed consent for research participation in assisted living residents, *Am J Geriatr Psychiatry* 16(1):83–91, 2008.

24. US Food and Drug Administration. *Clinical Research vs Medical Treatment*, 2018. Available at https://www.fda.gov/patients/clinical-trials-what-patients-need-know/clinical-research-versus-medical-treatment.

25. US Department of Health, Education, and Welfare: *National Commission for the Protection of Human Subjects of Biomedical and Behavioral Research, The Belmont Report: Ethical Principles and Guidelines for the Protection of Human Subjects of Research, 1979*. Available at https://www.hhs.gov/ohrp/sites/default/files/the-belmont-report-508c_FINAL.pdf.

26. Odwazny LM, Berkman BE: The "Reasonable Person" standard for research informed consent, *Am J Bioethics* 17(7):49–51, 2017.

27. U.S. Department of Health and Human Services: Office for Human Research Protections. 45 CFR §46, Revised January 19, 2017. Available at https://www.hhs.gov/ohrp/regulations-and-policy/regulations.

28. Carlson L: Research ethics and intellectual disability: broadening the debates, *Yale J Biol Med* 86:303–314, 2013.

29. Collaborative Institutional Training Initiative: CITI program mission and vision, 2019. Available at https://about.citiprogram.org/en/mission-and-history/.

30. Sihvonen R, Paavola M, Malmivaara A, et al: Arthroscopic partial meniscectomy versus placebo surgery for a degenerative meniscus tear: a 2-year follow-up of the randomised controlled trial, *Ann Rheum Dis* 77(2):188–195, 2018.

31. Beecher HK: The powerful placebo, *JAMA* 159:1602–1606, 1955.

32. American Cancer Society: *Placebo effect*. Available at http://www.cancer.org/treatment/treatmentsandsideeffects/treatmenttypes/placebo-effect. Accessed August 1, 2019. Last updated April, 2015.

33. Garrett T, Baillie H, Garrett R: Principles of confidentiality and truthfulness. *Health care ethics: principles and problems*, ed 4, Upper Saddle River, NJ, 2001, Prentice Hall, pp 111–135.

34. Puski A, Hovick S, Senter L, et al: Involvement and influence of healthcare providers, family members, and other mutation carriers in the cancer risk management decision-making process of BRCA1 and BRCA2 mutation carriers, *J Genet Couns* 27(5):1291–2130, 2018.

35. National Human Genome Research Institute: *Genetic discrimination*, September 24, 2019. Available at https://www.genome.gov/about-genomics/policy-issues/Genetic-Discrimination. Accessed October 15, 2019.
36. Reynolds S, Lou JQ: Occupational therapy in the age of the human genome: occupations therapists' role in genetics research and its impact on clinical practice, *Am J Occup Ther* 63(4):511–515, 2009.
37. Roth SC: What is genomic medicine? *J Med Libr Assoc* 107(3):442–448, 2019. doi: 10.5195/jmla.2019.604.
38. Juengst ET: FACE facts: why human genetics will always provoke bioethics, *J Law Med Ethics* 32:267–275, 2004.
39. Mahon SM: Direct-to-consumer genetic testing: helping patients make informed choices, *Clin J Oncol Nurs* 22(1):33–36, 2018.

Ethical Dimensions of Chronic and End-of-Life Care

12

Ethical Issues in Chronic Care and Disability

Objectives

The reader should be able to:

- List several common chronic medical conditions that necessitate clinical interventions over months or years.
- Describe four considerations a professional usually must take into account in arriving at a caring response in a chronic condition compared with an acute condition.
- Compare challenges to interprofessional care that present themselves in chronic care situations with those in the acute care setting.
- Discuss how and why quality-of-life considerations become a major feature of care for individuals with chronic conditions and disability.
- Identify several ways in which the professional-patient-family caregiver unit is an essential focus of decision making in situations that involve chronic conditions and disability.

New terms and ideas you will encounter in this chapter

chronic condition	disability	experimental treatment
multiple chronic conditions	specialty care team	health disparity

Topics in this chapter introduced in earlier chapters

Topic	Introduced in chapter
Ethics committee and ethics consultation	1
A caring response	2
Interprofessional care team	2
Moral distress	3
Quality of life	3
Utilitarianism	3
Principles approach	3
Nonmaleficence, beneficence	3
Communication	8
Shared decision making	10
Informed consent	11
Assent	11

Introduction

With more than 133 million people in the United States living with one or more chronic conditions, chronic care is demanding the attention of health professionals, families, and the healthcare system more than ever before.[1] Chronic diseases and conditions are a leading cause of death and disability and one in three adults lives with more than one chronic condition (or *multiple chronic conditions* [MCCs].[2] Many factors contribute to the increase in the number of chronic conditions and symptoms when compared with even a few years ago. Among these are an increase in adult longevity, advances in neonatal intensive care, health disparities, and the increasing incidence rate of long-term survival after stroke and traumatic brain injury across the life span. These are just some sources of this growing population of patients nationally and globally.

The term *chronic condition* (from *kronos*, which means "time" in Latin) focuses attention on long-term management of a condition in contrast to one that is either quickly addressed or at the end of life. It does not denote that the person eventually will die of the condition, although some do. The common denominator in chronic conditions is that the symptoms persist over time, some for months, years, or a lifetime. You may know someone (or be a person) with a chronic condition or provide care to someone who lives with symptoms of arthritis, diabetes, clinical depression, or cardiovascular disease. The presence of all these forms lends support to the idea that in your generation of the health professions, most of you will be deeply involved in the treatment of chronic symptoms and the functional impairment that often accompanies them.

Because chronic conditions often lead to disability, these two terms are commonly associated together; however, it is important to recognize that the two do not coexist. Individuals with disabilities do not always have chronic conditions, and individuals with chronic conditions are not always disabled. A *disability* is defined by the World Health Organization's (WHO's) International Classification of Functioning, Disability and Health (ICF) as "an umbrella term for impairments, activity limitations and participation restrictions."[3] Disability affects different people in different ways and can occur at any point along the life span. It is a dynamic interaction between individuals with a health condition and environmental and personal factors.[3] Some individuals are born with a disabling condition (e.g., spina bifida), and other disabilities are acquired (e.g., a spinal cord injury as a result of a diving accident). According to the Centers for Disease Control and Prevention, about 61 million people in the United States are living with a disability.[4] At approximately 13% of the population, people with disabilities are the largest minority group in the United States.[5]

There are various types of disabilities including those related to genetic disorders and conditions present at birth, associated with developmental conditions, related to an injury, or associated with a long-standing condition (e.g., diabetes).[6] Disabilities can affect a person's vision, hearing, mental health, social relationships, movement, and/or ability to think, remember, learn, or communicate. Take the example of an individual with spina bifida. This condition may result in a limitation of body structures and functions (lower extremity muscles) and functional limitations (moving one's legs) that influence performance in activities of daily living (walking, dressing); however, through adaptations and environmental factors, such as technology, equipment, support and relationships, services, policies, and the accepting beliefs of others, the individual can fully participate in society. As you can see, participation is key to health and quality of life. WHO's definition of health as a "complete state of physical, mental and social well-being, not just the absence or disease or infirmary" has helped health professionals over the years reframe care and better advocate for individuals with disabilities.[7]

Currently, the clinical management of patients with chronic conditions and disabilities often lacks coordination among providers and the healthcare system, providing plenty of room for you to become an advocate for improving the quality of care for such persons.[8] Individuals with chronic conditions and disabilities face a variety of moral decisions, including those related to identity, goals of treatment, advance care planning, who to involve in their healthcare decision making, adequate support throughout the life span, the desirability and effectiveness of life-sustaining treatment and technologies (both proven and experimental), and the moral implications of inherited disease (including the benefits and risks of genetic testing and screening).[9,10] This chapter focuses directly on the ethical tensions encountered in chronic care and disability and relevant details for achieving a caring response. A caring response is not unique compared with other types of conditions, but, at times, the challenges and opportunities present in slightly different forms. It is noteworthy that in almost all chronic conditions and disabilities the patient interacts with the usual interprofessional care team and sometimes also with a *specialty care team*, one specifically devoted to a particular disease or injury. This in itself creates an environment of multiple relationships that affect the patient and, very often, include the family or others who provide care along with health professionals.

 Reflection

Do you have a friend, family member, or colleague who has a chronic condition that necessitates ongoing clinical interventions? Perhaps you have one yourself. What are the major challenges that you think, or know, face this person? Are there regular disruptions in everyday activity? How are daily routines different from those of others? Jot down a few notes so that, as you go through the chapter, you can relate that situation back to the opportunities health professionals have to provide patient-centered care.

_____

_____

_____

_____

As you have experienced in previous chapters, to further help set your thinking, you have an opportunity to examine a narrative, this one of a family who is interacting with the healthcare system because one family member is in a situation that requires ongoing care.

 The Story of the McDonalds and the Cystic Fibrosis Team

The pregnancy had been without complication, and the delivery was much easier than Megan had imagined it would be. She and Gerald beheld the screaming newborn with the wonder that only new parents can feel. Mary Elizabeth McDonald had entered this world with all the gusto her parents presumed she would need as a second-generation immigrant in their adopted land.

And so it came as a shock to parents and clinical staff alike when, shortly after her birth, Mary Elizabeth had developed a bowel obstruction and respiratory distress. She was placed in the pediatric intensive care unit, and after a series of tests, the clinicians told the McDonalds that Mary Elizabeth had cystic fibrosis. The parents asked many questions about this condition, and little they heard sounded overly encouraging. The interprofessional care team in the intensive care unit, including a genetic counselor, social workers, and others, tried to console and encourage them, highlighting the great strides in treatment and longevity that individuals with this incurable chronic condition have enjoyed in the past several years. But Megan and Gerald feared that they had brought this long-awaited and beloved child into the world to endure a life of suffering.

That was 12 years ago. Today, Mary Elizabeth is a bright, beautiful child, small and thin for her age but with a happy spirit. Her inner vitality is a joy to all that meet her, although her life includes long periods of hospitalization and home care and home tutoring because of the seriousness of her symptoms. She begins and ends each day with bouts of severe coughing, sometimes for an hour at a time, and several times she has had bacterial infections and pneumonia so serious that the family's parish priest has administered the sacrament of Last Rites, provided only for persons who are believed to be imminently dying. Her school schedule is arranged so that only a few of her classmates know where she goes when she leaves daily for the school clinic for the vigorous chest percussion needed to loosen the thick brown mucus that continuously gathers in her lungs. The entire family agrees that it was worth the expense to move to a larger city where they have access to the ongoing availability of an excellent cystic fibrosis specialty care team. Given their repeated encounters with the healthcare system, they find the move was a wise choice. Among the most helpful is team member Betty Mortimer, a respiratory therapist whose own family has a history of cystic fibrosis and who has been on the team treating Mary Elizabeth for years.

Mary Elizabeth excels in school and is seen as a leader among her peers. Over the years, all three McDonalds have learned to live a day at a time to see what it holds for them as a family. Some days, Mrs. McDonald's activities are completely given over to tending to Mary Elizabeth; other times, she almost forgets that there is any difference between her daughter and other children. Gerald has taken a second job to help defray expenses. Currently, both parents are concerned that Mary Elizabeth is entering puberty and fear that the teen years will present her with new challenges exacerbated by her chronic symptoms. They have long belonged to a parent support group and know that some young people with cystic fibrosis have less difficulty than others making the transition into the teen and adult years, succeeding in their social life and studies, having satisfying careers, and finding a life partner. They also have learned more about the genetic component of cystic fibrosis and know that soon they will have to discuss with her the probabilities of her own children having the condition or being carriers of it. Given their strong religious position on abortion, Megan was shocked to overhear Mary Elizabeth say to a friend recently, "If I got pregnant, I'd have to have an abortion so my child wouldn't have to go through what I'm going through." Megan wept all day.

Unbeknown to the McDonalds, the cystic fibrosis team is having a crisis of its own. The head pulmonary specialist on the team, Dr. Abraham Levy, who has managed Mary Elizabeth's care for 8 years, is a world-renowned expert in the field. He announces to the team that he plans to persuade the family to put Mary Elizabeth on an *experimental treatment* in the form of an intravenous medication that the team has used in two other cases rather than having her undergo a lung transplant. The experimental treatment has passed the test of safety and effectiveness standards set by the federal government and has been tested on animals. Now it is being attempted on select patients as part of a phase II clinical trial. A visible pall falls over the room. Three members of the eight-member team assent to his decision, but the second most experienced physician on the team begins to argue with Dr. Levy about this decision. What all of them know is that, although this experimental intervention has been heralded in reputable journals and medical circles as a "miracle drug," decreasing the rate of breakdown of the respiratory system in some patients, the first time it was attempted at this institution, the patient died shortly after the treatment was administered. Since then, two additional serious deleterious responses to the drug have been reported in the literature. Dr. Levy says that Mary Elizabeth so perfectly fits the criteria for inclusion in the clinical trial that he feels confident of its success and, on that basis, the patient's informed consent will be easy to obtain. Some members of the team believe that he will emphasize the benefits of the drug choice only and overemphasize the (to be sure) serious risks of a lung transplant option for the patient.

The next day, Dr. Levy announces to the team that he raised the issue with the McDonalds and obtained their informed consent. Mary Elizabeth was there, assented, and was very excited. "Maybe I can play soccer like my friends!" he reported her as saying. Although the McDonalds were more cautious, he relayed, they decided to go ahead, hoping that she might be among the first to benefit from this new intervention. Mary Elizabeth also mentioned maybe being able to help other girls like herself who will suffer from the effects of cystic fibrosis in the future. Looking around the room and seeing their questioning eyes, Dr. Levy says, "Come on, you doubters. We all have the same goals in mind, and we have to pull together!"

After the team meeting that day, the five members who question Dr. Levy's decision lag behind in the lounge. To put it lightly, they are upset and unsure of what to do. They pride themselves in being a well-working team and have great respect for Dr. Levy and each other. They have traditionally made such decisions as a full-care team. Betty, in particular, is concerned; she recalls Mary Elizabeth saying that she saw a television program on which some doctors were experimenting on patients behind the patients' backs and that of all the things she could not handle, it would be that. They tried to assure her that situation seldom happens and is completely unethical. It would not happen to her here. She could count on that. They are aware that Dr. Levy has little time for what he calls the "armchair philosophers" on the ethics committee, and he prides the team in being able to work out their differences in a reasonable and respectful manner. So he will be upset with them if his decision goes to the ethics committee, an alternative one of them suggests. Another member thinks, in this case, it is appropriate for each of them to do more research on their own both about the effects of the experimental medication and about what the McDonalds were told. Because the treatment is not scheduled to begin until the next week, they agree to all go home and sleep on it and then reconvene after work the next day.

This interprofessional care team, the patient, and the family are in a relationship that is not unusual for patients with chronic conditions. Some characteristics of this type of team relationship are:

- The shared concern for and loyalty to the patient;
- The long experience of working with each other;
- The knowledge that the family caregivers are very much affected by the patient's condition; and
- The care being provided is by the interprofessional team, which is designed to provide compassionate, coordinated care (but also can lead to fragmentation at times).

In addition, the complexity and uncertainty that faces all of them about what to do next is not unusual. Chronic, long-term conditions always continue to evolve over time, unlike more acute conditions. Let us turn now to the challenges they face together.

The Goal: A Caring Response

The means by which the goal of a caring response in this situation can be realized is, in many regards, similar to those in any other type of situation. For instance, the care must be personalized to the needs of the patient's specific situation. However, as we already noted, a key consideration that distinguishes a chronic care situation from many others is that collectively the interventions extend over a long period, sometimes from the patient's birth until adulthood and old age. Fig. 12.1 outlines several dimensions of the range and possible lifelong duration of chronic conditions.

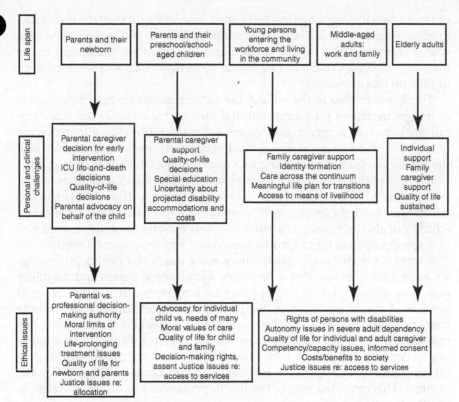

Fig. 12.1. Scope of chronic and long-term care issues. *(Modified with permission from a schema developed by Ellen Robinson and Ruth Purtilo to illustrate disability issues across the life span.)*

In Mary Elizabeth's case, she (and until she reaches adulthood, her parents) will be in relationships with health professionals on a regular basis. For her, the probability this will continue throughout her entire life is high.[11]

Several generic considerations apply to patients with chronic conditions.

First, for most patients, their expectations of the health professional or team is not to affect a cure, although if a cure would become known, the focus should shift in that direction.

Second, the point of accepting clinical interventions is to protect or improve the quality of life, whether through prevention of secondary symptoms, freedom from pain or other discomfort, or rehabilitation designed to help build or sustain important functions, relationships, and roles. The health-fostering and health maintenance interventions for the patient with one ongoing condition (complete with its evolving symptoms over months or years) casts the challenge in a somewhat different light than those directed to acute symptoms. It is a balance of periods of illness and wellness. Persons with a chronic condition have been found to experience challenges to life meaning, needing to balance freedom to do as they want and feel they need to do with loss of control.[12]

Third, and related to the second, the patient counts on the professionals to design treatment programs with the idea that the family (or other significant personal caregiver) is an essential consideration. More than in most other types of treatment planning, the interprofessional care team must take the family caregivers' well-being into account (see later for further discussion of this point). In Mary Elizabeth's or other children's situations, a parent or other adult guardian is the legal spokesperson. The same is true for adults with limited capacity, as discussed in Chapter 11. There are not only ethical but also economic and other practical reasons for making decisions that are appropriate for the family caregivers' and the patient's needs.[13]

Fourth, clinically and socially, the patient needs the health professionals to be acutely aware that individuals with chronic illness and disability may have difficulty harnessing appropriate long-term care medical or social services. A caring response on the part of the professionals must include concerted advocacy efforts designed to counteract and denounce such discrimination and dehumanizing experiences. This in turn may mean working to connect the patient with vocational counselors, social workers, or others whose base of operation may not be in traditional healthcare delivery settings. This extended role of the health professions is discussed more in Section V of this book.

 Reflection

Can you think of other considerations that should inform health professionals who are working with patients with chronic conditions but might not be as important in acute care settings? List them here.

_____

_____

_____

_____

Ⓢ **Summary**

In chronic conditions, a factor that affects treatment decisions is that cure often is not the goal, whereas quality of life is.

Again, the six-step process of ethical decision making can be called on for assessing and discerning an ethical course of action in chronic care situations.

The Six-Step Process in Chronic Care Situations

Let us return to the McDonalds and the cystic fibrosis specialty care team, picking up the story at the juncture at which the team has become divided about the decision made by the team leader. The first step is to gather relevant information.

Step 1: Gather Relevant Information

The team is paying attention to information that has caused them concern. They know that the experimental drug has been approved for human use in selected situations, such as Mary Elizabeth's case, and that the alternatives for Mary Elizabeth are few. They know all too well that a lung transplant is a high-risk surgery and that for some patients the symptoms of cystic fibrosis grow more serious during the changes of puberty and adulthood.

Evolving Clinical Status Over Time

Unlike most health professionals who work in acute care situations, the interprofessional specialty care team (in this case, the specialized cystic fibrosis team) is in a position to assess a patient's status over a period of time. The members have been working with the McDonalds for several years; therefore they have a reasonable understanding of Mary Elizabeth's current clinical condition compared with previously. Her condition can be characterized as stable, with the only big unknown being the patient's prepubescence; however, they can compare her condition with conditions of other similarly situated patients because their clinical expertise is in cystic fibrosis and respiratory disease.

Like many teams, they are now faced with a situation in which their certainty is faltering. They know that so far the team has been able to help the McDonalds manage Mary Elizabeth's symptoms. Unfortunately, at this pivotal moment in the team's relationship, they themselves are divided because of the uncertainty of what is best for Mary Elizabeth, a challenge that so often creates distress for teams whose skills focus on the treatment of chronic conditions. Their firsthand experience with the proposed course of action for Mary Elizabeth is limited to the serious negative outcome it had for one other patient in their practice, an 8-year-old child. They have to do their homework regarding this ongoing clinical trial and regarding the surgical option of lung transplant. Is the experimental approach appropriate for a young patient just entering puberty? There is no evidence of long-term effects because the intervention is so new. How does this weigh in the decision?

Team Effects

Fortunately, overall the professionals believe they are privileged to work with a group of outstanding colleagues in this practice, housed in one of the world's top academic medical centers that specialize in respiratory and pulmonary diseases. The team is a "dream team" (most of the time!), hitting the rough spots with their common goals to guide them and with deep respect for each other's competence.

It is relevant information that similar to most chronic care situations, the family caregivers have developed a deep trust in the team as a unit. The family must feel free to raise questions, express their emotions, and in other ways show their concern within the current situation. For the McDonalds' well-being, all activity should be pursued in a manner that allows that trust to be sustained, no matter the actual treatment approach, experimental or transplant. This, of course, means the team must be totally trustworthy (Fig. 12.2).

The entire team must reckon with the knowledge that this patient's immediate family is an excellent support system. Mary Elizabeth can count on both parents to be there for her. Knowing that, the team should use every means to discern the decision that will best keep this tightly knit family unit strong and optimally functional. Theirs is a long and arduous road ahead, and the opportunity for the patient to take the experimental medication is but a moment in their lifelong relationship. Not only is respect for the parents' wishes warranted, they also must be protected against any outside influences that will create needless guilt, unnecessary resignation, burnout, or other debilitating events in their life.

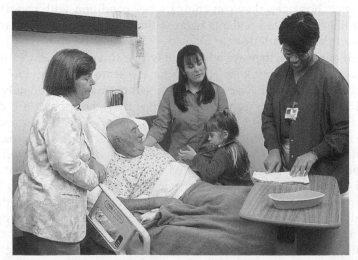

Fig. 12.2. The trust between the team and family is essential.

Quality-of-Life Focus Is Paramount

Team members who believe a patient's quality of life is being compromised by activity within the healthcare environment have good reason for consternation. In the story of the McDonalds, some members of their team are feeling stressed about the planned course of intervention. In part, this is an informed consent worry that the preteen and her family are not keenly enough aware of all the risks associated with the experimental treatment protocol, or of all the alternatives. The entire family's quality of life may be compromised by their not being fully informed agents in the type of important decision they are used to making as shared decision makers.

The team needs to get a better idea, if they can, about the full basis of the McDonald family's enthusiasm regarding the proposed experimental drug. Even if Mary Elizabeth fails to benefit appreciably in terms of her own physical symptoms, the entire family may feel better in the long run if each believes they also are contributing to ongoing research for a means by which the debilitating effects of the disease will be decreased.[14]

In taking quality-of-life considerations into account, each of the doubters must look beyond the specific symptoms of cystic fibrosis to consider the positive aspects of Mary Elizabeth's current situation. Examined in this more general context, they have consistently believed that Mary Elizabeth's quality of life is quite good; she appears to be successful academically, seems well accepted at school, participates in age-appropriate social and recreational activities, and has the benefit of devoted and capable teams both at the clinic and in her school system. However, she also is approaching an age at which her paroxysms of coughing, the exhaustion it can cause, and other signs of pulmonary compromise may make participation in the everyday activities that teens enjoy difficult for her. She may start to feel the negative effects of one who is viewed as "disabled" in some regard. In other words, as she becomes a teenager, she may experience greater teen pressure in her peer group because of her physical difference and may be discriminated against, openly or subtly, in the social activities appropriate for her age group. The International Classification of Functioning, Disability and Health: Children and Youth Version (ICF-CY) regards disability as neither purely biological nor social but instead as the interaction between health conditions and environmental and personal factors.[15,16] Mary Elizabeth may begin to experience participation restrictions, including social stigma and discrimination in the workplace if she looks for an after-school job, a common occurrence of the spillover between being viewed as having a chronic condition or a disability. None of these negative effects would be surprising because overall society has a tendency to show disrespect to persons with physical or mental impairments, no matter their age.[17]

Health Disparities

Evidence shows that individuals with disabilities experience various health disparities throughout the life span. A *health disparity* is a health difference, on the basis of one or more health outcomes, that adversely affects disadvantaged populations.[18] Race, ethnicity, socioeconomic status, sexuality, sexual orientation and identity, gender, skin color, and disability are all recognized as fostering inequities in healthcare and health outcomes. Adults with disabilities are more likely to be a victim of a violent crime, have cardiovascular disease, be obese, be a smoker, be restricted in leisure and work activities, and lack healthcare access.[19] Access to healthcare is a significant issue for individuals with disabilities. In addition to limited availability of services, there are physical barriers and inadequate knowledge and skills in health professionals who are providing care. A classic example of this is the case of a 21-year-old female with muscular dystrophy who is unable to access breast and pelvic exams because of the inaccessibility of height-adjustable examination tables and mammography equipment that cannot accommodate women who are unable to stand. You can already see that in this case being female and having a disability are both fostering inequities in health outcomes. This will be discussed further in Chapter 15, which focuses on compensatory and social justice.

External Factors

Interprofessional teams that care for patients with chronic conditions and symptoms associated with a disability need to have knowledge of the various financial supports available to patients and their families. Especially in the United States, but also in some other countries, insurance or other coverage can run out, either because the patient reaches a certain age, or school level, or because the source of coverage is capped at a certain financial figure. Moreover, a confusing variable in insurance coverage for different chronic conditions is that a diagnosis may slip from one coverage category to another. Cystic fibrosis often falls into that group. What is the McDonalds' situation regarding insurance coverage? Were any of these considerations taken into account, influencing both the physician's and the parents' decision? The team must have this information, too.

Reflection

Can you think of other information that the team members have—or if not, should have—in their reflection on Dr. Levy's decision? If so, jot them down here.

_____

_____

_____

_____

Step 2: Identify the Type of Ethical Problem

This story presents you with an interesting question about shared agency. There are several agents, namely, Dr. Levy, the other team members, the school system providers, and, of course, the patient's parents. Therefore on the one hand, there is a locus of authority consideration. Who should have the say about what? Medically and legally speaking, the physician in cooperation with the family of this preteen is responsible for the outcome. But the rub is that the proposed course of action appears to some other team members to be running slipshod over extremely important social and contextual considerations that they feel professionally qualified to follow up on further to be sure each is taken into account. The key players are at a point at which shared agency butts up against a team divided. Each member justifiably feels responsible as a moral agent whose specific expertise is informing their conflict with Dr. Levy's proposed course of action.

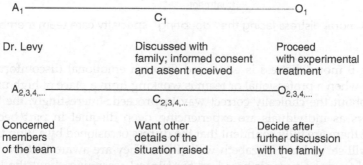

A_1 ———————————————————— O_1

C_1

Dr. Levy   Discussed with   Proceed
                            family; informed consent with experimental
                            and assent received   treatment

$A_{2,3,4,...}$ ———————————————————— $O_{2,3,4,...}$

$C_{2,3,4,...}$

Concerned   Want other   Decide after
members   details of the   further discussion
of the team   situation raised   with the family

Locus of authority considerations facing the entire care team.

It should be clear by now that the team also is facing moral distress. Now is a good time to go back and review the two types of moral distress. In type A, the moral agent or agents knows the right thing to do, but there are external (or internal) barriers to moving ahead to the ethically appropriate outcome. As you learned in the previous two chapters, an essential ethical feature of the health professional–patient relationship is shared decision making; this, in turn, depends on informed consent because this process ensures that the patient's autonomy has been honored. When the decision involves families, the challenge increases.[20] Type A moral distress in this situation is being generated by some of the team's doubt about whether Dr. Levy gave the McDonalds adequate information to make a fully informed decision. Without suggesting that he has been negligent or uncaring, it is not unreasonable for the doubting members of the team to raise this worry. With so many decisions about a patient over months or years (and often into older adulthood), the process of informed consent in chronic care and rehabilitation can get overlooked. As you recall from Chapter 11, there are distinct obligations for health professionals who find themselves in dual roles of care provider and research investigator.

Each member of the team has information they believe should be included so that the McDonalds' decision will incorporate all the areas of their life that may be affected.

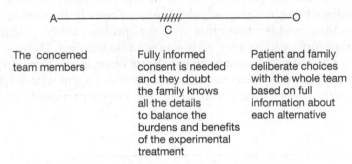

| The concerned team members | Fully informed consent is needed and they doubt the family knows all the details to balance the burdens and benefits of the experimental treatment | Patient and family deliberate choices with the whole team based on full information about each alternative |

Type A moral distress facing the "doubting" specialty care team members.

Type B moral distress is expressed through emotional discomfort and anxiety when a professional or team is working from a place of high uncertainty about the clinically correct way to proceed. Interestingly, the team members as individuals are experiencing deep disquiet in part because none of them are fully confident that the duress occasioned by a lung transplant will serve Mary Elizabeth well either. They are aware that Dr. Levy has had to make a wager based on his clinical reasoning about the likely best clinical course for this young patient even with a relative lack of data about the success of the experimental treatment and a known high risk of survival and thriving with a lung transplant. Because of all this uncertainty as it relates to the well-being of their young patient, the emotional upheaval and doubting carries the moral weight of their duty to affect the most positive outcome possible.

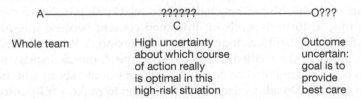

| Whole team | High uncertainty about which course of action really is optimal in this high-risk situation | Outcome uncertain: goal is to provide best care |

Type B moral distress facing the entire specialty care team about the best course to take.

Step 3: Use Ethics Theories or Approaches to Analyze the Problem

All the members of the team have learned that they need not remain in a state of moral distress. They can each reflect on the situation from the point of view of the ethics theories or approaches available to them.

Utilitarian Reasoning

The team members who are experiencing moral distress could appeal to their knowledge about the consequences they believe will be brought about by various courses of action and try to conclude which will bring about the most good overall. In so doing, they would be acting as utilitarians, trying to optimize the balance of benefits for everyone involved over the burdens brought about.

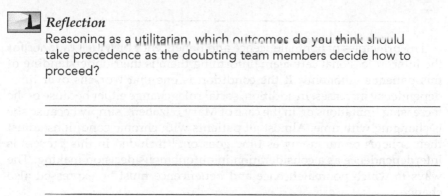

Reflection
Reasoning as a utilitarian, which outcomes do you think should take precedence as the doubting team members decide how to proceed?

_____

_____

_____

You may have listed such things as keeping the trust of the family on the heath professionals' judgment high, keeping a well-working team and giving the McDonalds every reason to believe they have all of the necessary information to make the decision. The overall desired outcome, of course, is to provide an ethically sound course of action based on the best available clinical evidence, the patient's informed values and preferences, and fully informed consent. In the case of this young girl, the parents are the decision makers, given what you have learned about the family, you can feel assured that her assent has been sought through discussion of the alternatives open to her.

Whatever your response, as almost always with a simple weighing of overall benefits and burdens, the team is faced with several unknowns about the consequences of their possible action. Reliance on this weighing alone seems insufficient to bring about the most morally supportable outcome. At the very least, the team members have the additional tool of ethical principles to help them in their ethical reasoning.

Principles Approaches
As you know by now, ethical principles can help you to determine the kind of action that your moral duties and attitudes require, not solely the outcome brought about.

Reflection
Name at least two principles you think the team can rely on in their deliberation about a course of action.

_____

_____

_____

_____

The principles of nonmaleficence and beneficence provide guidance for the interprofessional care team. Informing them is their understanding of this patient's autonomy. If the condition is one that worsens over time, dependency increases. In addition, social roles change either because of the increasing limitations or, in the case of Mary Elizabeth, simply because she is changing with time. Almost all patients with chronic conditions adjust their spheres of autonomy as time goes on.[21] Included in this process is interdependence as a consideration in autonomous decision making. The ways in which nonmaleficence and beneficence must be expressed also change.

The principle of nonmaleficence. As you may recall, the principle of nonmaleficence means that health professionals must "do no harm." In the discussion at hand, the obligation to do no harm requires the team members to look closely at the means they are using, not just the consequences. It includes not causing harm directly, removing it when it is present, and preventing it from happening. Each of these aspects of nonmaleficence is briefly examined.

Causing harm could result if the doubting members of the team engage in actions that cause the family, who needs the team over the long haul, to experience the direct harm of distrust. The McDonalds will be lost if they cannot trust the motivation and judgment of the team leader and members. Therefore nonmaleficence includes deciding how the family should be approached again, if at all, regarding the decision they have already consented to about the experimental treatment regimen.

Removing harm also is necessary. The doubters are worried that harm already has been done by virtue of the McDonalds acting on information that some team members believe is incomplete. If Mary Elizabeth and her parents have made their decision without all the available relevant knowledge, everyone on the team should be supportive in helping to rectify the short-coming. Viewed from this perspective, nonmaleficence also requires that Dr. Levy and the team members who supported his decision are willing to listen to the genuine concerns of the interprofessional care team and, if necessary, revisit his handling of the situation with the McDonalds. Each member has an opportunity and moral duty to act from a disposition of the compassion this family deserves.

In addition, harm must be prevented. In most chronic care situations, the health of the entire family is so intricately connected to the patient's well-being that the caregivers (in Mary Elizabeth's case, her parents) must never be put in a position to believe they have done anything but the best for the patient. This dimension of nonmaleficence supports the idea that the team collectively must ensure the parents have all the pertinent facts for true informed consent and give the McDonald family the support they need in their decision. At this juncture, the parents' autonomy as decision makers becomes a key to preventing harm.

The principle of beneficence. The principle of beneficence requires the professional not only to do no harm but also to seek the very best outcome possible for the patient. That is the job of the entire team. Again, the patient-family caregiver unit comes into central focus. The best possible outcome for the patient also must take seriously into account what constitutes the well-being of the family caregivers. This is true not only for instances such as the McDonalds, in which the patient is a minor, but for all situations of serious chronic and long-term care situations. Many people with chronic conditions live independently, but some need assistance with select aspects of their daily functioning. To complicate matters, many today are living at home with complex healthcare regimes and medical technologies. The health professional's advocacy designed to ensure that patients and family caregivers have the information they need for the operation of these "medical devices" is an important part of beneficence.[22] Caregiving in the home traditionally has fallen to women, and in the most recent estimate, upward of 75% of caregivers are women.[23] However, all families are structured differently. Caregivers are defined in terms of the commitments of ongoing support that individuals make to each other, rather than in terms of assigned attachments (husband, partner, mother) that happen to exist. In a recent project, the author helped organize a handbook directed to family caregivers. A part of it addresses the range of common stresses on them. A portion of it is shared in Box 12.1; it will give you insight into how to provide a caring response when family or other volunteer caregivers exhibit behaviors associated with stress.

In short, the "best decision" for the patient cannot be made in isolation from what will sustain and nourish the relationship of the caregiver as an individual and in relationship with the patient, whether the caregiver is a family member, friend, or other layperson.[24]

Box 12.1 Family Caregiver Handbook
A Helpful Outline for Addressing Family Stresses

Coping With the Stresses of a Prolonged Trajectory for Your Loved One
Prolonged illness situations, particularly where the outcome is uncertain,
are very stressful for family caregivers. An illness may present a variety
of stressors. Different individuals may experience stress differently
because of their personalities, their relationship with the ill person, their
role in the family, or their financial or employment situation. Sometimes
family members do not realize how stressed they are or why—they may
feel generally anxious or "just not right."

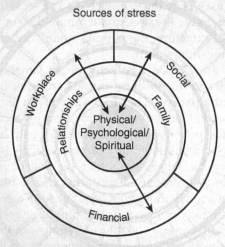

Sources of stress.

    The diagram shows different kinds of stressors. Psychological,
spiritual, and physical stressors are shown at the *center* because of their
role in our general well-being. The *arrows* show the interaction between
the layers of stress. The list below details different types of stressors. Take
a look at the list and try to identify the stressors you currently feel.

Types of stress
Physical

- Extra demand on time and energy
- Lack of sleep/altered sleep patterns; can lead to chronic overtiredness
  or exhaustion
- Changes in appetite: undereating or overeating
- Lack of ability to fight colds and illness
- Headaches, upset stomach, back and other body aches

Box 12.1   Family Caregiver Handbook (*Cont.*)

Psychological

- Anxiety
- Guilt
- Fear
- Anger
- Sadness, depression
- Helplessness
- Loss of control

Spiritual

- Anger at God, leading to feelings of guilt
- Feelings of being abandoned by God
- Life losing meaning
- Loss of faith

Family/Relationship

- Marital stress
- Children may act out in reaction to loss of time with parent
- Intrafamily fighting caused by family members seeing loved one's illness differently and feeling they would make different decisions

Social

- Decreased interaction with family/friends caused by lack of time or decreased physical and emotional energy
- Feelings of isolation
- Unwelcome increase in interaction with family/friends
- Less time/interest in usual recreational pursuits

Financial

- Loss of wages caused by absence from work
- Expenses related to hospitalization: travel, parking, meals out, childcare
- Anticipated cost of healthcare for loved one: hospital bills, potential home care

Workplace

- Missed work time
- Decreased ability to concentrate when at work
- Decreased job performance leading to decreased self-esteem
- Threatened loss of job

Adapted from "Coping with the Stresses of a Prolonged Trajectory for Your Loved One" from *Compassionate care handbook: a guide for families experiencing the uncertainty of a serious illness,* 2006. Reproduced with permissions from the MGH Institute of Health Professions, with special thanks to Dr. Ellen Robinson, managing editor; Marion Phipps, RN; and Mary Zimmer, MSW, contributing section authors.

Summary

Irrespective of disease or disability, all individuals are subject to health challenges during their life span. Weighing benefits and burdens of treatment interventions in a purely utilitarian fashion is insufficient as the situation must meet the test of taking into account specific harms and benefits *this* patient, *this* family, and *this* team face. The principles of nonmaleficence and beneficence provide a path to discerning the most morally supportable course of action and help to ensure the patient's and family's autonomy.

Step 4: Explore the Practical Alternatives

By now you know that one difficulty that professionals face in moral distress is deep emotional upheaval. Under such conditions, the range of alternatives often seems small. However, in your study of ethics, you have an opportunity to think broadly about the alternatives; hopefully they will prepare you for the real-life situations you are bound to encounter.

Several alternatives are available to the concerned members of the team.

1. Support Dr. Levy's decision unequivocally by letting the matter drop. What is done is done, and he is the one who will shoulder the ultimate burden of responsibility about the decision with this family.

2. Take the issue up with Dr. Levy again before the experimental drug is implemented so that the concerned team members can bring their concerns to the table and ask him for further details about the procedure, how his decision was made, and what he actually discussed in detail with the three McDonalds. As discussed in Chapter 7, showing team loyalty to Dr. Levy solely to keep the team running smoothly may not be a sufficient reason to let his decision rest without further discussion. An interprofessional care team must make the effort to understand the knowledge, expertise, ideas, and opinions of all members of the team.[25] In this way, the team is more effective, increasing the quality of care they provide. By synthesizing different facts and points of view, interprofessional care teams create new possibilities together and, irrespective of position in any hierarchy, can achieve shared goals that serve the patient.[26] Focusing on the McDonalds serves as an equalizer across each team member, in that the patient and family interests supersede the potentially competing interests of individual team members. To achieve the goal of a caring response, the team puts the patient first. This honors the tenants of patient and family–centered, value-based care.

3. If Dr. Levy will not meet with the entire team or they still feel unsettled after the meeting, tell Dr. Levy that they plan to request an ethics consultation so that an objective third party can help the entire team reexamine the doubters' causes for concern. Their goal is to help discern,

from an ethics point of view, which course most fully supports the principles of nonmaleficence and beneficence toward the patient. This consult also could provide insights into how they might coalesce around a mutually arrived at next step while maintaining team cohesiveness. The team can then follow up immediately with the results of the ethics consult as further guidance.

4. Each concerned team member goes directly to the McDonalds to express their specific concerns about the procedure and what they know about it and to give the McDonalds an opportunity to raise questions. This helps ensure that the McDonalds have an opportunity to directly provide feedback about the information they have and the conditions under which they gave consent or assent for the procedure. Then the team will be in a better position to decide whether to call an ethics consult before the experimental procedure is begun.

Reflection

List any other alternatives you think the team members can take to help ensure that the McDonalds receive the most appropriate caring response.

_____

_____

_____

Of all of the alternatives, including those listed and yours, which do you conclude is the most morally supportable course of action for the doubters to take?

_____

_____

_____

_____

Step 5: Complete the Action

The team has several alternatives from which to choose. Once the principles of nonmaleficence and beneficence are included in the mix of considerations, they will see that their course of action must fall on the side of the patient's (and her family's) best interests over the course of action that is the least stressful for the team. When push comes to shove, the team's comfort cannot be honored over the patient's well-being.

The first alternative of letting the matter drop is not advisable. There is too much agitation in this situation; letting it carry over into the treatment procedure cannot serve either the patient or the team well. This matter has to be addressed.

On that basis alone, the second alternative, with if necessary, the addition of the third, is the most morally supportable course of action. At the same time, the team is divided, and the more it becomes so, the more likely some other negative side effects of that division will spill over to the McDonalds. The doubters have a responsibility to approach Dr. Levy in a way that does not unnecessarily put him in conflict with the rest of the team. How they approach him, who approaches him, and when they approach him are relevant considerations to making the team meeting work to everyone's benefit.

What do you think about the fourth alternative, having each member of the team go directly to the family? It is a morally risky approach because the information that might be transmitted to the McDonalds may sound contradictory to them or become fragmented. The intent of the team may be positive, but this action will likely backfire, eroding the family's trust in the care team and disengaging them from the shared decision-making process. Care that is compassionate but not collaborative is incomplete. Moreover, Dr. Levy has a right to know that the information being provided to and evoked from the family is not unnecessarily raising doubts in the McDonalds' mind about the good intent that the entire team actually shares.

Support for the second and, if necessary, third alternative comes from some things you know about this situation. The team is a long-standing and well-working team with a liaison to Mary Elizabeth's professional support network in her school. They have their history of trust and mutual respect going for them, so the team members who have doubts now must muster enough courage to bring that trust into this difficult moment. They must be confident in their abilities to handle this difficult conversation using the communication skills introduced in Chapter 10. Compassionate, collaborative care is the gold standard of care in every healthcare encounter, organization, and system because it supports the resilience and well-being of the professional, the patient, and the family caregivers.[27] In addition, we have no reason to believe that Dr. Levy (or any member of the team) had ulterior motives in mind when recommending the experimental drug regimen. At the same time, the doubters have a right to be heard completely, too. We know how Dr. Levy feels about the ethics consultation, so he should certainly first be given an opportunity to meet with the team and then be informed that the doubting members of the team are exercising their right to take their concern to the ethics consultation service in the hospital if necessary.

Step 6: Evaluate the Process and Outcome

As in every difficult ethical situation, the team members should take time to reflect back on whatever does happen next and how their own dispositions, emotions, reasoning, and conduct played in the final decision. Because they will again have been reminded that in the end the care team's role is first and foremost to get behind the patient's best interests, they will have an opportunity to glean from their experience how those interests were honored and why, at times, they seemed not to be. It will serve them well to reflect on the special challenges of working in a setting where the patient, family or other caregivers, and healthcare team are together for a long time. A caring response to each other is as fundamental to the patient's positive experience as that response is to the patient directly.

ⓖ Summary

In the management of chronic conditions, team approaches dominate; therefore an effective team is essential to a caring response. An effective, efficient, and compassionate care team is one that always holds the patient's well-being as the gold standard against which all their activity is measured.

Summary

The increase in scope and number of patients who present to the healthcare system with chronic conditions and disability, together with the increasing range of interventions available to them, creates an opportunity for you to meet the goal of a caring response for this population. Actual interventions include prevention of new symptoms or decrease in symptom severity, rehabilitation and health maintenance within the constraints of the disease or injury, and vigilance not to assume every new symptom is part of the constellation of symptoms associated with the original chronic condition. Some key factors to take into consideration while arriving at a caring response are the persistence of the patient's symptoms and the generally predictable evolution of a specific chronic condition. The importance of nurturing the family or other caregiver relationships cannot be underscored enough. Promoting patient and family autonomy is a big factor. In Chapter 13, you will have an opportunity to carry some of these considerations over into the area of end-of-life care, demonstrating the similarities and differences when working with this population.

Questions for Thought and Discussion

1. Saul is 47 years old and has recently been diagnosed with Parkinson's disease. As a movie producer in Hollywood, he knows he has all the benefits of modern medicine at his disposal. Still, he slowly is acknowledging that

nothing he has read or learned from his sources of information promise him anything but increasing loss of physical and cognitive faculties over time. You are a therapist working in a sports center where a number of movie stars, producers, and other notables of the film industry work out. Saul has grown quite fond of you and often stays after his workout to chat, but today he is sad and depressed. He tells you of his diagnosis, about which you had not known, and asks you "as a member of the healthcare world" if you think there is any hope for him or whether he should just give up now. How would you respond to this man who is reaching out to you in your role as a health professional but who is not your patient per se? How would you help him balance hope and a realistic approach to what you know he may be facing? What, if anything, would you say to other people with whom you work that may help him through this initial phase of reckoning with his diagnosis?

2. A leading cause of pain and functional impairment in the United States is arthritis, which affects one of every five people. You are asked to serve on a national commission because of the role your profession plays in the clinical management of arthritis. The charge to the commission is to identify how social support, exercise promotion, and wellness counseling can contribute to a greater quality of life for individuals with arthritis. The commission has specifically been asked to consider how the use of virtual health agents (e.g., an automated virtual nurse that the client interacts with via a touch screen) can be successfully rolled out on a large scale with this population. Research has shown that virtual health agents can lead to increased accessibility, engagement, adherence, and retention in those with chronic conditions.[28] Examine how this innovative technology factors into the overall picture of symptom management in arthritis. What arguments would you bring to the commission on behalf of your profession and this patient population? What are the ethical considerations in the use of virtual health agents?

3. Chronic conditions and disability often are treated as one and the same. Still, many individuals with disabilities do not have illnesses or symptoms that necessitate healthcare interventions. One downside of this conflation of the two ideas is that persons with disability often are treated as if they are "sick." Discuss the problem from the flip side of the coin: namely, the ethical issues that arise when persons with a chronic condition are treated as if they have a disability, not an illness or clinical symptom. Name some chronic conditions in which there is likely also to be disability.

References

1. The National Center for Chronic Diseases and Health Promotion: *Chronic disease prevention and health promotion*, October 7, 2019. Available at https://www.cdc.gov/chronicdisease/index.htm. Accessed October 15, 2019.

2. Hajat C, Stein E: The global burden of multiple chronic conditions: a narrative review, *Prev Med Rep* 12:284–293, 2018.
3. World Health Organization: *Disability and health*. Available at https://www.who.int/en/news-room/fact-sheets/detail/disability-and-health. Accessed October 1, 2019.
4. National Center on Birth Defects and Developmental Disabilities, Centers for Disease Control and Prevention U.S. Census Bureau: *Disability and health*, October 25, 2019. Available at https://www.cdc.gov/ncbddd/disabilityand-health/dhds/index.html?CDC_AA_refVal=https%3A%2F%2Fwww.cdc.gov%2Fncbddd%2Fdisabilityandhealth%2Fdhds.html. Accessed October 26, 2019.
5. Drum C, McClain MR, Horner-Johnson W, et al: *Health disparities chart book on disability and racial and ethnic status in the United States*, Durham, NH, 2011, Institute on Disability, University of New Hampshire.
6. Centers for Disease Control and Prevention: *Disability and health overview*. September 4, 2019. Available at https://www.cdc.gov/ncbddd/disabilityan-dhealth/disability.html.
7. World Health Organization: *Constitution of the World Health Organization*, ed 45, March 2, 2018. Available at https://www.who.int/classifications/icf/en/.
8. Bodenheimer T: Coordinating care: a perilous journey through the health care system, *N Engl J Med* 358(10):1064–1071, 2009.
9. The Hastings Center: *Our vision*. Available at http://www.thehastingscenter.org/our-vision.aspx#End-of-Life. Accessed April 5, 2015.
10. Kirkendall A, Linton K, Farris S: Intellectual disabilities and decision making at End of Life: a literature review, *J Appl Res Intellect Disabil* 30(6):982–994, 2017.
11. Rothenberg L: *Breathing for a living: a memoir*, New York, 2003, Hyperion.
12. Delmar C, Boje T, Dylmer D, et al: Achieving harmony with oneself: life with a chronic illness, *Scand J Caring Sci* 19:204–212, 2008.
13. Blustein J: Integrating medicine and the family: toward a coherent ethic of care. In Levine C, Murray TH, editors: *The cultures of caregiving: conflict and common ground among families, health professionals and policy makers*, Baltimore, 2007, Johns Hopkins University Press, pp 127–146.
14. Sibley A, Fitzpatrick R, Davis E, et al: The family context of assent: comparison of child and parent perspectives on familial decision-making, *Child Soc* 32(4):266–278, 2018.
15. World Health Organization. *Early childhood development and disability: a discussion paper*, Geneva, Switzerland, 2012, WHO Press, World Health Organization.
16. Illum NO, Gradel KO: Parents' assessments of disability in their children using World Health Organization international classification of functioning, disability and health, child and youth version joined body functions and activity codes related to everyday life, *Clin Med Insights Pediatr* (11):1–11, 2017.
17. President's Council on Bioethics: *Taking care: ethical caregiving in our aging society*, Washington, DC, 2005, US Government Printing Office, pp 53–91, 95–150.

18. Alvidrez J, Castille D, Laude-Sharp M, et al: The National Institute on Minority Health and Health Disparities Research Framework, *Am J Public Health* 109(S1):S16–S20, 2019.
19. Krahn GL, Walker DK, Correa-De-Araujo R: Persons with disabilities as an unrecognized health disparity population, *Am J Public Health* 105(S2):S198–S206, 2015.
20. Weiss EM, Xie D, Cook N, et al: Characteristics associated with preferences for parent-centered decision making in neonatal intensive care, *JAMA Pediatr* 172(5):461–468, 2018.
21. Mars G, Kempen G, Widdershoven G, et al: Conceptualizing autonomy in the context of chronic physical illness: relating philosophical theories to social sciences perspectives, *Health (London)* 12(3):333–348, 2008.
22. Doherty R: The impact of advances in medical technology on rehabilitative care. In Purtilo RB, Jensen GM, Royeen CB, editors: *Educating for moral action*, Philadelphia, 2005, FA Davis, pp 99–106.
23. Family Caregiver Alliance: Caregiver statistics: demographics, April 17, 2019. Available at https://www.caregiver.org/caregiver-statistics-demographics, San Francisco, National Center on Caregiving.
24. Levine C: Acceptance, avoidance and ambiguity: conflicting social values about childhood disability, *Kennedy Inst Ethics J* 115(4):371–383, 2005.
25. Edmondson A: Teamwork on the fly: how to master the new art of teaming, *Harv Bus Rev*: 40: 72, 2012 (April).
26. ordon S, Mendenhall P, O'Connor B: *Beyond the checklist: what else health care can learn from aviation teamwork and safety*, Ithaca, NY, 2012, IRL Press.
27. Lown BA, McIntosh S, Gaines ME, et al: Integrating compassionate, collabortive care (the "Triple C") into health professional education to advance the triple aim of health care, *Acad Med: J Assoc Am Med Coll* 91(3):310–331, 2016.
28. Bickmore T, Schulman D, Lin L: Maintaining engagement in long term interactions with relational agents, *Appl Artif Intell* 24(6):648–666, 2010.

● 13

Ethical Issues in End-of-Life Care

Objectives

The reader should be able to:

- List six ways that a caring response can be achieved in end-of-life care.
- Define palliative care and give at least three examples of how it is expressed.
- Identify some practical means by which a dying patient's trust can be fostered and reasonable expectations can be met by health professionals.
- Discuss how abandonment affects people with life-limiting prognoses.
- Describe four guidelines that can help professionals continue to "abide with" a patient who is dying.
- Recognize some basic ethical concepts that have special importance in the treatment of patients at end of life.
- Discover three "faces" of the virtue of compassion.
- Discuss the professional's duty of nonmaleficence for its relevance in end-of-life care.
- Distinguish ordinary and extraordinary or heroic interventions, and list two criteria for deciding that an intervention is extraordinary.
- Explain the idea of medical futility and its role in the ethical debate about appropriate end-of-life interventions.
- Describe the ethical principle of double effect.
- List three mechanisms to assist patients and professionals in discerning the proper moral limits of intervention.
- Discuss the merits and limitations of advance directives.
- Summarize current themes in ethical debates about clinically assisted suicide and medical euthanasia.

New terms and ideas you will encounter in this chapter

life-limiting prognosis	hospice care	supererogation
end-of-life care	psychological	life-sustaining
palliation	abandonment	interventions
palliative care	abide	forgoing (withholding or
hospice	compassion	withdrawing)

extraordinary means
usual and customary
   treatments
benefit/burden ratio test
medical futility
killing

principle of double effect
advance care planning
living will
durable power
   of attorney for
   healthcare (DPAHC)

U.S. Patient Self-
   Determination Act
   (PSDA)
clinically assisted
   suicide
medical euthanasia

Topics in this chapter introduced in earlier chapters

Topic	Introduced in chapter
Ethics committees	1
Ethics consultation	1
Care and a caring response	2
Patient-centered care	2
Quality of life	2
Ethics-of-care approach	4
Virtue	4
Compassion	4
Benevolence	4
Fidelity	4
Nonmaleficence	4
Autonomy or self-determination	4
Six-step process of ethical decision making	5
Time-limited trial	5
Moral resilience	6
Hope	10
Do not resuscitate (DNR)	10
Shared decision making	10
Informed consent	11
Surrogate decision maker	11
Substituted judgment standard	11
Best interests standard	11

Introduction

Working with patients and their loved ones when the patient has a condition that carries a *life-limiting prognosis* poses special ethical challenges. A life-limiting prognosis sets a course that all expect to end in the patient's death. How should you, the health professional, treat such persons with the dignity they deserve? The terminology often encountered in the healthcare literature (e.g., terminal, fatal, irreversible, incurable) adds anxiety when health professionals use it in conversation with patients and their families. At the same time, your work with these patients can be the perfect opportunity to be a positive influence in their lives. For this and other reasons, this chapter addresses ethical issues that come sharply into focus when a person is going to die as the result of a medical condition. The current term used in the literature and in professional practice that you will encounter is *end-of-life care.*

Throughout this textbook, you have been reminded of the importance of care in the ethics of the health professional–patient relationship. In no situation does this apply more than in the treatment of persons who are coming to the end of their life. Most health professionals want to convey to patients who have incurable illnesses, "I care," and the examples in this chapter illustrate ways in which that message can be meaningfully conveyed. It requires a clear understanding of special ethical considerations that emerge in this type of situation, rigorous application of your technical competence, and personal adaptability to each patient. To help focus your thinking, consider the following story.

 The Story of Almena Lykes, Jarda Roubal, and Roy Moser

Mrs. Almena Lykes is 42 years old and was diagnosed with amyotrophic lateral sclerosis (ALS) about 18 months ago. When she was admitted to the hospital with severe pneumonia and shortness of breath, she had some movement in her arms and could get around in the wheelchair. Despite physical, occupational, and respiratory therapy and good nursing care, she has become weaker since being hospitalized. Test results indicate that the pneumonia probably developed because of weakness of the swallowing muscles (which allowed aspiration of mouth contents into the lungs). She is discouraged, knowing that her condition is going to get progressively worse and that she will eventually die. She also believes that her husband is not willing to care for her at home any longer, a fact that the staff cannot confirm because he has not called or appeared since she was admitted.

After a 2-week course of treatment, Almena's condition takes a decisive turn for the worse. Dr. Jarda Roubal, her physician, believes that she is not going to be able to bounce back from this pneumonia, even with vigorous treatment with antibiotics and respiratory therapy, because of rapid deterioration of her swallowing and breathing muscles. Dr. Roubal discusses the seriousness of her prognosis and the options open to her for interventions regarding her pneumonia (e.g., medications, respiratory therapy) and predicts that she is near to the time when she will have to make a decision whether or not she wishes to be placed on a ventilator. He answers all questions directly about the seriousness of her prognosis. He asks her nurse, Roy Moser, to place a respirator in her room for quick initiation of ventilator support should it be needed.

Yesterday evening, Mrs. Lykes asked Roy to sit down with her by her bed. Tearfully, she told him that she really was ready to die. She requested that her treatments in physical, occupational, and respiratory therapy be discontinued and that she not be placed on a respirator unless it would mean she would suffer less while she was dying. She said she had seen a movie in which a woman was given morphine to speed up the dying process and make it painless and explained that was what she wanted. She also requested a do not resuscitate (DNR) status. "Dr. Roubal means well, but he will make a vegetable out of me," she says, breaking down. Roy said he would talk to Dr. Roubal about her wishes related to the use or nonuse of life-sustaining treatments but that the final decision should be made in collaboration with her, her family, and her interprofessional care team. Then, Roy documented the conversation in her clinical record.

That evening when Dr. Roubal came through to check on the patients, Roy Moser took him aside and conveyed the entire conversation as best he could recall it. Dr. Roubal listened intently and said, "What do you think?"

"I think we should do what she suggests. She isn't going to get better."

After a moment, Dr. Roubal said, "Well, you are right about her not getting better, but I think she is depressed and once she gets on a respirator and over the pneumonia she will see it differently. She still has a lot of life in her." Dr. Roubal then went to visit Almena. He said to her, "The nurse has told me about your concerns. I would like you to think it over. There's still a lot we can do for you."

Later that evening, Roy went back to Almena Lykes's room. Almena looked extremely sad and alone, her eyes puffy from crying. Now she was dry eyed and made an attempt to lift her limp hand. "I don't know what to do," she said.

Before continuing, take a minute to think about Dr. Jarda Roubal's and Roy Moser's response to Almena Lykes.

Reflection

What is each doing to show a caring response to her problems? Do you think one or the other is more correct in their judgment about whether to continue treatment? On what do you base your opinion?

_____

_____

_____

_____

In this story, you can quickly discern by now that several important ethical dimensions of professional practice come into full view. As in previous chapters, the six-step process serves as a guide to highlight some of them; you may identify others.

The Goal: A Caring Response

Suppose that you are Dr. Jarda Roubal or Roy Moser. It goes without saying that Mrs. Lykes deserves all the respectful consideration from you that you would give to any patient. She needs to feel confident that you are competent because her life literally may be in your hands. In a word, she expects you to give her your best attention consistent with a caring response.

As discussed in previous chapters, caring is a balancing act. The very purpose of your professional role is to be technically competent and show the appropriate personalized nurturing also necessary for true care. This becomes even more important in end-of-life care. The health professional who is committed to patient-centered care at end of life does at least the following:

1. Maintains vigilant attention to evidence-based clinical interventions appropriate for the person's condition, whether preventive, rehabilitative, or comfort-enhancing. The diagnosis of an incurable condition does not mean that the entire range of interventions may be prematurely dropped from the clinician's resources for optimal treatment.

2. Takes enough time to communicate with the patient (and loved ones) to get a "feel" for the person's values, strongly held beliefs, habits, cultural and ethnic characteristics, and personality. This also helps facilitate discussion among patients, their support systems, and the care teams regarding how they would like to receive clinical information and handle shared decision-making tasks.

3. Listens carefully to what the person has to say. A focus on the patient's quality of life governs you in your attempt to create a warm, personal environment. Only the patient's (or if the patient is incapable of indicating preferences, the surrogate's) interpretation of what makes life worthwhile counts, not yours or anyone else's interpretations. Sometimes concerns that are important to the patient seem insignificant to a health professional and vice versa. Through simply listening, withholding judgment, holding space, and emotionally connecting, you communicate to patients the healing message that they are not alone.[1]

4. Stays in close contact with all members of the patient's interprofessional care team, even those who seem to be more tangentially involved with the patient's care.

5. Recognizes that a patient's perception of quality of life is fluid near the end of life. Many research studies (and clinical cases) verify the fact that

perception of quality of life often undergoes revision as an individual's condition evolves.[2] Patients should be given information, choices, and control whenever possible. Although a patient's concerns and desires may shift near end of life, the value of autonomy often remains. Autonomy allows patients the freedom to shape their lives in ways consistent with their values, character, and conviction.

6. Understands that the final phase of a condition brings with it a myriad of emotions. Patients facing end of life may experience shock, anger, fear, grief, denial, pain, and depression; others may express readiness or relief. In the words of Hank Dunn, "Facing the reality of death is like encountering a wide river that must be crossed…. None of us can force one another across."[3] And not all patients believe there is another side. These emotions take time to process and work through. Patients need your comfort, patience, and assistance to effectively do so.

Reflection

What do you expect weighs heavily on Mrs. Lykes's mind right now?

_____

_____

_____

How can you respond in a warm and supportive manner to her concerns?

_____

_____

_____

_____

Summary

A caring response in end-of-life situations requires apt attention to specific quality-of-life issues for the patient and family that may arise only in this final phase of the patient's life.

● Palliative Care

As one comes to realize that healthcare includes the provision of comfort measures to people who are dying, and attempts at curative and restorative treatments until they are shown to be futile, the notion of palliative care becomes integral to a caring response. *Palliation* means to reduce the severity of or relieve symptoms without curing the underlying disease.[4] *Palliative care* is patient-centered and family-centered care that optimizes quality of life by anticipating, preventing, and treating the physical, functional, psychosocial, and spiritual pain and suffering associated with life-threatening illness.[5] Palliative care is not limited to individuals with incurable conditions that lead to death, although that is the focus of our discussion.

Some objectives of palliative care include the following general guidelines:
- People with advanced, potentially fatal conditions and those close to them should expect and receive skillful and supportive care not focused on curing the patient.
- Health professionals must commit themselves to using their professional knowledge effectively to prevent and relieve pain and other consequences of a serious illness.
- Health professionals should regain awareness and humility about what modern medicine can and cannot do so that patients can deal with their own death realistically, not as the enemy but as a part of life.
- Health professionals must recognize that the patient's continuing downward course may be a time of anxiety for the health professional, too, which poses a challenge to the entire team.[6]
- Providing the best care possible means that as much imagination, competence, and energy must be directed to palliative interventions as would be devoted to care of a patient without an incurable condition.
- Palliative care is not setting specific. It can be delivered across all healthcare settings because it is based on patient and family's needs, not prognosis. The focus on assessment of symptom burden, functional status, and quality of life transcends organizations, inpatient hospitals, outpatient practices, health systems, home agencies, and providers.[7]

Throughout the patient's illness, the goal of providing the best palliative care possible includes giving emotional support to people closest to the patient. This helps encourage the patient, although you might find yourself frustrated with the patient's relatives and close friends because they are angry and confused or feeling intense sorrow and may transfer their feelings to you. Their demands, worries, questions, and interference with treatment can be disconcerting, especially when their actions call into question your own best judgment or exacerbate your own anxieties about the patient's plight. (This may be a good moment to review Fig. 12.2, which lists the sources of stress families experience when faced with caring for a loved one with a chronic condition. The sources are similar when end-of-life care goes on over a period of time.) Remember that any time the patient's most intimate sources of support are alienated or harmed, the patient also inevitably suffers deleterious consequences.

In palliative care, stopping intense efforts to affect a cure must be coordinated with an even more intense effort to engage in a regimen of interventions aimed at reduction of discomfort. The words of a talented physician, Ned Cassem, from over 40 years ago still have great relevance today:

> *Even when we decide that our advanced technologies are no longer indicated, we can still agree that certain extreme measures are indicated—extreme responsibility, extraordinary sensitivity, heroic compassion.[8]*

These words are especially valuable because often at the moment that you admit the person is indeed beyond medical intervention aimed at cure, you may momentarily feel at a loss as to how to continue to express your caring. We can imagine that Roy Moser had this feeling when he walked into Almena Lykes's room and noticed she had been crying or when she confessed she did not "know what to do." Your own imagination may be thwarted by the knowledge that the patient's time is limited. This could deter you from setting attainable goals that may be of importance to the patient. Tonight is the future. Tomorrow is the future. Mrs. Lykes can be encouraged toward the goal of using the bathroom unassisted tonight or sitting up to write some letters tomorrow. Sometimes, too, patients are hesitant to offer information about their desires because they fear the goal seems irrelevant or even silly to someone else. For example, one young woman confided to the chaplain that she longed to go to the chapel for religious services but was afraid it was too much work for the nurses to get her there. Another woman who needed large doses of pain-reducing medication told the medical technologist she was concerned that the "fuzziness" created by the medication would impair her judgment when her lawyer came to discuss her estate. The technologist relayed the information to the woman's physician, and the physician arranged to have the medication withheld during the lawyer's visit, with the grateful consent of the patient.

Another aspect of palliative care is to adjust your approach according to the probable time left before the patient's death. Because the human condition is specific to each person, one has to be an artist of "good timing." The person who senses that the end is near often asks to be left alone with only a few select people or, in some cases, with no one at all. To be cheerfully intrusive at such times denies a person the need to determine the use of last moments. In contrast, to treat persons who may live for months or years with a slowly progressing illness as if they are about to die at any moment robs those persons of the sense of belonging among the living. A balance is needed to plan and attend to life tasks amid what may be an uncertain disease trajectory. For example, a 16-year-old girl with a slowly progressing leukemia went into her local hospital for her monthly blood tests. A laboratory technician who had not seen her for several months greeted her by saying, "Well, hello there. Great to see you are still around!" The teenager's mother, who had accompanied her to this visit, later told her husband, "She was just teasing, but I know it made Haley (her daughter) feel funny—like maybe she was supposed to have died already or something."

Anyone who has experienced the ordeal of a loved one's prolonged dying knows that some of the tensest moments are those related to not knowing how long the person will be alive, to being afraid that one will prematurely die, and to not knowing how to make appropriate plans for the future. The art of palliative care includes being as sensitive as possible to the time frame the patient and family are living with and adjusting your own approach accordingly.

Hospice Care

One highly successful alternative for patients with conditions beyond medical cure is *hospice*, which originated in England and has spread to many countries in the world. *Hospice care* is focused on caring, not curing. It is considered the model for quality compassionate care for people facing a life-limiting illness, providing expert medical care, pain management, and emotional and spiritual support tailored to the patient's (and family's or other support network's) needs and wishes.[9] Hospice teams are interprofessional. They recognize the dying process as a part of the normal living process and provide support and care for the patient during this phase. Hospice programs provide a unique set of benefits for patients and their families. Evidence shows improved pain assessment and management, improved bereavement outcomes, decreased caregiver burden, improved quality of life, lower costs, and lower mortality rates among family members of patients who received hospice care.[10,11] Patients are generally eligible for hospice when they forgo curative treatment and have a life expectancy of 6 months or less, although as the concept continues to evolve, these regulations may change.

Summary

Palliative care has many dimensions, among them your concerted effort to maximize quality of life through decreasing physical, functional, psychological, and emotional pain and attending to the patient's own timing and life situation.

Now that the general groundwork has been laid for what a caring response entails in this type of situation, we let us turn to the familiar process of ethical decision making to consider Almena Lykes's story in more detail.

The Six-Step Process in End-of-Life Situations

The art of caring requires that health professionals are keenly aware of when the moral aspects of the relationship hit a snag and an ethical problem appears.

Reflection

Do you think Dr. Jarda Roubal and Roy Moser are faced with an ethical problem? If so, jot down why or why not and how their respective roles as physician and nurse are similar and different.

_____

_____

_____

_____

Given the seriousness of Almena Lykes's clinical condition, the health professionals face an ethical problem. The life-or-death decision about life-prolonging measures must be negotiated to her satisfaction, and her present anxiety must be taken seriously into account. Let us review the salient facts of her story to help highlight some details of the tensions in her particular situation.

Step 1: Gather Relevant Information

The most important fact is that Mrs. Lykes has a progressive, incurable condition, the pathology of which will continue to cause her muscles to grow weaker. She will experience greater functional impairment and ultimately failure of her lungs and respiratory muscles. She will lose control of her throat muscles, resulting in an inability to swallow. Eventually, she will die of her condition.

Dr. Jarda Roubal is monitoring this clinical course and trying to maintain her respiratory functions. Roy Moser is a central, coordinating figure of the interprofessional care team of therapists, technologists, and others who gauge how various interventions are helping to maintain her remaining health. They also are trying to stay in touch with her feelings and keep her optimally functional and comfortable. You know that all three of the key players in this story are at a crossroads. Should Mrs. Lykes's expressed wish to forgo ventilatory support now be honored, or should the health professionals listen to her confusion in the lonely evening hours and again encourage her to hang on? Dr. Roubal will be the one to make the final call, medically speaking, about how to proceed with technological and medical interventions. However, from an ethical viewpoint, that call must be made with as much certainty—and in as much accord with Mrs. Lykes's real wishes—as possible.

One key to her suffering is that she may be abandoned by her husband and may be (or already is) left alone by someone she deeply counted on. The fear and reality of such abandonment is common enough that it warrants your further consideration here. Almena, like many patients who face dying and eventual death, may fear isolation, pain, dependence, and the family's response to her deteriorating condition. Not only do patients experience betrayal from their own body, they often experience physical and emotional betrayal from those closest to them. Some patients like Almena with progressive neurological conditions may feel they are living with dying. This awareness of death can prompt one to reflect on life's meaning and to seek closure in personal, practical, and spiritual matters.[12]

Abandonment: A Patient's Reasonable Fear

Almena Lykes knows that things are not going to get better, clinically speaking. Sometimes spouses, other loved ones, and friends fall away during the patient's process of dying. Some challenges that face family and other loved ones in regard to their role during a long-term course were mentioned in Chapter 12. Mrs. Lykes has a life-limiting, disabling, and incurable condition. For whatever reason, Mr. Lykes has disappeared; whether his absence is because of fear, weariness, disgust, or anger at her situation or his own pathology is not possible to ascertain.

In addition to abandonment by loved ones, patients also sometimes detect that health professionals are distancing themselves, which exacerbates the patients' anxiety and suffering. Health professionals seldom physically abandon patients who have an incurable medical condition. Sometimes, however, they are caught in policies that prevent them from giving a patient as much of or the type of treatment the professionals believe that person needs.

Psychological abandonment is the greater danger that sometimes leads a health professional to physical neglect of the patient. Why? For one thing, their concepts of what healthcare interventions should accomplish may lead professionals to distance themselves because the patient continues to "get worse." Others are repulsed by the appearance, odors, or other disturbing manifestations of a patient's condition.[13] Psychological preparation for the pain of loss when a patient dies is advisable, and sometimes health professionals distance themselves to protect against the pain of that loss and feeling of failure. But psychological abandonment is distancing that far exceeds the use of necessary defense mechanisms. It follows that no matter what Mrs. Lykes's husband chooses to do, the responsibility for not abandoning her also falls on Dr. Roubal, Roy Moser, and the other members of the inter-professional care team.

 Reflection

Suppose you are Roy Moser that evening in Almena Lykes's room. What aspects of this situation might make you feel like fleeing? What steps can you take to help ensure this type of harm does not befall her? What additional information from Mrs. Lykes might be helpful or necessary to provide appropriate care for her, remaining faithful to your role?

_____

_____

_____

_____

Abiding: A Patient's Reasonable Hope

The idea of abiding with a patient may help you to think about what the opposite of abandonment looks like. To *abide* means "to endure without yielding," "to bear patiently," and "to remain stable."[14] Sometimes, good care simply requires digging your heels in and standing firm with the patient as his or her condition changes.

The following are some general guidelines that can help you to maintain an attentive position toward Mrs. Lykes that she will experience as you are abiding with her. You will recognize them as having themes similar to the ones you were introduced to as a part of personalized care and good palliative care in these situations. The guidelines include:

- Recognize your own feelings of fear, disgust, and repulsion. They are often embarrassing, and the inclination is to pretend that they do not exist. Denial does not make them disappear; you must muster the courage to be vulnerable to engage more fully with your patients.
- Make efforts to talk to patients so that you will know them better and can focus on who they are personally. In many instances, the troubling feelings become less important.
- Encourage sessions in your workplace in which everyone can share their feelings in a safe, constructive environment. These opportunities to discuss the impact of providing care promote well-being. As you recall from Chapter 6, an environment that supports resilience, self-care, and mutual support is essential for your long-term health and effectiveness as a health professional.

⑨ Summary
Physical or psychological abandonment of a person who is dying can be encountered by professionals who choose to abide with the patient. Professionals need mutual support and self-care resources in this situation.

Having touched on some salient features of the patient's situation, let us now turn back to the ethical decision-making process.

Step 2: Identify the Type of Ethical Problem

Both the physician, Jarda Roubal, and the nurse, Roy Moser, are faced with ethical problems that come from a high degree of uncertainty about the best course of action to take for Mrs. Lykes.

Moral Distress

At the point you enter the picture, Dr. Roubal has made a clinical judgment that he believes is in Almena's best interest, but he certainly is shaken by Roy's report. Roy, too, must be in a situation in which he cannot be sure what is going on. Both have additional work to do as moral agents; therefore the health professionals face moral distress. They, like she, are emotionally unsettled, apparently because of their own uncertainty about how to proceed. They know she is approaching the end of her life and has a right to request the discontinuation of therapies. However, Dr. Roubal and others also want to be sure she is not making an impulsive decision because the stakes of the outcome are literally life and death. Almena has stated that one of her concerns regarding this phase of her condition is that if Dr. Roubal puts her on the ventilator it will "make a vegetable out of her." Roy has worked with many patients with amyotrophic lateral sclerosis (ALS) who have chosen ventilation as a pulmonary support and who have done quite well. Some only need ventilation at night. Once Almena's pneumonia clears, she may be in this category. Would she be okay with this as an option? Roy Moser also wonders if Almena has ever seen other patients with ALS who use assistive devices such as computerized communication systems or environmental control units. Her knowledge of these technologies as possible options to help her live better in the end stages of ALS would ensure that she is has all the needed information to make a truly informed decision.

Locus of Authority

This juncture of their quandary is an apt place for you to consider a locus of authority conflict.

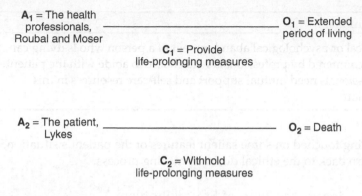

A_1 = The health
professionals,
Roubal and Moser

C_1 = Provide
life-prolonging measures

O_1 = Extended
period of living

A_2 = The patient,
Lykes

C_2 = Withhold
life-prolonging measures

O_2 = Death

A = Moral agent
C = Course of action
O = Outcome

Fig. 13.1. Locus of authority considerations.

You recall that considerations of locus of authority come into play when two or more moral agents in the situation need to decide which of them should be the final appropriate moral voice in the decision (see Fig. 13.1). To the extent that Almena Lykes is competent to make her own decisions, and the diagnosis of an incurable condition is confirmed, the ultimate answer is easy: She is. The physician has requested something that is potentially lifesaving, so we want to be sure she is not making a decision to refuse it on partial knowledge or because she is clinically depressed. She must not make a decision that she will regret and that is irreversible.

Talking to her further is an obvious next step the interprofessional care team will want to pursue. In Chapter 11, you were introduced to informed consent. The goal is to be sure that Almena is competent to make, and is making, an informed decision. Dr. Roubal believes she might be refusing the ventilator because she is depressed and that she will change her mind, suggesting that she will want to be put on the respirator when her depression lifts. Although many patients with chronic conditions suffer from depression at some point during their illness, this is not a judgment he should make lightly. A visit by the liaison psychiatrist can help ascertain whether she is clinically depressed to the point of being unable to make this important decision. The position he apparently is holding, that of a paternalistic authority who will try to talk her into accepting the respirator, should not be maintained without the additional information about her mental status.

⬤ 📖 *Reflection*

Recall that there are two types of moral distress. From the description we have given, is the team faced with type A or type B?

_____

_____

_____

_____

The uncertainty about the obvious best clinical way to proceed is so tied to the life and death consequences of their decision that they are experiencing type B moral distress. This often happens around end-of-life care, although one of the values of the ethical study you are engaged in is to decrease the margin of uncertainty with salient facts and the other steps of ethical decision making.

Step 3: Use Ethics Theories or Approaches to Analyze the Problem

What resources does each of these professionals need to arrive at a caring response in this type of situation? The ethics of care approach places virtues in a central place and provides a useful means of assessing the ethical issues here. Much has been written about the virtue of compassion in healthcare, and nowhere is it more important than when the patient has an incurable condition. The term *compassion* is defined as the emotional response to another's pain or suffering, involving an authentic desire to help.[15] When applied in the context of healthcare, treating another with compassion is not only the right thing to do, it is a moral imperative. Lown and colleagues summarized this well, stating that:

> *Without empathy and compassion, care may be technically excellent but depersonalized, and will fail to address the unique emotional, psychological and social needs of the person who seeks health and care.*[16]

As a result of scientific study of the effects of compassion on health, healthcare, and health providers, the new field of *compassionomics* has emerged. Overwhelming evidence exists regarding the effects of compassion on patient outcomes, patient safety, provider well-being, employee engagement, and organizational performance.[17] In short, compassionate care makes a difference. From an ethics perspective, you are invited to further examine compassion as a virtue, as a duty, and as going beyond duty.

Compassion: Three Moral Faces of an Idea

The three powerful components of compassion are[18]

*   The character trait or virtue of sympathetic understanding recognized as a virtue;
*   The willingness to perform your professional responsibilities toward the patient, recognized as moral duty; and
*   The readiness to go beyond the call of duty.

These dispositions are often observed in others but may not readily recognize them as compassion.

Compassion as a virtue. The virtues of kindness and benevolence are recognizable as promoting a desire to treat people with gentleness and to "do good" when it is in your power to do so. Research in neuroscience demonstrates that being able to do good depends first on the ability to notice another's suffering and resonate in some way with it so that you become aware of the needs and wants of the other person.[19] The word compassion comes from the Latin *passio* (suffering) and *con* (with). It entails the desire to treat others with empathetic understanding. It is from this root meaning that compassion usually is understood solely as a disposition toward others, a virtue.

Reflection

Knowing as little as you do about Mrs. Lykes's situation, what do you believe are some of her needs that warrant your empathetic understanding? To aid in your reflection, write them down.

_____

_____

_____

_____

The desire to be empathetic is a resource in itself. You might find it expressed in something as simple as a reassuring arm across her shoulder, knowing she is discouraged, or a telephone call to assist Mrs. Lykes in making contact with a close friend or a person in religious life who has been a source of guidance or comfort to her in the past. To do so with understanding increases the likelihood that you will get it right in terms of the way you choose to express your empathy. Compassion is a virtue that closely is associated with what it means to care. If you recall from Chapter 2, care is an opportunity but also is a burden. In other words, it goes beyond any superficial understanding of kindness or benevolence. The additional two components of compassion help to highlight this interpretation.

Compassion as willingly doing your duty. A form of compassion sometimes overlooked is willingness to perform your duties on behalf of the patient's best interests as you have discerned those interests through your empathetic posture. As compassion compels you to do what is right, you can see how two aspects of ethical thought (character traits and the deontological approach of duties) are brought together in an actual situation. Compassion, as a character trait in the type of person you want to be, aids you in the desire actually to do what you discern to be right. This helps you to keep to task, to pay attention to doing your work competently, and to not be careless about the well-being of the patient when you would rather be meeting a friend or golfing or even going about some other aspect of your daily work. In a word, it helps you to abide with the patient.

Compassion as going beyond duty. Finally, the motivating force of compassion positions you as a moral agent to exercise kindnesses that go beyond duty. In philosophic terms, acts that altruistically go beyond duty are called acts of *supererogation.* An example recalled by the author was of the recent death of a pediatric patient. The infant was in the neonatal intensive care unit for more than 7 weeks, during which time the ups and downs of his critical condition roller-coastered both the care team and the family through much uncertainty. The infant was withdrawn from life-sustaining treatment and died. The infant's funeral was attended by several of his care providers. This supererogative act brought tears to the parents' eyes to see such deep compassion actualized.

The Principle of Nonmaleficence

Your general duty of fidelity or faithfulness to patients includes the stringent principle not to harm them. Do you remember the more philosophical term for this duty? If you said "nonmaleficence," you are right. The deliberate and diligent efforts of many before you to put in place procedures to assist you in providing compassionate care is one indicator that your moral obligation not to harm has been taken seriously by health professionals and society.

Summary

Virtues and character traits guide the moral agent to act within an ethics of care approach. At the same time, the principle of nonmaleficence shows that the deontological approach also helps inform what is right in this type of situation.

To learn more specifically the forms that right actions might take in end-of-life care situations, let us proceed to the next step of decision making.

Step 4: Explore the Practical Alternatives

You have already noted that if you were in the shoes of Jarda Roubal or Roy Moser, an ethics of care and principle-based approach would have led you to explore what Mrs. Lykes really knows about the decision to be made, if she is too depressed to make an informed decision, and finally, what her considered choice is.

So, one alternative is to discuss your (and her) quandary with other members of the interprofessional care team who have been involved in her treatment across the healthcare delivery system: inpatient, outpatient, and home care. This activity will help decrease the amount of moral distress the team is experiencing. These discussions (along with the information gathering completed in step 1) will provide clarity to the locus of authority conflict and place the team in a better position to creatively problem solve alternatives together. This step is a place in which the *who* and *how* is broached with Almena once the decision is made about *what* is the morally correct course of action.

Once you have reached a point of greater certainty, you will have to assume a function appropriate to your professional role on the team involved in Almena Lykes's care in regard to life-prolonging interventions or, as they are often called, *life-sustaining interventions*. Life-sustaining interventions is that term applied to many technologies that assist in basic life functions, such as breathing, eating, and maintenance of vital organs that otherwise will shut down. Life-sustaining interventions range from cardiopulmonary resuscitation (CPR) to mechanical ventilation to nutrition and hydration to antibiotics, to name a few. Most of the difficult clinical and ethical issues arise around how far to go in *forgoing* these life-sustaining interventions, either in *withholding* their start-up or, if they have been started, in *withdrawing* them at a later time. The issues related to forgoing life-sustaining treatments are so important that you will learn more about them later in this chapter.

Assuming Dr. Roubal's referral to psychiatry has deemed Mrs. Lykes to be mentally competent, the team must determine. The proper moral limits of clinical interventions designed to support an extension on the length and quality of her life. Therefore one basic practical determination you have to make is whether interventions in this situation are "ordinary" or "extraordinary," according to what Almena Lykes believes is the balance of benefits over burdens she will receive by initiating them.

Employing Ordinary and Extraordinary Distinctions

Having introduced you earlier in this chapter to some problems that arise because health professionals stop treatment prematurely or psychologically withdraw, you now have an opportunity to consider the converse. Psychologically, withholding or stopping a treatment is sometimes difficult for a health professional. The development of do not resuscitate (DNR) orders some 40 years ago marked a pivotal change in healthcare delivery because it was the first order to directly withhold treatment.[20] The ethical notion of heroic procedures or *extraordinary means* has been developed to help protect patients, families, and health professionals from overzealous "do all that is possible" approaches.

From an ethical point of view, even *usual and customary treatments* (i.e., those considered the usual treatment regimen for conditions of this type) can, under certain circumstances, be judged extraordinary or heroic. The ethical criterion for considering a treatment heroic is that it may inflict undue physical, psychological, or spiritual harm on the person even as it serves to prolong the patient's life.[21] For instance, suppose that a relatively new treatment is being used successfully for ALS. It could add several months to Mrs. Lykes's life; however, it has disturbing cognitive side effects. Mrs. Lykes rejects it out of hand. You must honor a competent patient's wishes. On that basis, this new treatment becomes extraordinary.

⊙ Summary

Extraordinary treatment means that when a person makes a fully informed decision to refuse further treatment, that treatment is inappropriate, even though it may prolong life or have other beneficial physiological effects.

The ethical distinction between ordinary and extraordinary rests on the patient's informed decision, not the health professional's judgment. Any intervention, from the simplest and routine to the most technologically advanced, can be ordinary or extraordinary, depending on its fittingness for a particular patient. This is the most important thing you must bear in mind, not the fact of how "high-tech" or, in your view, invasive or expensive or experimental is the intervention.

The same test can be applied to an incompetent patient, but the surrogate decision maker bears the weight of deciding what the patient would have found an unbearable burden and what would constitute a benefit.

 Reflection
Now that you know more about the concept of ordinary and extraordinary measures, list some additional alternatives to help Mrs. Lykes and the team decide the next steps in her plan of care.

_____

_____

_____

_____

Applying the benefit/burden ratio test. Why do patients refuse certain treatments? Because they decide that treatments that may be promising from a medical point of view and that are administered routinely to others impose too great a burden on them to be worth it. Honoring the patient's assessment of benefits versus burdens in an intervention has been termed the *benefit/burden ratio test.* In the story you read, Almena Lykes said this at one point. Patients may refuse for many reasons. Some may detest the idea of a treatment that will cause memory loss, or will require amputation or other disfigurement, or has side effects that cause great discomfort, or is extremely costly to the family. At the same time, the reasons for refusal may be the benefit of gracefully "letting go." You can easily imagine two patients who would receive similar physiological benefits from a medical intervention but who would assign different weight to the personal, human benefits accruing from the treatment. Mrs. Lykes might weigh the benefit of the experimental intervention or even permanent use of the ventilator quite differently than you would because she believes she has accomplished what she hoped to in life and has a sense of being at peace with the nearness of death. She may have certain spiritual or religious convictions such as afterlife beliefs that guide her decision making. For these reasons, discussions around life-sustaining interventions must focus on the values and goals of care, rather than on specific treatments.

What happens when a competent patient refuses a treatment that the health professionals believe will be highly beneficial and effective? Health professionals are not required or allowed to override the patient's decision, even in this difficult situation. Competent patients can refuse any type of treatment, even one that is life-sustaining. Sometimes patients choose to withdraw from clinical care altogether and go home, an option they have a right to choose as long as it is an informed and competent choice.

Assessing medically futile care. The notion of extraordinary care also applies when there is no reasonable hope that patients will medically benefit from the care even though they may want it. The phrase around which discussion has evolved is *medical futility.* It addresses the flip side of the coin of the previous discussion of how patients have a right to refuse a treatment that health professionals think is medically appropriate. Sometimes patients (and more often families) demand interventions that health professionals judge are not designed to be of any benefit to the patient. In recent years, the idea of medical futility has become a point of lively sociopolitical debate and has raised questions of what medical and other clinical interventions actually are designed (and able) to achieve in life and death situations.[22]

At first glance, the idea of providing medically futile care seems ridiculous. Why does it even need to be discussed?

In many situations, interventions that did do some good initially are continued because to now withdraw them appears to the family or other interested parties to be harming, even killing, the patient. The discussion of medical futility has created helpful guidelines for judging when health professionals justifiably may withdraw previously helpful interventions on the basis that the patient's condition has changed.

Futility always has meant that something would not help. But today, with so many interventions available, there is a need for a clear understanding by everyone of what "helping" and "not helping" means. The discussion of medical futility has led to a refined understanding of when an intervention may be withheld even though a patient wants it. In recent years, some legal challenges have concerned how far to accede to a patient's, or surrogate's, demands in determining the degree or types of interventions that are warranted. The idea of futility has been useful in clarifying that medically useless treatments should be withheld or withdrawn, no matter how much a patient or surrogate wants them.

The ethically appropriate standard by which a procedure can be judged medically futile is the good of the whole patient, not that it can sustain a single organ or body system. The rationale for this should be clear because some medical interventions may allow an organ (e.g., the heart) to survive, but the patient's condition may otherwise be completely irreversible and devastating.

In today's exciting high-technology healthcare environment, the tendency to extend the arm of technical intervention can lead to a distortion of the art of clinical intervention.[23] From the earliest times, our professional predecessors warned about this type of abuse, counseling always that our practice follow not only the science but also what we know about the effect on the patient's well-being.

The standard for declaring an intervention medically futile continues to be the subject of debate. Questions regarding survival, prognosis, reasonable hope of recovery, and quality of life can be exceedingly difficult.[24] Many professionals assert that the values of a person's life that make intervention worthwhile are not for others to determine in these complex situations.

At least three measuring rods have been applied to the idea that an intervention can be called "futile," giving health professionals the opportunity to consider not honoring the patient's or family's wishes.

- *Physiological standard*. This approach is based on the clinical evidence that an intervention will not, or no longer will, have any appreciable beneficial physiological effect on the patient. An example is the use of antibiotics for a viral infection.
- *Probability standard*. A second approach is to try to quantify the probability that an intervention will have an appreciable beneficial physiological effect. Proponents of this position suggest that although the intervention could conceivably achieve the patient's goal, it is highly unlikely so it should be dropped as a realistic alternative for this patient.
- *Quality-of-life/qualitative standard*. In this standard, the goal is to develop either an individual or group standard of quality of life. The benefit is

framed in terms of the quality of life a patient would realize. For example, should an intervention that would bring a patient to the point of responding to light and sound but never to the point of responding to the environment in a more purposive fashion be judged futile? The risks of determining entire categories of persons who have qualities worth or not worth supporting with interventions should be apparent in this approach.

 Summary

Any treatment is extraordinary if it is also futile (i.e., offers no appreciable hope of benefit to the patient).

You will be joining the ranks of the health professions at a time when this important topic undoubtedly will continue to be debated. Currently, all three standards of futility are applied in different settings. Let us return now to the larger framework in which this discussion is placed; namely, the criteria of ordinary and extraordinary care. Whether the care will benefit this patient in this circumstance is the governing consideration.

Keeping the Focus on the (Whole) Patient

The ethical reasoning about the limits of intervention that are morally appropriate (including consideration of ordinary and extraordinary distinctions) requires a focus on the individual patient's well-being as a point of reference. There are several helpful mechanisms for approaching the difficult question of ascertaining when enough is enough; their goal is to provide a more humane approach to patients who are critically ill or have irreversible conditions that will lead to death.

The interprofessional care team, guided by the physician, who is the appropriate person to make the clinical judgment about the patient's medical status, should make the decisions, informed by the patient's wishes. However, as we have been discussing, the key considerations that arise are not solely about medical status.

Ethics committees are one mechanism to guide health professionals, patients, and their families in end-of-life care decisions. There is one important difference between what you (as a current or future health professional) must do and what an ethics committee or ethics consultant does. You are in a position to perform, or at least be on the team that performs, the action. The committee or consultant stops with identifying the practical alternatives with the distinctions you have been reading about in this chapter. Often, the decision involves whether to withdraw or withhold measures that, under other circumstances, would be considered usual and customary to use, or, in other words, would be "ordinary treatment."

Forgoing Life Supports

The function of withdrawing and withholding life-sustaining treatment was mentioned previously in this chapter as one way to approach the limits of what clinical care can and cannot do. On the positive side, when a condition is reversible, many technologies act as "bridges" between life-threatening symptoms and health, allowing the person to return to a healthy, or healthier, state. Further, when a condition is not reversible, medical supports and technologies sometimes act as life-sustaining bridges between severe episodes within the dying process but ultimately are a temporary bridge between life and death itself. Almena Lykes is faced with being put on mechanical ventilation. At this point, she is refusing this treatment, and Jarda Roubal and Roy Moser are concerned about the enormity of her decision. Her response indicates she is at a point where to continue to ply her with more devices to assist in various organ functions such as breathing is moving from life-sustaining to life-prolonging, raising questions about what it means to "prolong life." Sometimes, such prolongation begins to look like an assault on the patient as a person, overriding his or her values, quality of life, and judgment about whether the artificially supported organs are indeed "life."

The proper moral limits of medical intervention described in the preceding discussion provide a general ethical framework for forgoing life-sustaining treatment. An intervention that the patient (or the patient's surrogate) finds much more burdensome than beneficial may be withheld or removed ethically. A futile intervention that will not reverse the condition or symptom ("offers no appreciable hope of benefit") also may be withheld or withdrawn.

In such an act, you, the health professional, are not killing the patient. It is an ethically justifiable act, the end of which may be the patient's death, but it does not meet the criterion of "killing." *Killing* is a direct act of commission, meaning that you, the agent, intend to bring about a patient's death and actively intervene to do so. In other words, in forgoing a procedure, you are not engaging in the activity with the intention of ending the patient's life nor are you the direct cause of death. For example, in the case of Mrs. Lykes, she has a disease that will cause her death. Her death will probably come sooner without artificial, medically applied interventions to assist her breathing, heartbeat, kidney function, ingestion of nutrition and hydration, and other bodily functions, but eventually the medical condition directly will kill her. She does not have a ventilator to assist her in her breathing. Dr. Roubal, her physician, determines that she will die shortly without this medical intervention, but she refuses it anyway. Her death will be brought about by the illness within her. At best, her death can be delayed by your intervention.[25]

A decision to forgo a treatment should be made openly, communicated with the team, and documented in the medical record so that all health professionals involved in the patient's care are aware of the decision. A physician may, in private consultation with the patient or patient's family, decide that a patient will not receive a certain intervention, but if there is no documentation of this decision in the patient's medical record, the nurses, residents, or others on duty will feel obligated to initiate it in the event of a life-threatening episode.

 Summary

Forgoing (whether withdrawing or withholding) treatment is not to be confused with acts of directly ending a patient's life.

Decisions concerning limitations in life-sustaining treatments can be psychologically difficult for health professionals. The process of withdrawing the life-sustaining treatment of nutrition and hydration is especially challenging. Although professionals may know that from a scientific, ethical, and legal perspective there should be no differentiation between withholding and withdrawing artificial nutrition and hydration, emotionally it seems to feel true, nevertheless, when they disconnect the feeding tube.[26] All the team support mechanisms discussed in Chapter 7 need to be brought into play to assist colleagues in these difficult moments.

Principle of double effect. The *principle of double effect* is an ethical reasoning tool that can help you in situations in which you act with the intent of providing palliative care for a patient but, in so doing, have the unintended effect of hastening the patient's death. The most commonly cited example of this principle is the administration of a pain reliever (e.g., morphine) that has a side effect of compromising respiration. Because the patient becomes more and more tolerant of the medication, doses high enough to relieve the pain also suppress and at some point stop the patient's breathing.

The principle of double effect acknowledges that one act can embrace two effects: an intended effect and an unintended, secondary effect. The intended effect governs the morality of the act. In this case, the intended effect is the patient's comfort, with the professional acting on the presumption that the quality of life must be preserved. The inescapable but unintended secondary effect is that at some point in the continuum of this care the patient will die of the high dosage. Another aspect is that the increase in dosage must be the minimum necessary to achieve the patient's comfort. Finally, the unintended side effect cannot ever become the intended effect; that is, death cannot become the goal of the person providing the medication.

In summary, the most important thing for you to learn about this tool is that the intent is key. The intent to relieve the patient's pain or other serious discomfort governs the morality of the act, not the unfortunate and unintended secondary consequences (i.e., the patient dies). The second most important thing to learn is that the proportion of increase in the comfort-enhancing intervention must be only the minimum needed to achieve the intended effect; namely, the patient's relief of suffering from pain or other symptoms. Although only the prescribing professional has authority to order such medication, nurses almost always must implement the procedures, and other team members may be involved in ensuring the patient's comfort.

Steps 5 and 6: Complete the Action and Evaluate the Process and Outcome

Returning to the story as written, Dr. Jarda Roubal and Roy Moser have several considerations to take into account before they decide whether to withhold the ventilator and other life-prolonging measures. Their first action is to get Almena Lykes's wishes as crystal clear as possible through continued conversation with her and to take whatever steps are necessary to learn whether she is indeed clinically depressed so that she is not in a reliable state to know her true wishes. Further action regarding intervention cannot justifiably be completed without knowing her informed preferences. Once they know this important information, they will have an opportunity to work together with her and the team to continue each portion of her care motivated by the goal of a caring response.

Oftentimes, in cases such as Almena's, a time-limited trial of life-sustaining treatment is warranted. As introduced in Chapter 5, a time-limited trial designates the use of a life-sustaining treatment or other therapeutic intervention for a defined time period. The time period can range greatly depending on the intervention or agreed-on clinical outcome. The purpose of such a trial is to ascertain the true benefits and burdens of an intervention.[27] At each decision point, the team, in collaboration with the patient, is well advised to use the tools of evaluation and thoughtful reflection on the portion of the action they have just completed. These conditions help ensure that Almena does not become abandoned and that her care remains competent and personalized.

Assessment of Mrs. Lykes's circumstances and the health professionals' considerations should provide you with a good general framework for a caring response in end-of-life care. However, before leaving the subject, you will benefit from considering two additional facets of such care: first, informed consent in situations in which a patient clearly is no longer competent to make decisions; and second, a brief discussion of clinically assisted suicide and medical euthanasia.

Advance Care Planning in End-of-Life Care

What should happen when persons are, or become, incompetent? Recall from Chapter 11 that their wishes then are "heard" through the voice of an appointed surrogate. One modern societal mechanism to assist surrogates and professionals alike in important decisions under such circumstances is *advance care planning,* a process that includes discussing, determining, or executing treatment directives that are in alignment with patients values, preferences, and goals; appointing a proxy decision maker; documentation; and periodic review of advance care plans.[28,29]

Advance directives are processes accompanied by forms that have been developed to help reassure patients that their end-of-life wishes will be honored. They are a tool for ensuring that care providers and significant others know what treatment the patient would, or would not, want. Advance directives are legally binding in all 50 states and become effective only when patients no longer are able to make their wishes known regarding the types and extent of medical intervention that they think are appropriate.

Reflection
Because of their emphasis on the patient's wishes, what ethical principle forms the foundation for advance directives?

_____

_____

_____

_____

If you responded "autonomy" or "self-determination," you remember well what you have learned so far. If you did not answer correctly, now is a good time to go back and review the discussion of autonomy in Chapter 4.

There are basically two major types of advance directives, although some documents bear slightly different names or combine the two:
1. *Living will* documents are designed to enable patients to specify the types of treatment they would want to have and, more importantly, not have.
2. *Durable power of attorney for healthcare (DPAHC)* documents are designed to enable patients to specify a surrogate or proxy decision maker to make the treatment decisions when they are no longer able to make them. This document may also be called a healthcare proxy.

Reflection
As you look at these two types of advance directives, what do you think are the major strengths and drawbacks of a living will?

_____

_____

In comparison, what are the major strengths of a durable power of attorney? What are its major drawbacks?

_____

_____

_____

_____

Surrogate or proxy decision makers must use substitute judgment, addressed in Chapter 11, when deciding what their loved one would want. Recall that this means they must make a decision as the patient would have based on the patient's values and preferences, not their own. This is what makes proxy decision making so complex. Many surrogates say that they do not know what the patient would want. In such cases, surrogates are often asked to recall previous medical experiences that the patient went through and related discussions that the patient may have had regarding desired values, goals, and preferences. In absence of knowing what decision the patient would have made, a surrogate can collaborate with the interprofessional care team to use the best interest standard. This entails making a decision that is in the best interest of the patient. It is often used in pediatrics and in situations in which the patient was never competent. The living will and durable power of attorney are legally binding in all 50 U.S. states, but their wording may differ. You should familiarize yourself with those in the area where you live and work (and, by the way, where your loved ones live).

In January 1990, a nationally mandated *U.S. Patient Self-Determination Act (PSDA)* made it necessary for all patients in the United States to be asked on admission to a healthcare institution whether they have an advance directive or want to prepare one. For those who have one, it is placed in the patient's permanent healthcare record in that institution. If the person desires one but does not have one, the institution has forms for the person to complete. Other countries do not have similar nationally mandated mechanisms such as the PSDA, although many share the task of trying to ascertain what is best for the patient in our current era in which life can be prolonged almost indefinitely in some instances.

Although these forms are helpful in making an incapacitated patient's wishes known, far more important is that the patient talk to loved ones and professionals long before the moment of decision making arrives. Advance care planning conversations that occur too late (or not at all) can result in care that is invasive, expensive, and not aligned with patients' wishes.[30] For this reason, advocates of advance care planning suggest that the best place for these discussions to take place is in the primary care or home setting. This setting provides opportunities for end-of-life discussions because its outpatient, noncrisis environment can best set the stage for defining patient values, goals, and expectations. To encourage healthcare professionals to initiate advance care planning discussions, Medicare began reimbursing for advanced care planning in 2016.

Patients and families often look to health professionals to bring up these difficult conversations. As a future health professional, you should seek to develop strategies for talking with your patients and families about this topic. In the words of Atul Gawande: "If end of life discussions were an experimental drug, the FDA would approve it."[31] It is difficult at times to balance prognostic realities with hope; however, asking important questions such as "who would you want to speak for you if you can't speak for yourself" and "if time becomes short, what is most important to you?" are recommended places to start.[31,32] Good communication regarding goals of care is an essential skill for a caring response and a high priority for the delivery of quality care at the end of life.

Clinically Assisted Suicide and Medical Euthanasia

No modern discussion of end-of-life care is complete without a discussion of clinically assisted suicide and medical euthanasia.

Although assisted suicide often is called "physician-assisted suicide," the words *clinically assisted suicide* are purposefully used in this chapter because almost all health professionals who have interactions with patients could face patients who are contemplating this course of action and ask for assistance. Some health professionals, such as nurses, social workers, and pharmacists, work directly with doctors in the chain of events that lead to a patient's suicide when it is treated as a medical option in end-of-life care.[33] Many health profession organizations have issued position statements affirming their opposition to the practice on the basis that it is incompatible with professional ethics.

In the United States, the most decisive cases against this type of action occurred over a decade ago. In 1996, the Supreme Court ruled on two cases involving physician-assisted suicide and ruled against the rationale set forth for permitting assisted suicide in these instances.[34] What many people do not understand is that although the rulings are important in setting precedents against this practice, they do not (and did not) preclude individual states from passing legislation permitting clinically assisted suicide. In fact, legislation permitting it currently exists in the states of California, Colorado,

Hawaii, Maine, Montana, New Jersey, Oregon, Vermont, Washington, and the District of Columbia.

Most ethical debate identifies intent and consequences as key factors, distinguishing withdrawing and withholding life-prolonging measures from assisted suicide and direct euthanasia.[35] In all these cases, the patient dies after the act. As you now know from previous discussions in this chapter, the intent is a morally relevant distinction between withdrawing or withholding life supports with death ensuing and those interventions designed to end a patient's life mercifully. In the former, the intent is not to cause the patient's death but rather to honor the patient's right to have certain invasive, life-prolonging interventions withheld or stopped. In assisted suicide, the health professional is the direct agent of administering the means by which patients can effectively end their own life. The most commonly discussed form of clinically assisted suicide is the health professional who provides information about and a prescription for the lethal dose of a medication. In actual cases, the health professional may or may not be physically present at the suicide. The question then is how involved the health professional must be to be judged an agent in the patient's death. More fundamentally, the ethical debate steps back to a discussion of whether assisted suicide should be permitted at all.

Proponents of clinically assisted suicide probably are in a minority among health professionals, although it is impossible to ascertain how strong the support really is. Those in favor of legislation that decriminalizes assisted suicide argue that respect for a patient is determined, first and foremost, by a respect for the patient's autonomy. They also argue that the health professional promises to abide with patients, show compassion, and be committed to providing comfort when cure is no longer possible and that these commitments extend to helping patients gain information or access to the medical means to take their own life.

Reflection

Suppose Mrs. Lykes requests that Dr. Roubal give her the information and means necessary for her to effectively end her own life. What might her reasons be?

_____

_____

_____

_____

If you said things such as, "she cannot imagine going on in this condition; for her, life is no longer worth living" or "she knows it is going to get worse and she can't take it," you would be identifying the reasons given by patients and the themes that therefore often are used in support of this procedure.

Opponents argue that lethal prescriptions should never substitute for compassionate, palliative end-of-life care.[36] They object to the idea that respect for persons is embraced fully by honoring their wishes, important as they are. Respect for persons must entail a respect for life, and the appropriate moral role of the health professional is to save life, not to assist in any way in taking it. Choosing to become an advocate of death is a distortion of the age-old ethical mandate of the health professions to save life. Neither faithfulness nor nonmaleficence can be honored once the line between being an advocate of life and being an advocate of death has been crossed. Opponents also assert that compassion never can be expressed by having a part in intentionally ending a patient's life.

Medical euthanasia, that is, ending a patient's life with medical means administered by a physician, requires the direct moral agency of the physician.

The patient is truly a "passive bystander" while the health professional's intervention is carried out with the goal of ending the patient's life.

Assisted Suicide

1. The physician provides the medical means (a prescription).
2. The physician is necessary but not sufficient for the act to be completed.
3. The patient needs to do the final act (take the lethal medication).

Medical Euthanasia

1. Physician directly commits the act by medical means.
2. The physician is necessary and sufficient for the act to be completed.
3. The patient's condition provides the context.

Proponents and opponents in the ethical debate about medical euthanasia draw on arguments similar to the ones described previously regarding assisted suicide. Proponents also often draw the line between voluntary medical euthanasia (in which a competent patient requests euthanasia) and involuntary medical euthanasia (in which requests cannot be made because the patient is incompetent). In countries where medical euthanasia legally is permitted (e.g., the Netherlands, Belgium), proponents reject advance directives as a legitimate mechanism for continuing such a request into a period when a patient no longer can speak for himself. Opponents add to their other objections that voluntary euthanasia inevitably slips into involuntary euthanasia.

Concerns from opponents to both types of procedures are that the trust health professionals accrue from their willingness to take the patient's life seriously when others devalue the patient will be fatally compromised and that health professionals themselves may become less diligent in seeking comfort measures for a dying patient if it is permissible, instead, to assist a patient in "ending it all." There also are serious concerns that minority patients and other socially marginalized members of society will be encouraged to end their lives (or have them terminated), whereas others will be offered alternatives. Alternatives in the form of diligent end-of-life care that stops short of assisted suicide then become the mandate that guides a professional's approach.

Summary

Decisions about life and death in the health professions are among the most challenging from an ethical and a practical viewpoint. As a health professional, you must be introspective about your feelings toward death. This will help you gain insight into your role as humble mediator between life and death, sickness and well-being. By so doing, you will learn how the ethical tools of character traits and duties based on principles of nonmaleficence, patient autonomy, and faithfulness can help to build and sustain the moral foundations of compassionate care in these challenging situations. Conceptual distinctions, such as ordinary and extraordinary, withdrawing and withholding, double effect, and the role of the health professional vis-à-vis allowing or intending death, can help. The ethics of care counsels each of us to keep the lens of professional treatment focused on what constitutes a caring response.

Questions for Thought and Discussion

1. Laura Penman works in a nursing home with a specialty in dementia care. She floats from the units that provide care to patients with mild dementia to the locked floor for those with severe end stages of the disease. Today she is assigned to care for Sandra McKendrick. Sandra is an 82-year-old woman with end-stage Alzheimer's disease. Laura remembers her from when she was admitted to the facility several years ago. Last month, Sandra's daughter, Kate, agreed to placement of a feeding tube to get her mom through an acute hospitalization for flu-related pneumonia. She completed her course of intravenous antibiotics, but her cognitive and self-care (particularly feeding and eating) abilities have not improved. Kate is visiting tonight and says "I don't know what to do for my mom. I wish I never agreed to the tube. She is not better, but if I ask the doctors to take it out now, my sister says I will be inhumane because my mom will starve. I don't know why my mom picked me

as her healthcare proxy. This whole situation stinks!" How would you respond to Kate's statement? Is it ethical for the family to withdraw the feeding tube? What would you say to Kate's sister during this difficult situation?

2. It has been said that the values you espouse should be the values you practice. To truly understand the process of advance care planning, begin the process of completing your own advance directive. To do so, you might start by looking at information on several websites, including the conversation project (www.theconversationproject.org) or five wishes (https://fivewishes.org). Next, investigate your state regulations. What are the provisions for advanced care planning documents? What is the legal significance of such documents, and how does that differ from its psychological and ethical significance?

3. You are at a dinner party and the topic of a ballot question in the state you live in regarding legalizing physician-assisted suicide is raised. Basically, a yes vote would legalize physician-assisted suicide in the state, a no vote would mean no change to the laws in this area. Your neighbor turns to you and says, "In an era of healthcare costs spiraling out of control, I don't know why anyone would not be in support of this. We are more compassionate to our pets than we are to humans nowadays." The neighbor then turns to you and says, "You're a health professional, how are you voting on this one?" Write/talk out a potential response. Include in your response some of the important ethical considerations that you should communicate.

References

1. Brown B: *Daring greatly: how the courage to be vulnerable transforms the way we live, love, parent, and lead*, New York, 2015, Avery.
2. Dresden SM, McCarthy DM, Engel KG, et al: Perceptions and expectations of health-related quality of life among geriatric patients seeking emergency care: a qualitative study, *BMC Geriatr* 19(1):1–8, 2019.
3. Dunn H: *Light in the shadows: meditations while living with a life-threatening illness*, ed 2, Herdon, VA, 2005, A and A Publishers, Inc.
4. Stedman TL: *Stedman's medical dictionary for the health professions and nursing*, ed 6, New York, 2008, Wolters Kluwer/Lippincott, Williams and Wilkins, p 1144.
5. World Health Organization: Definition of palliative care, 2019. Available at https://www.who.int/cancer/palliative/definition/en/.
6. Geller G, Harrison KL, Rushton CH, et al: Ethical challenges in the care of children and families affected by life-limiting neuromuscular diseases, *J Dev Behav Pediatr* 33:548–561, 2012.
7. National Consensus Project for Quality Palliative Care: *Clinical practice guidelines for quality palliative care*, ed 4, Richmond, VA, 2018, National Coalition for Hospice and Palliative Care. Available at https://www.nationalcoalitionhpc.org/ncp.

8. Cassem N: Treatment decisions in irreversible illness. In Cassem N, Hackett T, editors: *Massachusetts General Hospital handbook of general hospital psychiatry*, St. Louis, 1978, Mosby, pp 573–574.

9. NHPCO Facts and Figures: *Hospice care in America*, Edition Revision 7-2-2019, Alexandria, VA, 2018, National Hospice and Palliative Care Organization. Available at https://www.nhpco.org/wp-content/uploads/2019/07/2018_NHPCO_Facts_Figures.pdf.

10. Kleinpell R, Vasilevskis EE, Fogg L, et al: Exploring the association of hospice care on patient experience and outcomes of care, *BMJ Suppo Palliat Care* 9(1):e13, 2019.

11. Ware OD, Cagle JG: Informal caregiving networks for hospice patients with cancer and their impact on outcomes: a brief report, *Am J Hosp Palliat Med* 36(3):235–240, 2019.

12. Casaret DJ, Quill TE: I'm not ready for hospice": strategies for timely and effective hospice discussions, *Ann Intern Med* 146(6):443–449, 2007.

13. Toombs K: Review essay: taking the body seriously, *Hastings Cent Rep* 27(5): 39–43, 1997.

14. Abide. In Random House, editor: *Webster's unabridged dictionary*, New York, 2001, Random House, p 4.

15. Goetz JL, Keltner D, Simon-Thomas E: Compassion: an evolutionary analysis and empirical review, *Psychol Bull* 136(3):351–374, 2010.

16. Lown B, McIntosh S, McGuinn K, et al: *Advancing compassionate, person- and family-centered care through interprofessional education for collaborative practice: compassionate, collaborative care model and framework*, 2014. Available at http://www.theschwartz-center.org/media/Triple-C-Conference-Framework-Tables_FINAL.pdf.

17. Trzeciak S, Mazzarelli A: *Compassionomics: the revolutionary scientific evidence that caring makes a difference*, Pensacola, FL, 2019, Studer Group, LLC.

18. Dougherty C, Purtilo R: The duty of compassion in an era of health care reform, *Cambridge Q* 4:426–433, 1995.

19. Engen HG, Singer T: Compassion-based emotional regulation up-regulates experienced positive affect and associated neural networks, *Soc Cogn Affect Neurosci* 10(9):1291–1301, 2015.

20. Burns JP, Truog RD: The DNR order after 40 years, *New Engl J Med* 375(6): 504–506, 2016. doi: 10.1056/NEJMp1605597.

21. Prendergast TJ, Puntillo KA: Withdrawal of life support: intensive caring at the end of life, *JAMA* 288(21):2732–2740, 2002.

22. Prince-Paul M, Daly BJ: Ethical considerations in palliative care. In Ferrell B, Paice J, editors: *Oxford textbook of palliative nursing*, ed 5, New York, 2019, Oxford University Press. doi: 10.1093/med/9780190862374.003.0070.

23. Cassel C, Purtilo R, McFarland E: Ethical and social issues in contemporary medicine. In Dale D, editor: *Scientific American medicine*, vol 1, New York, 2003, WebMD, Inc, pp 3–7.

24. Mentzelopoulos SD, Slowther A-M, Fritz Z, et al: Ethical challenges in resuscitation, *Int Care Med* 44(6):703–716, 2018.

25. Randall F, Downe R: The moral distinction between killing and letting die. *Palliative care ethics: a companion for all specialties,* ed 2, New York, 1999, Oxford University Press, pp 270–277.

26. Barrocas A, Gepper C, Durfee SM, et al: A.S.P.E.N. ethics position paper, *Nutr Clin Pract* 25(6):672–679, 2010.

27. Vink EE, Azoulay E, Caplan A, et al: Time-limited trial of intensive care treatment: an overview of current literature, *Int Care Med* 44(9):1369–1377, 2018.

28. U.S. Department of Health and Human Services National Institute on Aging. *Advance Care Planning: Healthcare Directives,* January 15, 2018. Available at https://www.nia.nih.gov/health/advance-care-planning-healthcare-directives.

29. Aasmul I, Husebo BS, Flo E: Description of an advance care planning intervention in nursing homes: outcomes of the process evaluation, *BMC Geriatr* 18(1):26, 2018.

30. Pelland K, Morphis B, Harris D, et al: Assessment of first-year use of medicare's advance care planning billing codes, *JAMA Intern Med* 179(6):827–829, 2019. doi: 10.1001/jamainternmed.2018.8107.

31. Gawande A: *Being mortal: medicine and what matters in the end,* New York, 2014, Metropolitian Books, Henry Holt Company, p 177.

32. Rushton CH, Kaylor BD, Christopher M: Twenty years since Cruzan and the Patient Self-Determination Act: opportunities for improving care at the end of life in critical care settings, *Am Assoc Crit Care Nurs Adv Crit Care* 23(1):99–106, 2012.

33. Altman TK, Collins SE: Oregon's death with dignity act (ORS 127.800-897): a health policy analysis, *J Nurs Law* 11(1):43–52, 2007.

34. *Quill v. Vacco,* 80 F3d 716 (2nd Cir., 1996); and *Compassion in Dying v. State of Washington,* 79 F.3d 790 (9th Cir. 1996) (en banc).

35. American Academy of Hospice and Palliative Medicine: *Position statement—withholding and withdrawing non-beneficial medical interventions,* Glenview, IL, 2017, American Academy of Hospice and Palliative Medicine. Available at http://aahpm.org/positions/withholding-nonbeneficial-interventions.

36. Snyder SL, Mueller PS: Ethics and the legalization of physician-assisted suicide: an American College of Physicians position paper, *Ann Intern Med* 167(8):576–578, 2017.

Ethical Dimensions
of the Social Context
# of Healthcare

14

Distributive Justice: Rights, Resource Allocation, and Policy Considerations

Objectives

The reader should be able to:

- Understand how the concept and function of distributive justice affect the healthcare environment.
- Describe what a caring response involves in situations that require the allocation of scarce resources.
- Compare the concepts of microallocation and macroallocation.
- Distinguish the contexts in which fairness and equity considerations apply to everyday professional practice.
- Describe some situations in healthcare in which fairness considerations are relevant for a just allocation of resources.
- Evaluate the function of procedural justice in the context of healthcare delivery.
- Discuss the relevance of the philosophical starting point of deliberation in distributive justice: treat similar cases similarly.
- Identify three aspects of policy based on the concept of equity in allocation decisions.
- Compare the ideas of allocation based on a right to healthcare, on need, and on merit.

New terms and ideas you will encounter in this chapter

allocation of resources	data-driven decision making	positive rights
distributive justice	data banks and patient registries	healthcare as a commodity
macroallocation	formal principle of justice	negative right
microallocation	material principles of justice	merit justice
principle of fairness	entitlement	very important person (VIP)
"first come, first served"		parsimonious decisions
procedural justice		financial stewardship
principle of equity		

Topics in this chapter introduced in earlier chapters	
Topic	*Introduced in chapter*
Hippocratic Oath	1
A caring response	2
Moral agent	3
Moral distress	3
Ethical dilemma	3
Principle of justice	4
Clinical reasoning	4
Deontology/duty reasoning	4
Rights	4
Principle of autonomy	4
Principle of beneficence	4
Moral resilience	6
Health professional well-being	6

Introduction

We humans are beings that have needs, values, desires, and hopes related to our understanding of what makes life worthwhile. We also are beings that face inevitable limitations in our striving to achieve those ends. Some are internal limitations such as fears or responsibilities that result in us putting aside a single-minded goal of achieving personal fulfillment. Others are imposed by external circumstances (e.g., shortages in natural resources and those imposed through policies and practices over which we seemingly have no control). It is this fact of limitation in the human condition that gave rise to the idea of justice.

Like individuals or groups, nations also face questions of limited re-source. These issues worldwide create ethical challenges that involve the *allocation of resources*. Allocation is a term that suggests intentional decisions about how a good is distributed. In ethical deliberation, such challenges fall within the category of distributive justice, the topic of this chapter, and com-pensatory justice, discussed in Chapter 15.

Distributive justice purports that humans have the capacity to make non-arbitrary, reasonable bases for allocating goods and services that are in at least moderately scarce supply but desired by many. Healthcare resources are among those goods and services.

The concept of justice itself has been the subject of rich discussion from the beginning of Western ethics. Generally speaking, justice has been thought of as an arbiter, useful for analyzing and resolving ethical problems regarding what is rightfully due each individual or group who presents a claim on resources and what proportion of the burden should be borne by whom. Conditions that clue you into the fact that you are in a situation re-quiring justice are

- There is a good or service that more than one person or group wants,
- There is a scarcity of the good or service, and

- The moral agent has an obligation not to allocate the good on an arbitrary basis.

Some justice-related decisions require that different types of societal goods be compared, with the recognition that a society does not have infinite resources to cover all of them. For instance, allocation decisions may involve trade-offs between more children having access to free dental care, or roads being built, or military installations provided with better facilities for troops, or existing national parks made available to more people by decreasing the cost to enter and camp in them. These judgments are called *macroallocation* decisions. Although these decisions are extremely important, we leave this aspect of your study to other courses.

Other justice issues involve trade-offs among goods and services within one value arena, such as healthcare. The resulting decisions about who gets what, and why, are termed *microallocation* decisions and are the focus of this chapter.

Some of the most critical issues regarding allocation of healthcare resources take place at the level of national, local, or institutional policy in which whole groups of similarly situated people are implicated. For instance, in the United States and globally, current lively policy debates surround such issues as how to distribute limited supplies of medicines or medical products when there are disruptions in the supply chain, immunizations in times of epidemics or pandemics, and organs for transplantation.

Still others are best addressed by examining your direct caregiving role. For example, you may be faced with a personnel shortage in your workplace or you may work where not enough equipment, space, or money is available to fully satisfy what your best effort requires. In operating under that extenuating circumstance, you are forced to make decisions about how to spread out the desired good or service within healthcare.

 Reflection

To help you reflect on the concept of distributive justice, consider the following frequently debated question. Do you think a person whose liver has been damaged by alcohol-related liver disease should have the same chance for a transplant as someone whose equally serious liver damage was caused by other reasons?
Yes____ No ___
Why? If yes, make a list of any conditions you would impose and supports that should be in place to ensure the "fairness" of allocating scarce organs, knowing that the success rate depends in part on abstinence before and after the transplant. If you think that the patient should not be given exactly the same priority as anyone else

with similar medical need, take a minute before reading further to write down some reasons why you feel this way.

_____

_____

_____

_____

Currently, in most countries where liver transplants are offered, individuals with substance use disorder have a waiting period to show that they are successfully abstaining from substance use, a criterion that appears to reduce the recidivism rate among those fortunate enough to be allocated an organ. Debates regarding the priority list for allocation of scarce resources revolve around considerations of urgency and likelihood of survival benefit, and they often include considerations of lifestyle.[1] The example of organ transplantation points out that, in the allocation of healthcare resources, conscious choices are made, and the choices do make a difference in the lives and well-being of entire groups of similarly situated people.

---

⑥ **Summary**

Distributive justice helps us apply morally justifiable criteria for the distribution of desired and needed resources. Macroallocation involves decisions among different types of valued societal goods or services; microallocation focuses on the distribution of one good or service.

The following story will assist you in your thinking about your role in these complex practice and policy issues.

💗 **The Story of Christopher Lacey and the Contenders for an Intensive Care Unit Bed**

On Monday mornings, the interprofessional care team in the intensive care unit (ICU) has their weekly meeting to review the past week and project what lies ahead given the hospital census and the status of the patients currently in the ICU. Dr. Sidney McCally, the head of the team, reports that once again they are in the unhappy position of not only having the ICU beds still filled to capacity but also at this moment having three critically ill patients waiting for a bed. She proposes that the patient most likely to be able to be moved out of the unit is Christopher Lacey. The team agrees, although some more reluctantly than others, that if a bed is available in the step-down medical unit, his symptoms can be managed. This will not completely solve the problem, but it will open up one ICU bed. Dr. McCally says that she will speak with the family and make the necessary inquiries as to the availability of a bed for this patient.

Later in the day, John Krescher, a critical care nurse specialist, is going back into the ICU after his lunch break when he is stopped by Christopher Lacey's sister, a nurse. John often sees her and her husband at her brother's bedside, although he has not had any lengthy discussions about Christopher with them. This morning, Mr. Lacey's sister says angrily that Christopher's physician is planning to transfer her brother prematurely to the step-down medical unit. She believes the transfer is because Dr. McCally is being urged to do so by the hospital utilization committee and the case manager for Mr. Lacey's medical coverage plan. She and her husband are threatening a lawsuit against the hospital unless her brother is allowed to remain in the ICU and receive what she believes is optimal medical care for him there. She rushes away, apparently on the verge of tears.

John goes over to Christopher Lacey's bedside and puts his hand on the man's shoulder. He studies the patient's face for some sign of response but finds none. John's mind is flooded with thoughts. Mr. Lacey is a 28-year-old, divorced postal employee with no children. "He is only a year older than I am," John thinks. Initially, Christopher was admitted to the hospital with severe, acute abdominal pain. After several days of tests that yielded no clues, the physicians did an exploratory laparotomy.

At that time, an ischemic segment of bowel was resected. In the postoperative suite, Christopher experienced respiratory arrest for reasons the doctors could not explain and was transferred to the ICU under the interprofessional care team's care. Since that time, 3 weeks ago, his condition has been fluctuating neurologically, and he has never fully regained consciousness.

In fact, Christopher Lacey has had a stormy course characterized by multiple serious medical complications. A systemic infection developed immediately after surgery at which time it was thought he would die. He was treated with massive doses of antibiotics and appeared to be recovered, but the antibiotics were severely toxic to his kidneys. He now shows signs of kidney failure, which may necessitate renal dialysis.

Some members of the interprofessional care team have become progressively more pessimistic about Christopher Lacey's prognosis. In the ICU rounds a week earlier, Dr. McCally shared with the ICU team that she had had several discussions with the patient's sister and had tried to explain to her the likelihood that his condition would not improve. "But," Dr. McCally said, "she and her husband want aggressive treatment as long as there is any hope of meaningful recovery or survival." Mr. Lacey had left no living will or durable power of attorney and had never expressed an opinion about long-term life support.

John goes over to the ICU desk where his colleague, Janet Cumming, is at the computer entering data in the patients' medical records. Janet says, "Mr. Lacey's sister is really upset because Dr. McCally has decided to transfer him to the step-down medicine unit later today." John says, "I know. It makes me anxious that she is so upset."

The Goal: A Caring Response

Discerning a caring response in situations of distributive justice creates special psychological and ethical challenges for health professionals. Some bioethicists have suggested that the demands of justice are at odds with the demands of professional care because the former focuses on the well-being of entire groups and the latter on an individual patient, like Christopher Lacey. You can hear the concern of the two professionals who are confronted with Christopher's distressed sister. However, in his recent assessment of the challenge, ethicist Leonard Fleck[2] placed his hope on the democratic process in a society that has both justice and caring as two of its founding values and assumptions. We cannot be a just society if we leave out care, and we cannot effectively care if we focus on the individual only without taking into account the affect our decision has on other similarly situated individuals. If Fleck is correct in embracing the good news that we can arrive at a caring response while taking microallocation decisions into account, the task is to apply our clinical and ethical reasoning about what is best for an individual patient from the perspective of also acknowledging the limits on the overall resources available. This does not only include reimbursement limits for services offered to the patient but also limits in your own energies, clinic schedule–imposed limitations, availability of clinical modalities or professional expertise, and space. The strength of this perspective is that it keeps us crisply cognizant of what can best be done within the reality of human limitations. It uses all aspects of a health professional's clinical reasoning discussed previously in this text, with a balance of the larger contextual elements of the situation.

You have before you the story of Christopher Lacey, his family, and the interprofessional care team. A seemingly healthy young man becomes a victim of a series of events that leave him septic, unresponsive, and dependent on extensive medical supports for his life and sustenance. On an individual patient basis, a widely recognized goal for his interprofessional care team is to do whatever is clinically and ethically best for him, and the entire team understandably has been working to ensure that Christopher Lacey is receiving the most caring response consistent with the professional skill that each is able to provide. It is what we expect of the health professional–patient relationship.

But this chapter confronts you squarely with the reality often faced by moral agents; namely, that what one actually can offer him threatens to fall short of the optimum either for him or for other equally qualified patients. In the story as written, Dr. McCally has not clearly indicated her reasons for moving Christopher Lacey out of the intensive care unit (ICU) to a general medical unit, but there is no reason to believe that this physician has a less than pure intent. Maybe she is being pushed by the bed utilization committee of the hospital because his medical coverage will no longer support ICU-level treatment, or maybe she judges deeply that a disproportionate amount of extremely expensive life support measures are being expended on him in view of his serious prognosis. She may be haunted by the knowledge that three other patients who may benefit more from ICU interventions are waiting in the wings for a bed to clear. All of these reasons fall within the purview of justice considerations that this team is facing. You can again rely on the six-step process of ethical decision making as a tool to assess ethical problems that arise when viewed through the lens of distributive justice to arrive at the best possible course.

The Six-Step Process in Microallocation Decisions

Of the many issues involved in this situation, consider the following that are related to the broad questions regarding the allocation of healthcare resources directed to a single patient:

- Should care be continued in the ICU for patients whose progress is uncertain (e.g., whose conditions may worsen if they are transferred out but do not seem to be getting any better in the ICU)?
- Should patient care be continued in the ICU because the family has a right to require continued treatment of this sort?
- Mr. Lacey's regimen is based on pooled data derived from many other people in his health plan who were in circumstances similar to his. Should Mr. Lacey be transferred out because his health plan dictates that he has used up his fair share of the plan's resources?
- Should Mr. Lacey's financial situation in relation to other patients who are waiting for an ICU bed be a factor at all in deciding whether or not he stays?

In recent years, the direct relationship between health professional and patient has become strained by institutional constraints, some of which were addressed in Chapter 8. Traditional healthcare ethics, with its emphasis only on the private transaction between the professional and the patient, often has not addressed the larger institutional questions. For instance, nothing in the Hippocratic Oath, or even in most professional codes of ethics today, provides guidance for how to allocate healthcare resources fairly and equitably. The challenge is heightened when the allocation involves a scarce resource.

Step 1: Gather Relevant Information

As you can see, patients such as Christopher Lacey bring the troubling aspects of resource allocation keenly into focus. Costs are often a major consideration. Although, as Chapter 13 suggests, many people with clinically compromised conditions can be kept alive almost indefinitely, the reality in most Western countries is that the technology needed to keep patients on life support is extremely expensive and resource intensive. Callahan[3] made the argument that it is in fact the high cost of medical technology that makes our current healthcare system unsustainable. He noted: "In a rare instance of consensus, healthcare economists attribute about 50% of the annual increase in healthcare costs to new technologies or to the intensified use of old ones."[3] One piece of highly relevant information is determination of the likelihood of which ICU technologies will be the bridge to help patients recover functions essential to life and a higher quality of life.[4] It does not appear that Mr. Lacey is "getting better" in the ICU, but some uncertainty exists about whether his condition will deteriorate further if he is removed from the unit. His sister believes it will, in contrast to the ICU team's assessment.

The limited number of ICU beds is another consideration. We do not know the full clinical status of the patients in line for the ICU bed currently occupied by Christopher Lacey, but according to Dr. McCally, they are patients who are equally if not more clinically compromised. It does not appear in this instance that professional staff or medical equipment and supplies on the medical unit of the hospital are in short supply to compound the allocation challenge.

When viewed from the standpoint of how justice enters into such decisions, the ideas of fairness and equity are ethical tools that assist in ethical decision making. Each are examined here.

Fairness Considerations

An understanding of what often is called the *principle of fairness* in justice discussions requires you to explore two issues raised by Mr. Lacey's situation.

"First come, first served" and procedural justice. First, there is the idea of *first come, first served*. As noted, the treatment (and related resources) Mr. Lacey is receiving may keep someone else from receiving life-sustaining therapy in the ICU. Generally speaking, once patients are in an ICU, they are not removed for other similarly situated persons who come along afterward. Fairness considerations often rely on this culturally derived first come, first served idea as a device of arbitration. The assumption is that there is something in the nature of the procedures we adopt that have a moral prescription in them. Procedures for determining who gets priority attention in a queue (when everyone's need or desire is judged to be similar) is understood to lend insight into the deeper aspects of an overall just society. In the United States and most Western cultures, the *procedural justice* rule is accepted whether queuing up for an ICU bed, standing in line for concert tickets, or taking a number at a deli counter. If you happened to get there first, you have constituted a moral claim on the spot, something like a "squatter's right." You can see how this rule can help to mitigate constant bickering over a resource that would equally benefit many who want or need it.

There is a caveat here. Although "first in line" covers a lot of people who present for healthcare services, it is not always the case. The idea of who should have top priority may fall to the eldest, to tribal leaders, or to others, not to whoever happened to get there first. In each case, however, the procedural justice idea that the person with top priority should be able to remain in place seems to hold.

The identified one versus the as-yet-unidentified many. Consider a second type of fairness issue. Theoretically, resources that Mr. Lacey is using to be sustained in his bodily functions could be channeled into other kinds of programs that could save the lives of hundreds or at least improve their level of well-being (e.g., in screening or immunization programs).

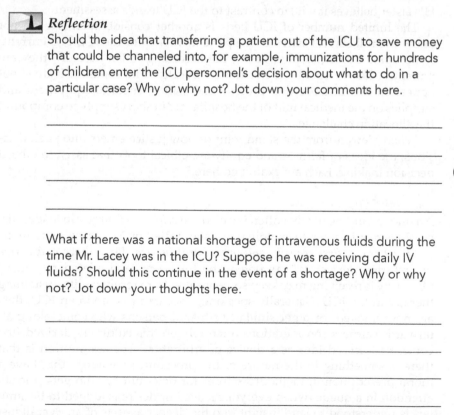

Reflection

Should the idea that transferring a patient out of the ICU to save money that could be channeled into, for example, immunizations for hundreds of children enter the ICU personnel's decision about what to do in a particular case? Why or why not? Jot down your comments here.

_____

_____

_____

_____

What if there was a national shortage of intravenous fluids during the time Mr. Lacey was in the ICU? Suppose he was receiving daily IV fluids? Should this continue in the event of a shortage? Why or why not? Jot down your thoughts here.

_____

_____

_____

_____

In everyday circumstances, this type of reasoning that pits the identified patient against an unidentified many in a group is a morally questionable guide for action at the level that decisions are made about a particular patient by the healthcare team. You have learned that a fundamental promise of professional ethics is that the individual patient's well-being is your appropriate focus; therefore your patient cannot be placed in a faceless pool with risk for jeopardy. For one thing, the healthcare team cannot ensure that funds and other resources "saved" by removing Mr. Lacey from the ICU will be channeled into saving more lives or increasing the level of healthcare overall because of the fragmentation that exists in the policies of healthcare financing. Even if that assurance existed, the respect for this person's dignity as a human should preclude the health professional's willingness to compromise a single patient's well-being for the sake of others "out there."

Whatever the strength of procedural justice reasoning, almost anyone would agree that in healthcare these good guidelines taken alone leave too much unaccounted for if used as the sole criterion for determining the fate of Mr. Lacey or the other identified patients in dire need of the ICU resources.

Equity Considerations

Health professionals must take institutional and other policies into account when faced with allocation decisions. From a justice standpoint, the *principle of equity* means that policy decision makers must make every effort to set guidelines that treat each person in a similarly situated circumstance alike, with differences among them based on criteria that are ethically acceptable. Therefore often the debate about who receives services does not only take into account the access of one patient or group over another. It also addresses the other two sides of what has been traditionally known as the triangle of considerations: access, cost and quality (Fig. 14.1).

Different government and other policy-making bodies take different sides of the triangle as their focus. There have been notable changes in professional debates as a result of shifts in U.S. healthcare policy over recent years. From fee for

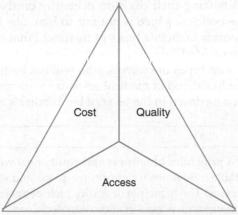

Fig. 14.1. The triad of healthcare policy.

service, to managed care where there were capitated payments and financial incentives for care, to the promotion of accountable care organizations to contain costs, to the current value-based care model that emphasizes reimbursement based on patient outcomes and payment linked with performance.[5,6]

Another popular angle of policy analysis today relies on aggregating outcomes to drive data-driven decision making and ensure quality patient outcomes. *Data-driven decision making* is the use of collected and analyzed data to support systematic reasoning and decision making.[7,8] Through collection of data from many like-situated patients, optimal clinical care outcomes can be advanced for all members of the group. In healthcare, this supports the implementation of evidence-based practice for tailored, client-centered care. It improves patient outcomes through integrating quality measures into practice. In short, it supports the triple aim. *Data banks and patient registries*, along with electronic health records, are used to collect, analyze, and disseminate mass amounts of data to be used for this purpose in health plans, within professional organizations, and by government agencies.[9] As you can see, there is less direct emphasis in this approach on access, but the implication is that those with authentic needs will be given optimal quality of care that is evidence based at a reasonable cost.

Critical analysis of such themes as the difference between policies based on insurance companies' assessments of what equity requires and those based on more traditional notions of professional ethics is helping everyone understand better what an "equitable" course of action requires.[10]

In Christopher Lacey's case, the interprofessional care team in the ICU should not have to—and will not have full prerogative to—take his situation from scratch and try to figure out who is and who is not eligible for what on the basis of relative clinical need alone. Policies that help guide their decision may be in the form of federal or other government or institutional policies, as well as evidence-based position papers published by professional organizations. Mr. Lacey's sister, a nurse, is concerned that Dr. McCally and her colleagues are making their decision primarily on the basis of institutional or insurance policies, which is not fair to him. She knows that these policies have the power to dictate types of treatment that will or will not be covered by insurance, Medicare, or other third-party payers, or they might provide guidelines for types of patients who will not be treated because of excessive cost or unlikelihood of medical response to treatment. The triad of health policy has come down to the level of her brother's treatment.

ⓢ Summary

The justice-related principles of fairness and equity deal with determining ethically supportable guidelines for allocating goods and services among individuals or groups. The principle of equity includes considerations of cost and quality along with access in allocation decisions.

● Step 2: Identify the Type of Ethical Problem

Despite the fact that the ICU interprofessional care team surely knows that some factors outside of their control are figuring into the decision about Mr. Lacey and the others immediately in need of immediate ICU care, they are still in a position to experience emotional distress. First and foremost, they are health professionals; therefore, in their deliberation, they are pushed back to rely on their foundation of ethical reasoning from the standpoint of professional ethics. Fundamentally, their problem is more deeply rooted in the competing clinical claims that they face from other similarly situated patients who are waiting to be admitted to the ICU. In other words, they have butted up against the most challenging aspect of whether care and justice are reconcilable. In Chapter 3, you were introduced to the schematic representation of the basic type of ethical problem that addresses justice-related issues.

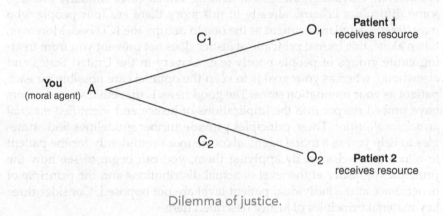

Dilemma of justice.

This was identified as one type of ethical dilemma.

⌐L *Reflection*

To refresh your memory, describe what makes an ethical dilemma different from a moral distress.

_____

_____

_____

_____

An additional ethical consideration in ethical problems is locus of authority. It, too, is present here insofar as you have learned that cost and other external considerations may be playing a role in the decision about what to do in this situation.

Step 3: Use Ethics Theories or Approaches to Analyze the Problem

Once the ethical problem has been identified as a dilemma with locus of authority considerations, the interprofessional care team members can move forward in their ethical reasoning. To sort out the dilemma, the professionals again can go back to the concept of justice. It is so highly regarded in the history of ethics that the principles approach includes it as one of the basic ethical principles. In justice situations, the starting place for assessment, called the *formal principle of justice*, is that similarly situated persons must be treated similarly. You will recognize this stance as the conceptual basis from which the notions of fairness and equity, discussed previously, are derived. Obviously, the idea of treating similar cases similarly presents some difficulties because already in this story there are four people who may deserve similar treatment as the one to occupy the ICU bed. Moreover, taken alone, this formal principle of justice does not prevent you from treating entire groups of people poorly (e.g., slavery in the United States and elsewhere), whereas your goal is to keep the optimal care possible for each patient as your foundation stone. The good news is that ethicists and others have probed deeper into the implications of justice and identified *material principles of justice*. These principles provide further guidelines and strategies to help you as a moral agent advocate more confidently for the patient in allocation decisions. By applying them, you can begin to see how the principles of justice at the level of actual distributions and the principle of beneficence at the individual patient level are not opposed. Consider three key material principles of justice described here.

Healthcare as a Right

As you recall, ethical principles often have the deontological function of duties. Justice is one example. Duties are related to rights. A right is a stringent claim on another to respond in a certain fashion consistent with one's ethical (or legal) duty. The stronger the claim as a right, the more an agent (whether a person or society) has a duty—and must accept responsibility—for addressing the claim. Therefore to treat healthcare of all individuals as a right means that no one can be dismissed at this basic level of ethical critique. This is important. At the same time, it does not differentiate how much and what kind of healthcare each individual or group is entitled to receive.

 Reflection

From what you know about the current policies regarding healthcare in your country, do you think healthcare is viewed as a right or privilege? Why? Explain here.

_____

_____

_____

_____

   Your answer may depend in part on your understanding of the idea of rights. The concept sometimes used in discussing a rights approach is that of _entitlement_. A person deserves the good or service simply by being a member of a group with a basic claim on a share of a prized good or service. A _positive right_s approach, adopted by many countries in the world, supports policies that make everyone eligible to receive basic healthcare benefits. At a minimum, access has to be universally available at the level of basic services, either free of charge or provided for a very modest price. In this way of thinking, one could argue that people such as Mr. Lacey and the other patients who need ICU beds should be able to have them. Ideally, the societal challenge is to find money to support an adequate supply of ICU beds and train adequate numbers of ICU personnel so that this basic resource is available for those who will benefit from this type of care. But as you are learning in this chapter, not even the stringency of a rights approach means that everyone qualified for a bed (or other good or service) necessarily receives one. Considerations of equity in the face of limited resources must also guide such decisions. An essential function of viewing healthcare as a right is that it empowers health professionals to be strong advocates for policies and practices that optimally benefit their patients.

Healthcare as a Response to Basic Need
A second material principle of justice that can help to identify different types of resources that are appropriate for different patients is to allocate goods or services based on relative need. This also has a deontological foundation. Healthcare offers a universal human good: the means to healthfulness. Therefore everyone who lacks it ought to receive a beneficial response to this need, and those in a position to provide it have a duty to do so. In this approach, healthcare can still be viewed as a right, but even that does not necessitate that everyone receives the same treatments. Moreover, not all who hold a needs-oriented position base it on the idea of human rights. As you can imagine, one of the greatest challenges in this type of reasoning is to define the relative severity of need and likelihood of benefit among different individuals or groups. How does one compare the need for functional gait training with pain relief for end-stage bone cancer with eye surgery for a detached retina? Another challenge is to determine what constitutes a truly clinical need.

⬛ *Reflection*

Currently, debate exists about whether cosmetic plastic surgery should be covered as a basic healthcare need. What reasons can be given for the position that such surgery is morally appropriate as a healthcare intervention? What reasons for such surgery based on health or medical need do you find unacceptable?

_____

_____

_____

In spite of difficulties, the basic premise that humans have varying types of need to maintain or restore a higher level of healthfulness seems to be a humane and reasonable position. Professional ethics rests largely on the idea that those with more need should have greater priority unless evidence shows that the expenditure of resources on this group would not yield positive results. Chapters 12 and 13 addressed the fine line that sometimes exists between responding to medical need that can hope to lead to an improved quality of life or effective relief from pain and others that cannot be justified based on that criterion. Here the interprofessional ICU care team basically agrees with Dr. McCally's clinical assessment of Christopher Lacey, proposing that she felt this patient could continue to be treated optimally outside of the ICU setting on the basis of his current clinical need. An assessment to determine which of the three "candidates" waiting to come into the ICU bed currently occupied by Mr. Lacey will also be essential to the process. Again you can see how the clinical expertise of the health professionals becomes an important, and often the governing, criterion for allocation decisions that affect others as well.

Healthcare as a Commodity

This perspective moves away from the previous foundational ethical assumptions that healthcare is an entitlement right and at least that clinical need is a sound ethical criterion on which to base allocation. In each of these traditional understandings, the principle of beneficence is viewed as being satisfied in the face of the unavoidable limits on resources. *Healthcare as a commodity* takes a different line of reasoning, advocating that healthcare should be viewed ethically as any other type of product in a free market society. Healthcare is something to be purchased, like a summer vacation package, new car, or computer tablet. The informed consumer decides and makes choices. This interpretation does not embody the idea of a duty of beneficence based on a right or relative need. The assumption is that citizens are free, autonomous individuals who make choices consistent with their own values and that in doing so are contributing to the type of society that maximizes the greatest amount of well-being for the most people overall. At the individual patient level, the principle of autonomy governs the choice to receive healthcare services.

Reflection

What aspects of this approach, if any, do you ascribe to? What are its strengths from an ethics point of view?

Rights language sometimes is brought into the argument that healthcare is a commodity but that it is a different type of right than a positive right of entitlement to a good or service based on a duty of beneficence. This is the idea of a *negative right*, that is, the right to an opportunity to purchase a good or service. Money is the key resource that governs who buys what. In this approach, it is not the responsibility of others in society to provide money (or vouchers or employee-based health insurance plans) to help people pay for healthcare. Everyone buys what they need and want and, in addition, can afford. Assuming that the treatment Christopher Lacey needs is out of reach for him and his family financially, the benefits he derives from treatment inevitably are at the expense of pooled financial resources in the form of revenue from taxes, his and others' insurance premiums, and other common aggregated funds that are distributed according to criteria established by the fund holders. Of course, he has worked since he was 16 years old, so he also has contributed to some of these pooled funds over the years. Even if his insurance denied this level of ICU care but the family could pay the full amount out of pocket, other justice considerations are facing the professionals because more than one patient can benefit from the bed he currently occupies.

Sometimes this way of reasoning about justice does include a component that places a claim on government and other pooled societal resources. It is recognized that, even in a free market society, some interventions are well beyond the personal means of most individuals. In such instances, societal resources should be spent on individuals or groups viewed as a "good investment." In the context of justice discussions, this "investment approach" falls into the idea that *merit justice*, rather than justice according to relative medical need, is the key to allocation decisions. Western societies often see merit not only in a person's societal contributions and wealth, but also in other things such as fame.

One topic that often arises in healthcare institutions is that of *very important persons (VIPs)* and specialty treatment. A VIP may not only be given the best bed in the facility and preferential treatment by staff but also may jump to the head of the line for precious resources. VIPs sometimes are literally royalty but more often are popular public figures who are given high social status: government officials, rock or movie stars, chief executive officers of major corporations, major league athletes, and so forth. What is your feeling response to professionals and institutions who assign merit to famous or powerful people?

Even when one takes the VIP situation out of the picture, merit reasoning based on social criteria of worth poses a challenge. For example, who is the better investment in the following case?

Two men are brought into the emergency department of a community hospital in a small town after the crash of a small plane that was carrying 16 passengers. Both need emergency life saving surgery immediately, but only one operating suite and team are available. Mr. A, a brilliant 26-year-old PhD researcher, is on the brink of making a major breakthrough in Alzheimer's disease research. His ability to pay for care is limited because of the burden of his large student loans. Mr. B, who is 75 years old, is a wealthy, world-renowned, retired concert pianist who is now showing the first stages of Alzheimer's disease and is in the process of completing a bequest to endow a world-class Alzheimer's research unit at Mr. A's facility.

Reflection

What qualifications does each man have that might influence the type of thinking that an "investment" or merit approach to allocation would take? Do you agree with this approach? Why or why not?

_____

_____

_____

_____

In brief, three basic perspectives on the way to address ethical dilemmas of justice are presented here in somewhat "pure" form: rights, need, and merit being the governing criterion. However, they are presented as if they are completely distinct from each other. In fact, practices and policies often are based on many factors and may include components of each of them. For instance, a healthcare benefits package that takes shape from the basic premise that healthcare is a right may be founded primarily on assessments of relative need among different groups as determined by the collection of aggregate data and also include a sliding scale of "copayments" according to the difference in people's ability to pay for care.

⟳ Summary

In situations of moderate scarcity, justice decisions about the distribution of goods depend on material principles of justice that include assessments of rights, relative need, and relative merit to determine a patient's or group's moral claim on goods and services.

As you can see, there is not always agreement about how the ethical requirements of justice best can be served. As you begin practice, you can help maintain your professional integrity by actively engaging the issues of justice as part of your clinical reasoning and decisions.

Step 4: Explore the Practical Alternatives

In previous chapters, the application of step 4 almost always placed you and the interprofessional care team solely in the moral role of advocate for an individual patient and acting in accordance to what an optimal care plan will entail to achieve a professional caring response. That is the role the ICU interprofessional care team members have maintained throughout their relationship with Mr. Lacey and Mr. Lacey's family up to this point. Now they are faced with an allocation decision that takes them beyond this as the sole context of their search for an optimal solution. Some of their alternatives take them squarely back to Christopher's well-being:

- They can check to be sure there has been an attempt to wean Christopher from some of the life-supporting interventions in the ICU to see his response instead of transferring him.
- If it becomes a concern for any of them, they can inquire further regarding what specific services can be made available in the step-down unit to which he may be moved soon. If needed, they can advocate for an alternative temporary staffing model to ensure that Christopher's medical needs are met in the step-down unit.
- The team can acknowledge that Christopher Lacey's sister is a clinically informed source as a nurse. She can be an important ally, and as a loved one, her concerns about her brother warrant attention.
- If their further diligence raises serious questions for them, they can try to make a strong case for keeping this patient in the ICU until their concerns are met.

All of these alternatives to quickly moving the patient have the benefit of assuring themselves and his sister that, as professionals and therefore patient advocates, they feel as confident as possible that Christopher Lacey will continue to receive treatment consistent with a professional caring response due to each patient.

Step 5: Complete the Action

Once having addressed the need to follow up on one or more of the alternatives that arise out of their professional duty, the interprofessional ICU care team is as ready as possible to participate fully in the decision about moving Mr. Lacey and accepting who will be admitted if he is moved to a step-down unit. In short, unless they become convinced that he cannot continue to receive appropriate care, they can accept his move.

At the same time, their challenge has involved understanding that some aspects of the decision may be out of their hands because of equity concerns that include costs and the sources of reimbursement (if any) for this intensive level of interventions. Acknowledgment of such extraprofessional limitations has been seen by some as an opportunity to make *parsimonious decisions:* recognition of the wisdom of realizing the overall value of honoring limits that do not hold professionals hostage to the traditional professional ethic in which an identified patient's right or need becomes the sole criterion for decisions in the healthcare arena.[11] In fact, one current theme that has emerged is an emphasis on cost-effectiveness. In keeping with the previous discussions of the shift to value-based care, health professionals now have a responsibility to attend to clinical effectiveness in combination with cost-effectiveness and value to deliver quality care effectively and efficiently.[12,13] This shift has also been articulated in health professionals codes of ethics, moving attention to justice in resource allocation from a consideration to an ethical imperative. In a recent article, one interviewee put it, "The new care paradigm is all about value. And if you're doing things that increase costs without improving outcomes, you're not adding value."[14] In previous policy discussions, this idea might have been seen as "cost-effectiveness." However, by emphasizing an intrinsic value of taking costs and quality of outcomes seriously into account, some are steadily moving toward an ethic of care that involves decisions based not only on patient well-being but also on *financial stewardship.*[15] Financial stewardship advances the idea that clinicians ought to play a more direct role in controlling healthcare costs.

Thinking clearly about these alternatives allows you to bring the concerns of care and justice more fully into alignment.

Step 6: Evaluate the Process and Outcome

The expression "The proof is in the pudding" means that only if the pudding tastes as good as it looks or smells should one conclude that the chef has succeeded. The team must now engage in a reflective review of what Mr. Lacey's situation has taught all of them for future dilemmas of justice. The proof of a caring response to Mr. Lacey is that he has received the best clinical care available within reasonable constraints on resources, which are being allocated according to nonarbitrary procedures based on justice considerations.

The ICU team's reflection can also serve as an incentive to become more involved at the level of policy making and review in their institution and otherwise. The alternative of passively letting others make policy decisions and then reacting to them distorts the role of the professional as a moral agent today. As you recall from Chapter 7, living ethically as a member of the interprofessional care team includes participating in shared governance and collaborative decision making for safe, efficient, and effective care delivery. Some alternatives to the team members for policy advocacy include:

- The interprofessional care team should volunteer to be involved in developing ICU policies in their institution. Their participation supports discussion on the much-debated topic of the need to move resource allocation decision making from the bedside to the policy level.[16] This can help them minimize their justice dilemmas even if they cannot totally eliminate them.
- Allocation policy often is set by insurers, government bodies, and other extrainstitutional bodies. The ICU team members can be willing to participate in commissions, review committees, and other public forums, taking advantage of their opportunity to contribute considered opinions and provide documentation and data regarding their experiences.
- Individually or together, this interprofessional care team can also contribute to the work of national organizations that publish white papers, position statements, or other consensus opinions on the topic of resource allocation. Front-line clinicians are in an ideal position to contribute to such work. The American Geriatric Society Position Statement on feeding tubes in advanced dementia[17] and the American Occupational Therapy Association (AOTA)/American Physical Therapy Association (APTA)/ American Speech-Language-Hearing Association (ASHA) consensus statement on clinical judgment in healthcare settings[18] are two such examples of interprofessional statements that provide opinions, guidance, and recommendations based on a consensus of research evidence, expert opinion, best practice, and clinical expertise.

All the "Mr. Laceys" are the beneficiaries of the interprofessional care team's reflections, so that whatever the outcome in Mr. Lacey's immediate situation, the team members can rest assured that they have done the best they can for him and created an awareness of the vicissitudes of limitations imposed by scarce resources. Despite this assurance, the emotional burden of allocating resources can be high, and the interprofessional care team must attend to their own well-being. As you recall from Chapters 6 and 7, reflection and support from one's team supports provider resilience and well-being. In their randomized control trial comparing protected time alone to protected time with small-group discussions covering elements of mindfulness, reflection, and shared experience, West and colleagues found significantly increased levels of workplace engagement and empowerment

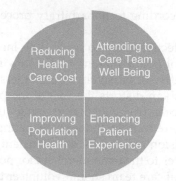

Fig. 14.2. The Quadruple Aim.

in nurses and physicians.[19] Attending to the experience of providing care has been referred to in the literature as the fourth, or *Quadruple Aim*[20,21] (Fig. 14.2). Attending to, and improving, the work life of health professionals and staff ensures that care providers are more resilient and better prepared to cope with disruptors in healthcare, such as evolving regulations and reimbursement structures and complex patient–family relationships.[22] By reflecting on care, health professionals attend to their own emotions and are empowered to care for themselves so that they can provide enhanced care for others. A professional resilience mindset is not only key to preventing burnout, it is the vehicle to the Quadruple Aim. As a resilient health professional, you will be able to add your insights into current debates about whether healthcare is a right, should be a resource to respond to basic need despite ability to pay, or is a commodity. In other words, in allocation decisions, your moral agency can be effective at both practice and policy levels to ensure the delivery of compassionate care.

Summary

Discussion of the proper moral response viewed from the lens of what distributive justice considerations require raises many questions regarding the most morally desirable way to proceed with professional care. A caring response may counsel one course of action, but real limits may require a different course.

What individual professionals and interprofessional care teams decide to do that is the most consistent with a caring response is based on clinical *and* policy considerations. In the ethical dimensions of the decision, they are faced with the issues of fairness and equity. They need moral courage to act on their decision in addition to wisdom to decide well. They also see the wisdom of participating in policy formation and review to try to minimize the harm that may result in situations of scarcity. Policymakers who take seriously what equity means in these types of situations help health professionals do the morally correct thing.

Understandably, much thought should go into determining ethical allocation policies to help health professionals implement good decisions. You are entering the healthcare environment in an era in which "evidence-based" outcomes of treatment based on aggregate data and notions of parsimonious decision making and values that include financial stewardship in clinical decisions challenge traditional ideas of professional ethics that do not take the larger context of policy fully into consideration. Your ability to think critically about unique patient cases is essential to implement best practices and sustain moral resilience.

Questions for Thought and Discussion

1. This exercise can be performed as an individual or group exercise.

   You have an opportunity to advocate for services that you judge should be included or excluded in your state's healthcare plan for allocating healthcare resources to Medicaid recipients (i.e., persons in the United States whose financial burdens qualify them for government-assisted healthcare). You take this task seriously for many reasons, but one is that the federal government has given your state the opportunity to develop an allocation plan for Medicaid reform nationally.

   Now the real crisis has come because several important services that the members of this interprofessional task force hoped could be included are not. You now have to decide among yourselves how to make the final cuts but not tinker with the list created by the first part of the process that has received approval. The task force has before it six possible services that could be added for the state's 20,000 Medicaid recipients (all estimated costs are annual, and the task force has $46,136,000 to adjudicate). Rank order, with highest priority number 1 and lowest 6, and write your rationale below each one. When you have reached $46,136,000 you have exhausted the remaining available funds.

   a. Preventive dental care for children ages 2 to 6 years. Includes a yearly check-up and teeth cleaning. Does not include fillings, orthodontics, or other acute dental or surgical services. Estimated cost: $3,760,000.

   b. Outpatient behavioral/mental health services (initial evaluation and up to 12 visits) for children and adolescents (ages 4–19 years). Does not include medications or hospitalization. Estimated cost: $8,000,000.

   c. Smoking-related asthma treatments. Estimated cost: $8,860,000.

   d. Liver transplantation and follow-up. Estimated cost: $12,200,000.

   e. Mammograms for women younger than 50 years. Estimated cost: $6,900,000.

   f. Coverage for pain management for patients with chronic back pain, including medications, rehabilitation, and pain centers, but not including surgery, which could be covered in another surgical category that ranked higher on the list of services. Estimated cost: $21,040,000.

2. A close friend of your mother has a rare progressive, life-limiting, and eventually fatal disease. In the course of your work, you discover a highly experimental but potentially lifesaving medication that is being tested as a clinical trial at the institution where you are employed. You make a few inquiries and now have serious doubts about whether your mother's friend will be able to get into the study because the waiting list already is much longer than the experimental protocol allows. Still, you think the caring thing to do is to at least let her know that such an intervention is available. Knowing her, she will definitely want to go for it and will push you hard to try to influence your colleague to get her into the study. While you are thinking about these things, the clinician conducting the protocol calls you back to say that on the basis of your being a fellow employee, she may try to rearrange the queue to get your mother's friend into the study. No promises. Now you find yourself wondering if it is fair to those who are already waiting in the queue if your influence does work and your mother's friend jumps ahead in the line.

   How do you go about deciding what to do in this situation that brings to your doorstep both your care for someone close to your mother with a medical need (although not a patient of yours) and your reflection about others eligible for inclusion in the study who may end up being ousted?

3. You are a physician assistant in a private clinic. Your receptionist asks if you can see an unscheduled new patient who is crying in the waiting room. You glance at the back-to-back appointments for the afternoon, sigh, and ask your assistant if he can get a better idea of what brings her here today with such an urgent need to see you.

   He interviews her, and after your next patient, you get this report: The patient, 26 years old, explained haltingly that her headaches began around the time she began rationing her insulin dosage. She then burst into tears saying, "My mother said once I turned 21 I was on my own. I can't afford the copays until my next paycheck in 2 weeks, so I started to decrease my dosage each day to make the vials go further." You know this woman needs help; her anxiety is overwhelming her, and she is at risk for ketoacidosis. She needs a more thorough endocrine workup, and a social work consult, neither of which you will be able to arrange for today. You have begun to see this trend in the clinic. Insulin prices have more than doubled over the last 5 years. A single vial is around $250 and general use for an individual with type 1 diabetes is two to four vials a month. You are genuinely concerned about her but also conscious of the full waiting room outside your door.

   What considerations of a caring response and the claims of distributive justice come into consideration in your deliberation about what to do? What will you do? Why?

References

1. Mellinger JL, Volk ML: Transplantation for alcohol-related liver disease: Is it fair? *Alcohol Alcoholism* 53(2):173–177, 2018.
2. Fleck LM: *Just caring: health care rationing and democratic deliberation*, New York, 2009, Oxford University Press.
3. Callahan DT: *Taming the beloved beast: how medical technology costs are destroying our health care system*, Princeton, NJ, 2009, Princeton University Press, p 2.
4. Doherty R: The impact of advances in medical technology on rehabilitative care. In Purtilo RB, Jensen GM, Royeen CB, editors: *Educating for moral action: a sourcebook in health and rehabilitation ethics*, Philadelphia, 2005, FA Davis, pp 99–106.
5. Ubel PA: Why it's not time for health care rationing, *Hastings Cent Rep* 45(2):15–19, 2015.
6. Martin DR, Moskop JC, Bookman K, et al: Compensation models in emergency medicine: an ethical perspective, *Am J Emerg Med*, January 2019. doi: 10.1016/j.ajem.2019.158372.
7. Faller P, Hunt J, van Hooydonk E, et al: Application of data-driven decision making using Ayres Sensory Integration® with a child with autism, *Am J Occup Ther* 70(1):1–9, Jan/Feb 2016.
8. Bärring M, Lundgren C, Åkerman M, et al: 5G enabled manufacturing evaluation for data-driven decision making, *Procedia CIRP* 72:266–271, 2018.
9. APTA: *Physical therapy outcomes registry*. Available at www.ptoutcomes.com/. *Uniform data system*. Available at www.udsmr.org. *Medical data systems*. Available at www.cms.gov/. *National Quality Forum*. Available at http://www.qualityforum.org.
10. Hoffman S: Actuarial fairness vs. moral fairness in health insurance, *Law Bioethics Rep* 1(4):2–4, 2002.
11. Tilburt J, Cassel C: Why the ethics of parsimonious medicine is not the ethics of rationing, *JAMA* 309(8):773–774, 2013.
12. Rosoff PM: Who Should Ration? *AMA J Ethics* 19(2):164–173, 2017.
13. Gurwitz JH, Pearson SD: Novel therapies for an aging population: grappling with price, value, and affordability, *JAMA* 321(16):1567–1568, 2019.
14. Hayhurst C: Putting data to work, *PTinMOTIONmag* 7(2):3436, 39-42, 2015.
15. Ubel PA, Jagsi R: Promoting population health through financial stewardship, *N Engl J Med* 370(14):1280–1281, 2014.
16. Persson E, Andersson D, Back L, et al: Discrepancy between health care rationing at the bedside and policy level, *Med Decis Making* 38(7):881–887, 2018.
17. American Geriatrics Society Ethics Committee and Clinical Practice and Models of Care Committee, American Geriatrics Society: Feeding tubes in advanced dementia position statement, *J Am Geriatr Soc* 62:1590–1593, 2014.
18. American Occupational Therapy Association, American Physical Therapy Association, and American Speech Language and Hearing Association: *AOTA, APTA, ASHA Consensus statement on clinical judgment in health care settings*.

Available at http://www.aota.org/Practice/Ethics/Consensus-Statement-AOTA-APTA-ASHA.aspx#sthash.say1opqG.dpuf.

19. West CP, Dyrbye LN, Rabatin JT, et al: Intervention to promote physician well-being, job satisfaction, and professionalism: a randomized clinical trial, *JAMA Intern Med* 174(4):527–533, 2014.
20. Bodenheimer T, Sinsky C: From triple to quadruple aim: care of the patient requires care of the provider, *Ann Fam Med* 12(6):573–576, 2014.
21. Fitzpatrick B, Bloore K, Blake N: Joy in work and reducing nurse burnout: from triple aim to quadruple aim, *AACN Adv Crit Care* 30(2):185–188, 2019.
22. Fink-Samnick E: Professional resilience paradigm meets the quadruple aim: professional mandate, ethical imperative, *Prof Case Manage* 22(5):248–253, 2017.

Compensatory and Social Justice: Essential Equity and Inclusion Considerations

Objectives

The reader should be able to:

- Distinguish some key differences and similarities in distributive justice, compensatory justice, and social justice perspectives.
- Identify a range of policy options that could be adopted in situations in which compensatory justice is being considered as an appropriate response to a group that has been harmed.
- Describe some considerations that must be taken into account when social justice approaches are applied toward the goal of a more equitable society.
- Discuss the "dilemma of difference" in regard to labeling and its effect on a just allocation of resources.
- Evaluate why stigma and social marginalization are barriers to creating just healthcare policies based on the ideals of social justice.
- Discuss how inclusion and inclusive practices serve to guide professional duties and inform opportunities to promote social justice in healthcare.
- Recognize how the notion of solidarity shifts the focus away from individual autonomy in the ethical analysis of justice issues.
- Examine how health disparities figure into discussions of justice from a social justice perspective.
- Identify and evaluate the role of personal responsibility for health maintenance from the standpoints of compensatory and social justice perspectives.

New terms and ideas you will encounter in this chapter

inequality	interdependence	intersectionality
inequity/inequitable	altruism	privilege
compensatory justice	reciprocity ethic	socially marginalized
social justice	social need	solidarity
stigma	labeling	inclusion
worker's compensation	the dilemma of	personal responsibility
collective responsibility	difference	for health
communitarian approach	vulnerability	

Introduction

One only needs to browse the pages of any major U.S. newspaper or watch the newsfeed across the globe to hear headlines such as divided nation, wealth gap, and health disparity. These publications and media outlets share the common goal of bringing attention to structural injustices that are pervasive in our country and in many places around the world. When considering the juxtaposition of tremendous wealth beside abject poverty and the other vast disparities, we begin to reflect on inequality and inequity. By definition, an *inequality* is when persons or groups have an equal claim on basic resources that will support their opportunity and well-being but one group has realized an unfair share that puts the others at a serious disadvantage. This disadvantage can be a disparity of distribution or opportunity. An *inequity* is an instance of injustice. *Inequitable* is the term that has been adopted to underscore political, social, or cultural processes that have been adopted to the detriment of those who are being treated unfairly to the point that policies and practices put them at an even greater societal disadvantage. Thus these publications and media outlets highlight that the way basic goods and services are allocated go offtrack from the kind of distributive justice reasoning introduced in Chapter 14, resulting in further disadvantage to those in the more vulnerable societal positions.

Well-intentioned people through the ages have been concerned with how to justly distribute basic goods and services, knowing that different persons or groups do begin life at different starting blocks, some with more barriers or opportunities for "success" than others. Some disadvantageous inequalities, it is argued, arise from unfortunate accidents of fate to which no one can be held accountable, and others are the result of unjust laws, policies, and practices constructed to consciously benefit a select group. Attempts to deal with these situations have given rise to two additional interpretations of justice: compensatory justice and social justice. These concepts mostly overlap with those introduced in Chapter 14 but with some noteworthy differences.

Their distinction is that compensatory and social justice take into account the person's or group's relative disadvantage in society overall as a source of claims on societal resources. This goes beyond distributive justice reasoning that some persons have particular needs (such as the need for healthcare) and that justice concerns about their claim comes from that particular circumstance. *Compensatory justice* and *social justice* reasoning hold that, regardless of specific need for a particular good or service such as healthcare, it is simply the individual's or group's societal disadvantage overall that creates their claim for any specific service. One might say that it goes "upstream" from a claim that arises among a group who has a specific type of need to one that arises because of societal disadvantage overall. The shared assumptions, sometimes more fully articulated than others, are that there is a positive right to basic goods and services, there is a duty to respect everyone as worthy of a share of society's resources, and society must try to make adjustments according to need. At the core of the issue for our study here is the question of whether some groups of people in an economically or other type of societally disadvantaged position have a claim to healthcare goods and services on that basis. Most of the study in this chapter is devoted to compensatory justice but also demonstrates how it is one aspect of the broader concept of social justice, the latter of which focuses on serious, often systemic disparities in health and healthcare microallocation.

The story of the Maki brothers is an example designed to help you focus on how societal position factors into compensatory justice considerations and how you, the health professional, are involved.

🌱 The Story of the Maki Brothers

Mr. Eino Maki is a miner who emigrated from Finland to the United States in 1985. He was born into a poor rural family that lived in a small remote village near the Russian border. Eino did not attend school in Finland after the first grade because he was a "slow learner" and could not keep up with the other students. Although most students in his country received excellent educations, his family refused to send him to a special school in Tampere, some 300 miles away, saying they needed his help on the farm.

One dreadful morning in 1982, a fire destroyed the family's home and Eino's parents perished in the fire. Eino and his younger sister went to live with an aunt and uncle in Helsinki where he stayed for 3 years. At the age of 18 years, he could not find work in Helsinki given the decrease in asbestos mining and exportation, so he immigrated to the United States to live with his unmarried older brother in an area where there are many coal and mineral mines. The community where his brother lives is about 50% Finnish.

When Eino arrived in the United States, his brother John attempted unsuccessfully to find him a job in the railroad construction company in which he was employed as a section worker. After several months, Eino did secure a job in a nearby mine. With the company's assistance he was able to secure a work permit that would eventually lead to U.S. citizenship.

Eino has been employed by this same mining company and has held essentially the same position for the past 35 years. Although he still suffers occasional teasing by his coworkers associated with his being "slow" at grasping ideas, he is an excellent employee and participates in the social life of the community. Many evenings at the local bar, the men spend time reminiscing about the "good old days" in Finland, and everyone talks about going back. Privately, however, John and Eino agree that it is unlikely they will ever return.

In the past 2 or 3 months, Eino has had increasing difficulty breathing. Occasionally, he has coughed up blood-tinged sputum. He often has pains in his chest when he awakens, but the pains disappear after he has been up and around for a couple of hours. At first, he does not say anything to John, but one November morning he realizes that he cannot make it to work. He asks John to take him to the company physician.

Eino has never liked doctors. In all of his years of employment, he has visited the company clinic only for the required routine annual physical examinations and once when he suffered a dislocated shoulder in a fall from a mine platform. He has always passed the physical examinations with a "clean bill of health."

After the examination, the physician assistant who conducted the initial tests tells Eino that some further tests are needed and that he will have to be admitted to a hospital, which is about 120 miles away. Eino is angered at this news but realizes that he cannot go back to work feeling the way he does. He tells John he wants to rest at home until he feels better, but John, seeing the trouble his brother is having breathing, insists he goes and drives him there.

Eino is admitted and 5 days later his condition takes a sudden turn for the worse. John is called and drives back to the hospital. When he arrives, he is met by Dr. Kai Nielson, a young physician who looks to John as if he cannot be a day older than 16 years. Dr. Nielson invites John into a little room next to the nurse's desk and closes the door. "Mr. Maki, I'm afraid I have some bad news," he says. "Your brother has not been told yet, but he has cancer and has had it for quite some time. Ideally, we should start treatment immediately. Unfortunately, the case manager tells me that Eino's company's health plan does not fully cover the type of treatment I have recommended."

So far, John has barely been hearing what the young doctor is saying. His mind is racing wildly. He vaguely recalls Eino's report of a discussion at a union meeting a year or so ago regarding a rumor that work in some coal mines causes cancer and that their union was looking into it. This concerned John greatly, but Eino brushed it aside and said it was "a bunch of hogwash" and he was "healthy as a horse," refusing to discuss it further. Later he told a friend, "You know that Eino is not only healthy as a horse but stubborn as a mule. What could I do? I let the matter drop."

Finally, John realizes that Dr. Nielson has been talking to him. "We could do the treatment, but unless Eino has additional insurance coverage, the treatment is going to cost him a lot of money."

John tells the physician that they own a small cottage together, with about two acres of unfarmed land around it. They have no savings, only the pension that their respective companies provide, but that benefit cannot be realized until Eino is 65 years old. Dr. Nielson replies sympathetically, "Well, there is a chance your brother will be eligible for federal assistance, but, unfortunately, it may mean you will have to sell your house to become eligible for it once you've expended the earnings you'd realize from that. I don't know exactly how it works, but I'll have the social worker talk to you. Of course, we can't guarantee that the treatment will beat the disease, but we feel reasonably sure that it would at least slow down the rate of growth of the cancer cells."

There is a pause. Then he adds, "It is, of course, a big decision. It is entirely up to you and your brother what you decide to do. We haven't talked to him or, rather, been able to talk to him. He doesn't like doctors much. Why don't you two talk it over with the social worker here or the physician assistant he saw back at his company clinic? Remember, it's your decision and your brother's. But don't take too long in deciding... I think every day counts. Now what questions do you have for me?" John shakes his head "none." "Well," Dr. Nielson concludes, "if you do after talking with the others I've recommended, have them set up an appointment for you to see me again."

As John stands, Dr. Nielson extends his hand and John shakes it warmly. John glances up into the doctor's face and sees genuine compassion in the young man's eyes. John blurts out, "Was the cancer caused by the mines?" The young doctor drops John's hand and studies his own hands as he answers, "Mr. Maki, the cause of cancer is often complex. It can be the result of a combination of factors. But the type of cancer that your brother has is the same type that coal miners get at a higher rate than the general population. Primarily it attacks the lungs."

John thanks Dr. Nielson. Outside the doctor's office, he wanders over to a window and stares outside into the snowy darkness for a long time, his hands in the pockets of his cargo pants. He has not cried since their brother Matt was killed in a tractor accident many years before, but he feels a lump rising in his throat now. He feels totally unable to move, as if he is glued to the floor. He struggles to think clearly, but his mind remains a blank.

The story of John and Eino Maki raises numerous ethical questions. For instance, some people reading this story have questions about confidentiality. Why is Kai Nielson sharing all of this information with John when Eino, a competent adult, is the patient? What about Eino's informed consent? Is it appropriate for the physician to put the burden of sharing the bad news with Eino on John's shoulders? What should the role of the physician assistant and social worker be? These are certainly important ethical questions.

However, the lens in this chapter focuses on the justice issues that patients in similar situations to Eino's raise. Their basic similarity is that they are among the members of society who are dismissed or even disdained by those in society who have security that their healthcare and other needs will be met.[1]

The Goal: A Caring Response

Eino Maki, a seemingly healthy, hard-working man, becomes a victim of circumstances that leave his health compromised. A caring response by health professionals requires that they do whatever is "best" or, in the language of ethics, is beneficent for this patient. In the story, the physician assistant and Kai Nielson have been doing exactly that in their attempt to get at the clinical root of Eino's symptoms, and they each make strong recommendations about what he needs to do. Other members of the interprofessional care team (the case manager Kai mentioned, a social worker, a respiratory therapist, and a team of nurses) are also involved in his care during this 5-day hospitalization. At the same time, they know that matters are fast slipping out of their hands. There is an environmental source of his cancer, a death-dealing cancer we presume, triggered by his employment in a company in which he likely has been exposed to toxic levels of carcinogens over a prolonged period of time. Mr. Maki's decision about what to do for his cancer treatment will depend in part on the availability of funds from his employing company or a government source to help pay for them. If the professionals think this through to its logical conclusion, they will realize that they have an opportunity to try to help build and strengthen institutions and societal arrangements that support individuals in such predicaments. Such policies are not designed only for one person (e.g., Mr. Maki) the way a treatment plan is created for a specific patient but outline a program that covers him and others like him. A subgroup of institutional and societal arrangements addresses legal mechanisms to compensate persons for harms incurred in the larger environment, whether workplace, home, or publicly shared spaces. Compensatory justice deals with this reality from an ethical and legal standpoint, and it is those ethical considerations that are addressed here.

The Six-Step Process in Compensatory Justice Decisions

As the introduction described, Eino Maki is carrying out a type of work that is dangerous to his health, but he remains in a job available to him and others who have similar low social and economic status in society. You might respond that others who are at more financially and socially secure levels of society have an opportunity for this kind of work, too. True, but this reasoning is akin to the French political philosopher during the French Revolution who observed that "both the rich and the poor have an equal right to sleep under the bridges of Paris at night." Eino's autonomy to select a safer or more pleasant work environment is greatly diminished or absent. Thoughtful individuals have pondered the role that such societally determined differences among patients should play. To help elucidate some of their thinking, let us first consider the relevant information in the story of the Maki brothers.

Step 1: Gather Relevant Information

For the purpose of encouraging you to think about compensatory justice situations, it is assumed that Eino's situation is caused by his work environment. However, in an actual clinical evaluation, your gathering of relevant information first requires clarifying further his stage of lung cancer and whether tests substantiate that the source is the carcinogens to which he has been exposed as a mining company employee.

Another relevant piece of information is how much responsibility the company took to help prevent undue exposure. The way risks were presented and action taken to minimize them could make a difference in how we view this situation.

You do know that Eino, and others like him, perform labor tasks that are needed for the society to function well but often are not valued in other ways and may carry high risks to the workers. Of course, some high-risk situations are respected, and individuals who perform the tasks are given extra financial benefits and are held in high regard. Examples are firefighters, members of a police force, or U.S. Navy Seals. Others, like Eino, are relegated to greater risk and less desirable jobs because of their overall lower social status, often accompanied by poverty or other characteristics that carry a societal stigma with them. *Stigma* in this social sense is a term first used by Goffman,[2] a sociologist, to depict persons held in low regard because of qualities they have or functions they play in society. Status comes into being when mainstream society members, those in control and authority, make arbitrary judgments about the value of different kinds of lives and assign low priority to some whom they devalue. The most explicit negative effect on stigmatized groups comes through their disproportionately small allotment of the society's goods and services or opportunity to access those goods and services. It can be argued that even if Eino did have the full cognitive capacity to comprehend the danger he encountered in his life in the mines, he would have been able to do little to change his situation.

Step 2: Identify the Type of Ethical Problem

The idea of "compensation" at the root of compensatory justice issues arises out of society's consciousness that it is the morally right thing to be fair. But not everyone has the same chance at basic lifesaving or life-enhancing benefits from the get-go. You are probably familiar with the idea of a "handicap" among competitors in the sports arena. In that environment, good sportsmanship dictates that the handicapped player be given additional "points" to try to make up for the disadvantage. There is an intuitive correctness about this attempt to "even the playing field." But this compensation activity is not always the case in the larger society, so it is not surprising that the problem it raises is characterized as a dilemma of justice.

Compensatory justice acknowledges due regard for groups of individuals by offering them compensations for disadvantages to which they are exposed. It is a means of ensuring justice.[3,4] As for Eino, we have reason to believe that his work in the mines led to a life-threatening, industry-related condition. If the company management knowingly placed workers in harm's way by neglecting to provide adequate safeguards in an effort to benefit the company's bottom line, their responsibility as moral agents to redress this wrong squarely can be placed on them. If they, too, are surprised by this bad news, society's understanding of the wisdom of compensating individuals in such a situation has led to certain mechanisms for spreading the cost of the compensation across the larger society with taxes and other common resources. (In the United States, *worker's compensation* grew out of this idea originally but since has come to be considered a protection for anyone injured on a job, regardless of their social status, economic security, or other variables.) Sometimes the wisdom of providing compensation has come from pressure by interest groups, such as unions or other organizations (e.g., nonprofits run by various religious groups), that try to provide a voice for those who are not in a position to speak effectively against such wrongs themselves. In recent years, concern has arisen in the literature that labor unions' effective voice may be suffering from divided loyalties within the unions themselves.[5]

However voiced, the idea that a moral claim for compensation should influence how resources are allocated makes this problem an ethical dilemma of justice, which was introduced in Chapter 3.

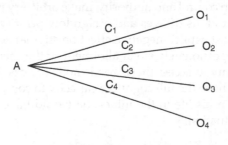

A = Moral agent
C_1 = Action taken on behalf of claimants whose societal "handicaps" are added to their medical need
O_1 = Outcome is priority on allocation of resources to those whose societal "handicaps" are added to medical need
C_{2-4} = Action taken on behalf of other claimants
O_{2-4} = Outcome determined by priorities on basis of claimants in 2–4

Compensatory justice ethical problem.

Similar reasoning has been applied to priority setting for shelter, food, or other basic goods of society, with the underlying assumption that not everyone comes equally supported by society to adequately take part in life's basic benefits.

> ### ◎ Summary
>
> Compensatory justice assumes that the allocation of resources should be made to address healthcare problems of an individual or group on the basis of more than medical need alone. Their relatively disadvantaged position in society also is a relevant factor.

Step 3: Use Ethics Theories or Approaches to Analyze the Problem

In Chapter 14, you were introduced to the principle of equity and the idea of positive rights as ethical concepts that are critical for analyzing the morally appropriate allocation of resources according to distributive justice reasoning. The concepts are useful for analysis here too, along with the principle of nonmaleficence.

To review, equity begins with the formal principle of justice that every effort must be made to treat each person in a similarly situated circumstance alike, with allowance for departures from that baseline of equality on the condition that differences are derived from ethically acceptable criteria. Policy based on equity also takes into account costs and quality of care that are inherent in policy formation.

Mr. Maki works in a dangerous environment that is not highly regarded as a career line for mainstream members of society. Other miners are "similarly situated." They are in a class all their own, equal with each other but not with mainstream society. A compensatory justice approach takes into account that members of mainstream society have more opportunities and resources to deal with crises such as Eino faces. So, "similarly situated" means that all like him fall within the same general category of need for claimants on healthcare resources. The compensation in the idea of compensatory justice is that there is a moral pull on a just society to respond to the disadvantages that Eino faces as one who is lower on the rung of the social and economic ladder of society through no fault of his own. Priority standing or more societal resources may be necessary to be sure he receives quality care equal to his mainstream counterparts with similar clinical need. The fact that he is contributing an important service that others usually do not choose adds to the argument that those with more resources have a moral responsibility to help the larger society stay intact through compensations to those like Eino who are less well-off economically or socially.

Where does healthcare as a positive right fit into the compensatory justice framework? It certainly helps support the idea of compensatory justice if healthcare is viewed as a right that everyone should have access to in

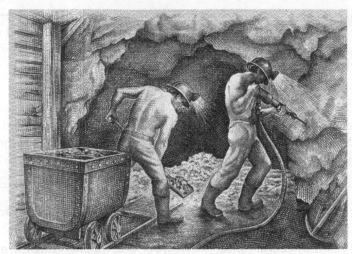

Fig. 15.1. Mine workers are one example of people whose jobs carry significant dangers to health and safety. *(Copyright iStock.com/GeorgiosArt.)*

contrast to the opposite idea that healthcare is a commodity like all other products to be bought by those who can afford to do so. In some cases, the right may necessitate that those who are better off as members of mainstream society are required to do whatever is needed to support access for all.

The principle of nonmaleficence also figures in this analysis. The principle of nonmaleficence, "do no harm," highlights that there should be a commitment to prevent harm and remove harm when possible. In Mr. Maki's case, a compelling argument in favor of supporting his medical treatments financially is not only that he has a terrible medical condition but that he has the condition because he is in a job that carries with it the albatross of a carcinogenic agent. It seems wrong, from a compensatory justice point of view, that he should have to suffer the ravages of a debilitating, painful, and incurable disease because he has been working in a setting that economically disadvantaged individuals are more apt to accept because it is one of the only options open to them even though it carries a life-threatening hazard with it (Fig. 15.1). Compensation is a positive response to Eino's harm. For many, this case for compensation is strengthened by the possibility that the company might have known about the risk to the miners and failed to take humane measures and strong precautions on their behalf.

⊚ Summary

Compensatory justice holds that some persons are at a societal disadvantage in ways that require the larger community or some aspect of it to respond to medical or other harms that occur because of the person's or group's disadvantaged financial or societal position.

Step 4: Explore the Practical Alternatives

Societal disadvantage today creates disparities in health status, and access to healthcare resources are limited for disadvantaged groups.[6] The compensatory justice issue can be highlighted by comparing several policies that might be adopted by companies, governments, or other policy-making bodies. All but one of them suggests that there is a *collective responsibility* by a company or government agency to respond to harm in situations such as Eino's. You have an opportunity to explore six major alternatives from an ethical standpoint informed by reasoning about compensatory justice. In each case, you can choose whether you support or do not support the policy and provide reasons to help you defend your decision.

---

1. The mining company should offer Eino, and all similarly situated employees, a sum of money equal to that which would pay for their treatment and provide early retirement with all retirement privileges if they are unable to return to work. The affected employees can decide whether to spend the money on treatment or something else.
   Support _____ Do not support _____
   Consider:
   - The most caring response to all similarly situated employees
   - Eino's rights, autonomy, and moral responsibility
   - The company's rights and moral responsibility
   - The larger society's involvement

2. The company should pay for the employees' treatment with the understanding that, if medically able, the employees will return to work and, if unable, they will be retired with full privileges of retirement that would have accrued if they had worked until regular retirement age.
   Support _____ Do not support _____
   Consider:
   - The most caring response
   - Eino's rights and moral responsibility
   - The company's rights and moral responsibility
   - The larger society's involvement

3. The company should pay for the employees' treatment with the understanding that they will return to work if medically able. If unable, the persons will be terminated with whatever retirement has accumulated up to the time of termination.
   Support _____ Do not support _____
   Consider:
   - The most caring response
   - Eino's rights, autonomy, and moral responsibility

(Continued)

- The company's rights and moral responsibility
- The larger society's possible involvement of supplementing Eino's income if he has little or no retirement income (society as a "safety net")

4. Federal or state funds from tax dollars or other public sources should provide Eino (and all similarly situated people) a sum of money equal to that which would pay for treatment and arrange to supplement his current retirement earnings up to his company's full retirement level if he is unable to return to work. The affected persons can decide whether to spend the money on treatment or on something else.
   Support _____ Do not support _____
   Consider:
   - The most caring response
   - Eino's rights, autonomy, and moral responsibility
   - The company's lack of involvement for compensation beyond what Eino has already earned
   - The larger public's collective contributions and assurance of being able to be supported in Eino's situation

5. Federal or state funds from tax dollars or other public sources should pay for full medical coverage for people like Eino but not offer them a cash equivalent. That is, the compensatory considerations are limited to medical treatment directly related to the disabling medical condition that resulted from employment in the dangerous environment. The understanding is that such persons will return to the former employment if medically able. If unable, they will be retired by the company with full privileges, and the company will receive a subsidy from the government.
   Support _____ Do not support _____
   Consider:
   - The most caring response
   - Eino's rights and autonomy
   - The shared moral responsibility of the company and the larger public and how it is divided (society as provider of medical compensation, retirement "safety net" covered by the company)

6. No company or public compensation should be provided for Eino or similarly situated people.
   Support _____ Do not support _____
   Consider:
   - The most caring response
   - Eino's rights, autonomy, and moral responsibility
   - The company's rights, autonomy, and moral responsibility
   - The public's rights, autonomy, and moral responsibility

As you can see, each of these six alternative courses of response provides a variety of possible conflicts of interest or opportunities for community-wide solidarity efforts. The conflicts may be seen as the competing interests of the similarly situated harmed individuals, the private sector of society, and the larger public sector of society. Questions of the most caring approach (all things considered), rights, autonomy, and the sphere of moral responsibility should be taken into account in the analysis of any of them. Options 1 through 5 support the compensatory justice position that compensation should be provided for the harm suffered by people such as Eino Maki, although the form, amount, and source of compensatory funds differ according to the political and social context in which the compensatory mechanisms are situated. Many ethicists who address healthcare issues support the position that at least a basic safety net of healthcare benefits should be provided by federal, state, or local governments (the public sector). The position that the entire community of society should work together to find common solutions because it will, in fact, more likely benefit all is called a *communitarian approach.*[7] Although there are several varieties of communitarian thinking, they reflect a basic theme of *interdependence.* We are fundamentally not autonomous after all, and at some time, each of us depends heavily on others to help sustain us.

The first five options all have elements of such thinking. Each provides some compensation for Eino and other people made vulnerable by circumstance. The tradition of the United States has carried some communitarian themes in it but is largely based on the individual autonomy of persons living within structures and institutions in which markets drive what each individual or group will justly enjoy.[8] Canada and many European countries take a more communitarian approach. Eino and John Maki are good examples of people who want to "earn their own way," the hallmark of this type of thinking. There also are several varieties of this liberal approach within modern society. The sixth option most fully conveys the extreme of the liberal society free market approach, which treats healthcare as a commodity as discussed in Chapter 14. In this reasoning, Eino, like anyone else, should not be provided for by company or public funds. He does have a job and like anyone else may have to spend what he and his brother believe is a disproportionate level of income on necessary or desired goods and services. Proponents of this argument feel that Eino chose to work in the mines, perhaps even knowing the risks involved. As you can see, this latter approach in its bare form leaves no room for the idea of compensatory justice in healthcare.

⑥ Summary

Compensatory justice approaches require an assumption of interdependence of people in society. This assumption does not preclude shared responsibility for some compensation benefits by the private sector (i.e., the company), the individual, and public resources.

The previous discussion illustrates that compensatory justice cannot be discussed apart from determination of who in the population should bear the burden of costs incurred as a result of policies based on compensatory reasoning. For example, the first three options suggest that the cost should be borne privately—in this case, by the company. Options 4 and 5 remove the responsibility from the private sector. Taxes to pay for compensation plans come from those people who, under the U.S. doctrine of personal liberty, have been able to become and remain self-sufficient. As taxes increase for the purpose of supporting groups or individuals with situations such as that of Eino Maki, compensatory justice may be viewed as impinging on the personal autonomy of people who currently are not ill or in need of medical services. This hits deep in the North American psyche. As one colleague in the United States reflected recently, autonomy has a monopoly on our moral attention. Resistance grows out of anger that one has earned the means to pay for healthcare and then, because of an unfair societal mandate to help support basic needs of strangers, has to forgo being financially able to send children to colleges they otherwise would choose, put additions on their homes, buy sports and exercise equipment to keep fit, or, for some, even heat their homes properly. The question of the conditions by which each of us is our brothers' [and sisters'] keeper currently is being debated as yet another round of national healthcare reform measures are placed before the U.S. public and legislature.

Step 5: Complete the Action

To arrive at a policy that supports public financing in whole or in part for Mr. Maki, policymakers must decide how much personal liberty the more societally advantaged members of society are willing to contribute toward mechanisms that allow compensatory justice to be upheld. Those in favor of the community-oriented spirit of compensatory justice argue that it is a "contribution" instead of a "sacrifice" or loss. One example is that such a contribution yields the rewards of altruism. *Altruism* is the act of doing something on another's behalf with no thought or expectation of return, a concept that is found in almost every major religious tradition.[9] Another is the idea of a *reciprocity ethic*. In the latter, a contribution to someone else's well-being creates a societal environment in which others are willing to contribute to one's own well-being when the need arises. Those who have written the most extensively from this orientation as an ethical approach emphasize its similarity to the Golden Rule of the Christian Bible: "Do to others what you want them to do to you"—a basic idea with analogues in many other religious and philosophical traditions.

 Reflection
Having considered all the ramifications, suppose that you are a member of a policy-making committee that must vote on the six

policy options discussed. You have already made your personal selection by completing the exercise. Now you are confronted with committee members who hold different views from your own. Of the arguments opposing your choice, which ones do you think will be the most powerful?

_____

_____

_____

_____

Although you have been a responsible committee member, what (if any) lingering reservations do you have regarding your own choice?

_____

_____

_____

_____

In participating in this type of policy decision process, you have exercised your ethical reasoning in a manner similar to that which you will need to use in the policy-related aspects of the practice of your profession. In your process of coming to a decision, you have had an opportunity to engage in the step-by-step process of ethical decision making. You have brought to consciousness the expressions of caring, considered the relevant facts, dealt with the ethical dilemma of justice in the situation with which you are faced, considered the alternatives, and, through that, arrived at your decision.

Step 6: Evaluate the Process and Outcome

Although much can be said in support of compensatory justice, the determination of groups in society to be singled out for preferential treatment requires that they be designated as a special class. This raises at least two important caveats: one emerges from the double edge of labeling, and the other is from the specific label of "vulnerability." Let us shift our attention from compensatory justice situations alone to the larger context of social justice. The topics that follow will show the ways in which compensatory justice and social justice approaches are related.

Social Justice, Social Need, and Respect for All

By focusing on Eino Maki's situation and the type of contribution he makes as a worker, we can begin to see how a person's societal position impacts a deeper understanding of what justice requires. However, there are some important shortcomings in relying solely on the fact that a person is contributing to the workforce as the means of triggering the wheels of justice. *Social justice* questions in bioethics and political science circles focus on discussions of societal responsibility, such as government-sponsored policies that provide access to healthcare (or other basic goods and services) for disadvantaged or impoverished members of a society.[10] Impoverishment is not only financial; it also includes lack of opportunities for participation in other health-supporting aspects of society.

Health professionals in many fields are becoming more aware of how health disparities are an issue of social justice that they must help to alleviate. As you recall from Chapter 13, a health disparity is a particular type of health difference that is closely linked with social or economic disadvantage.[11] Race, ethnicity, socioeconomic status, sexual orientation and identity, gender, skin color, and disability are all recognized as fostering inequities in healthcare and health outcomes. Importantly, from a social justice perspective, these identities do not exist independently, rather in *intersectionality*. They are interconnected and cannot be separated from each other. Intersectionality is a framework for conceptualizing "a person, group of people, or social problem as affected by multiple discriminations and disadvantages."[12] An excellent example of an initiative to document health disparities through patient reported outcomes and care utilization is being undertaken by rehabilitation professionals at the national level.[13]

It embraces situations like Eino's but goes further to tackle the issue of serious and pervasive racial and educational disparities in health that persist among millions of people in the United States. Although it goes beyond the scope of this text, it is important to highlight some of the pressing issues in health disparities as they relate to social justice. For example, racial and ethnic disparities in mental health have been well documented in healthcare. Black and Latinx patients frequently experience greater rates of persistent mental health disorders, yet are less likely to receive guideline-based care and novel treatments than whites.[14] Individuals with disabilities are more likely to experience lower education levels, lower employment rates, fewer household resources, and poorer health than people without disabilities.[15,16] They also experience delayed diagnosis in chronic conditions, which result in restrictions in participation. For this reason, public health interventions are critically important.[17] As you recall from Chapter 2, health disparities are complex and there is often no single cause for differences. As research in this area continues to advance, it is clear that several factors maintain and further these disparities at the patient, provider, and systemic or institutional level.[17] As a member of the interprofessional care team, you have the knowledge, skills, and responsibility to recognize the impact of health disparities on care delivery and the moral obligation to make every effort to eliminate such disparities.

Some argue the folly of allowing these disparities from a utilitarian approach. Nobel Prize–winning economist Amartya Sen[18] submitted that we cannot realize the benefits of a healthful society overall until we uncover the devaluation of stigmatized groups who simply by virtue of skin color, ethnicity, physical or mental condition, age, or gender bear the brunt of discrimination. He shows convincingly that our fate is intertwined and that, without respect for the capacities that every single member of society brings to the society, all eventually lose.[18] By disentangling "capacity" from the Western ideal of societal worth measured by "contribution," he honors the life situation of all, whatever the societal interpretation of their economic worth. As you can see, the principle of interdependence is embedded in this utilitarian conception of society. In short, the disproportionately small allotment of the society's goods and services to devalued members of society arises from prejudices that threaten to trade the idea of equality and respect for all at the price of well-being for everyone.

Others argue, similarly to the reasoning in compensatory justice, that disparities are just plain wrong from the standpoint of the ethical standards of equity, the notion of rights, and the principle of nonmaleficence. To counter the negative effects of inequality, the concept of social need is a useful tool.

Social need means that a person is in a societal environment that is not friendly to basic needs being met to the same degree that mainstream society enjoys. How social need is established then becomes a key consideration. Two societal tools to do so are presented for your consideration: labeling and vulnerability.

Labeling: A Double Edge

Labeling is an important mechanism used to help identify significant similarities among members of a group. Labeling was designed to help ensure that by grouping such persons their needs better could be met and often has been helpful in identifying great need. However, in her now classic work, Martha Minow[19] pointed out that "Difference... is a comparative term... different from whom? I am no more different from you than you are from me... The point of comparison is often unstated..." She says that at the root of this issue is *"the dilemma of difference."*[19] Labels can succeed in identifying differences among groups and assist in seeing that justice is done, but they can also be a barrier: "When does treating people differently... emphasize their differences and stigmatize or hinder them on that basis? And when does treating people the same become insensitive to their differences and likely to stigmatize them or hinder them on that basis?"[19] As you read in Chapter 12, persons whose chronic conditions receive a genetic label often find themselves disadvantaged with insurers and others because of the label. Labeled groups are not always given the positive treatment promised them and may be even further discriminated against.

A case in point is an extensive screening program for sickle cell disease that was initiated in the United States in the latter quarter of the 20th century. The important point from a social justice perspective is that sickle cell disease affects primarily African Americans, a group that traditionally has suffered stigma and oppression, with the resulting discrimination on many fronts. Sickle cell is a painful condition that manifests itself in infancy and continues throughout a shortened life span. Symptoms associated with it include infarction of the soft tissue and bone, which causes acute pain. It also affects the spleen, liver, and kidneys.[20] Screening designed to identify affected individuals and therefore identify them as a group deserving of special attention was conducted. However, once labeled, these individuals did not realize the benefits of large-scale treatment programs. Instead, in many instances, African Americans identified through the screening process found that insurance, employment, and other records carried stigmatizing information regarding their status as carriers of the sickle cell trait.[21] It is historical injustices like these that lead to mistrust of health professionals, contributing to ongoing health disparities.

Summary

Labels are designed to identify specific needs or characteristics for the purpose of providing priority consideration on the basis of respect for human dignity in all of its forms. However, populations who have been societally disadvantaged and experienced previous social wrongs do not necessarily benefit from placement in a labeled group alone.

The "Vulnerability" Criterion

Vulnerability or "vulnerable populations" are general labels applied to establish a stigmatized group's disadvantageous societal circumstances. Again, the intent is to provide a way to determine special needs that befall some members of the group and to respond positively. Some at-risk groups include older adults; children; individuals with disabilities; people whose incomes are below the federal poverty threshold; groups of people in racial, ethnic, and gender minorities; individuals who are undocumented; and other people who are burdened by homelessness, oppression, marginalization, or powerlessness.[22,23]

Vulnerable groups are *socially marginalized* compared with mainstream society and collectively are excluded at disproportionately high rates from desired opportunities and the goods and services of society, a state of affairs that many argue also removes them from opportunities to contribute to the common good to the detriment of all in the future.[24] Many marginalized groups face structural inequities that are deeply rooted in the past and carried into the present. Legal mechanisms to help minimize the discrimination against them are helping to provide some opportunities for fuller participation. The concept of *privilege* defined as "special rights, advantages, or immunities granted or available to a particular person or group of people" requires your attention as a health professional as well. Privileges contribute to oppression and injustice in groups and populations.[12]

The idea of social need focuses priority on the societal situation of the relatively less well-off and detaches it from the idea that some deserve to have less than others. The idea of vulnerable groups goes deeper into a kind of "no fault of their own" assumption that takes people where they are no matter what the reason is for their landing in this place. Their need is medical need for healthcare services, but the additive factor of societal disadvantage is best captured in the idea of social need. If the demands of social justice are to be met, there is an urgent onus on society to be more aware of our biases, to eliminate health disparities, and to foster inclusivity. As you recall from Chapter 10, the onus is on the health professional to strive for cultural inclusivity, honoring dignity and respect for all.

Summary

Mainstream society plays a major role in social marginalization with resulting serious health disparities. The appropriate moral response must be found in paying attention to how labels and the criterion of vulnerability may result in allocations that do not address social need or bring about social justice. A commitment to more inclusive societal arrangements is essential.

Justice, Inclusion, and Solidarity

Elizabeth Anderson[25] in her article "What Is the Point of Equality?" critiqued some of the thinking that has supported social justice policies. The compensatory and larger social justice goal for such individuals having drawn a so-called short straw in the natural lottery of life is to mitigate or eliminate the negative impact of their predicament. But ultimately, Anderson rejected this concept because, she argued, there is no way around an assumption embedded in it that the disadvantaged group has inferior basic worth, is "sadly inferior." In contrast, she proposed (with other thinkers today) that a more considered understanding of justice would work toward the aim of creating "a community in which people stand in relations of equality to others" based on true and deep respect (Fig. 15.2).

Silvers[26] emphasized that this can be achieved by giving priority to societal arrangements that allow everybody to optimize their freedom at all times, no matter their capacity. The basic conceptual underpinning is captured in the sociopolitical notion of *solidarity*. Groups who make claims on another could do so through virtue of their socially recognized equality with mainstream groups.

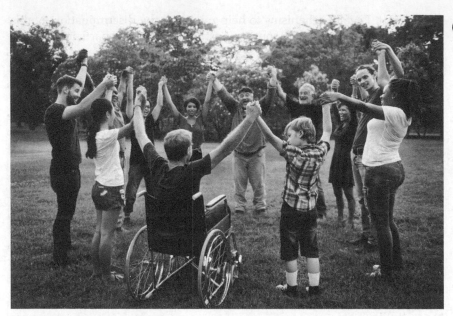

Fig. 15.2. True respect for all strengthens everyone in society. (*Copyright iStock.com/Rawpixel.*)

The construction of an inclusive social environment may be viewed by some as utopian, but substantive changes that already have been made show it to be an essential goal to pursue. *Inclusion* is a key element in honoring and achieving diversity in society. Health professionals who integrate inclusive practices are able to foster acceptance and support to maximize patient engagement for optimal health outcomes. Inclusive health care delivery cultivates belonging, respect, and value for all. Together, inclusion and solidarity can lead to collective action and collective health.[27] From a cost-quality approach alone, neglect and exclusion of entire groups of people are bad ideas. Health professionals are in a good position to be an important voice advocating for social justice in healthcare. For this reason, you will note that many profession's codes of ethics now include language outlining one's responsibility to advocate for changes to systems and/or policies that are biased or discriminatory or that unfairly limit/prevent access to health care services.

Individual Responsibility for Health Maintenance

Now we come to a potential snag in the evolving compensatory and social justice reasoning and a more solidarity-oriented approach to allocation. As noted previously, there is an idea that vulnerable populations who are socially marginalized when it comes to the allocation of goods and services may be disadvantaged through no fault of their own. Although the idea was embedded in some of the alternatives, the question of Eino's responsibility, if any, to prevent his current ill health was not fully addressed. Eino was a hard-working miner in a dangerous environment, and at least some people who read his story probably are sympathetic toward him. However, we also know that he may have refused to admit earlier that he was having symptoms that warranted medical attention. And some would ask whether he had really had no other choice but to work in the mines.

Today, there is a lively discussion about how the societal responsibility to allocate resources justly must be balanced against each individual's *personal responsibility for health*. As you read previously in the chapter, there is a strong ethos of autonomy in the United States and other Western societies that supports the idea that each of us has the freedom to be responsible for maintaining our own health.

The subsequent example illustrates some of the complexities that arise in the process of trying to exercise justice for everyone in a society. In the story you meet Jane who has a life-threatening condition (emphysema). Her story was chosen in part because, like Eino, she is having difficulty breathing and the condition will get worse without intervention. Viewed from a social justice standpoint, she is vulnerable. But her situation is different from Eino Maki's in some striking ways, too.

💗 The Story of Jane Tyler and Sam Puryo

Jane Tyler, a 32-year-old single woman and mother of three children (5, 8, and 12 years old), has been living on public assistance since her first child was born. Jane lives in a small apartment above her mother's in a high-crime area. Her mother helps with light housekeeping and child care. Now that all three children will be in school, Jane has successfully applied for a grant from the local Woman's Fund, a private organization, that will allow her to train to become an information technology assistant so that she can make a living for herself and her family. Receiving this award was a tremendous boost to her self-esteem, and she sees it as a bright doorway out of her current life situation. The one nagging anxiety she is experiencing is a severe shortness of breath at times and unusual fatigue. Before taking on this additional load of schooling, she decides to have a checkup at her neighborhood clinic.

It comes as a devastating blow to her to learn that she has emphysema. She has been threatening to stop smoking for a long time, but her daily smoking habit has had a strong grip on her since she was a teenager. She went from a two-pack-a-day habit to using electronic vapor products after the birth of her second child. It is an even greater shock to learn that, although the emphysema is only in the beginning stages, she may not be eligible for state-of-the-art surgical treatment because she is on public assistance. The state legislature presented to the voting public the opportunity to decide priorities for high-cost interventions provided through public funds by sending a questionnaire to a sample group. (Some readers will recognize this general approach from an exercise you were given a chance to participate in at the end of Chapter 14.) Three physicians concur that Jane's smoking is a direct cause of her emphysema. One of them believes there may be cofactors that lead some people to actually manifest the symptoms of emphysema, whereas others do not. The other two are completely convinced her smoking directly has created her serious health problem. Because two of the physicians of the three are needed for this policy to take effect, she is able to receive only noninvasive medical treatment. Her only opportunity for treatment by the surgical option is for her to find some way to pay for it.

Sam Puryo is a caseworker in the public assistance office. Jane has been one of his clients for several years. He is upset at what he judges to be the apparent injustice of the laws that have put her in her current unhappy situation. He tries to call his state senator to see whether there are any loopholes in the law that could help her or whether an exception can be made for this woman who Sam sees as exceptional. The senator is not encouraging; she is sympathetic but knows of no loopholes and is pessimistic about an exception being made.

During a coffee break, Sam gets into a discussion of the new rulings with his colleagues at the public assistance office. His fellow social worker is strongly in favor of the approach taken by the legislature. All the people at lunch agree that it is important to be willing to consider the arguments.

 Reflection

Now is your opportunity to join Sam and the others in their discussion. Consider the following questions. What is morally due Jane Tyler and other people in similar situations? More importantly, how should her situation be approached to ascertain what she should receive, if anything?

_____

_____

_____

_____

Viewed from a justice perspective, at least three variables are relevant in trying to sort out what, if any, support for her treatment is due Jane Tyler. One is her medical need, a second is her smoking habit that apparently has contributed significantly to her health condition, and the third is her low economic status.

Medical Need and Individual Responsibility

The first variable, her medical need, is relevant from the perspective of distributive justice. Therefore if you view Jane's predicament solely as a distributive justice question based on her symptoms, you have to conclude that optimal medical care is due her on the basis of her medical need. The state legislature obviously has not made their judgments strictly on the basis of medical need, which means Jane's situation is not only a distributive justice allocation decision.

Personal Habits and Individual Responsibility

Now comes the complication of her smoking-induced condition. From a social justice standpoint, this does not factor in as a strike against her. However, you can see compensatory justice reasoning working against Jane Tyler. Most of us believe—in theory, if not in practice—that responsible citizens should positively contribute something to society and attempt to refrain from destructive behaviors. Now she is viewed tacitly, if not explicitly, as doing harm through her smoking habit. The harm is not only the destruction of her lungs; she may also be viewed as causing harm to others by using societal resources and contributing to a drain on tax money that might be needed for her care and that of her small children as her condition deteriorates. Finally, some would argue that given mounting evidence of the harm of secondhand smoke, she is putting her children at risk for ill health.

One defining factor is the extent to which Jane is in a position to be held accountable for her tobacco dependence now and the ensuing difficulties it has brought on her. Distinguishing among individual disadvantages, and those that result from external forces over which individuals or groups have no or little control is not easy to do. Most readers know that a person's conduct develops in early childhood and is reinforced by one's cultural, ethnic, and socioeconomic group (to name some influences on adult behavior). However, many join society's individualism-based judgment that all she would have had to do to break her habit was "just say no." Moreover, many aids to stop smoking are on the market.

L *Reflection*

Do you think that Jane is voluntarily harming herself and others, or is this an example of blaming the victim? What reasons support your judgment about her conduct?

_____

_____

_____

_____

Economic Disadvantage and Individual Responsibility

Finally, Jane's low socioeconomic situation and being an urban, unemployed, single mother with three children ensures that she is vulnerable.

Her stigmatized status tends to exclude her from beneficial societal supports, a factor that is relevant from a social justice perspective. At the same time, she is not totally excluded because she has been receiving publicly funded assistance to help sustain her and her three children. But even this support is against a backdrop of her poverty. Jane has the capacity and the right, but not the opportunity. Her economic status may become another decisive variable because of the following lines of observation:

- Poverty can put individuals at a disadvantage in their opportunities to acquire an education and, through that means, increase their range of choices regarding careers, where they work, and how much money they make.
- Women and single mothers in poverty are more economically disadvantaged than men.
- Finding an avenue to a skilled worker position through education could be an important turning point in her life and in her children's welfare. She has found funds for bettering herself, but now her health needs may be the barrier.

You can see how social justice reasoning adds these economic considerations that go well beyond medical concerns taken alone.

Reflection

Do you think that these social factors should influence your decision about Jane's eligibility for the optimal healthcare for her medical condition? Why or why not?

_____

_____

_____

_____

You now have three perspectives on individual responsibility all tied up in this one case, leaving you to make the final decision about whether she should be eligible for the surgical care for her worsening emphysema. This discussion and your responses are germane because you are entering the health professions at a time when there is much debate about how much responsibility individuals must take for their own health.[28-30]

Individual Responsibility and a Caring Response

Although you cannot help but have opinions and personal feelings about issues related to others' habits and behaviors, in policy the relevant arguments are general, not specific. Therefore a caring response to a group in deciding what role their behaviors should play in the allocation of publicly generated resources for healthcare (or other basic goods) must begin with

• humility toward the complexity of disparities in health status. Although it cannot be reasonably expected that the larger society will support any and all types of ill-advised choices, the prior moral responsibility is to get to the root causes of a group's behavior. This cannot be accomplished without sound research data combined with skills that allow for culturally informed approaches to the variety of situations we find ourselves in whenever allocation decisions are being made.

ⓖ Summary

Currently, there is much debate about the role each individual must play in assuming responsibility for one's own health. Such assessments must be made within the larger societal context in which individuals reside to ensure that injustices in policies do not result in further disadvantages and health disparities.

Summary

The compensatory and larger social justice issues raised in this chapter have no easy answers, theoretically or in their practical application. In your professional practice, you will have ample opportunity to reflect further on the implications of how distributive justice, compensatory justice, and social justice approaches foster the larger societal goals of a caring response and health equity for all. The underlying concerns presented by social determinants of health and the complementary roles that individuals, their institutions, and the larger public should play in upholding the tenets of a flourishing society all are relevant considerations in implementing just policies. Only when just policies are in place can individual health professionals and others be confident that just practices will be possible.

Questions for Thought and Discussion

1. Some have argued that, because the extent to which people value health in relation to other goods (such as food, shelter, clothing, a car, living where there is fresh air, and so on) varies from person to person, the most just healthcare resource distribution would be to give the same amount of money to all citizens (a "voucher" or "savings account") and let them spend it however they choose over a lifetime. Discuss the strengths and weaknesses of this arrangement from the standpoint of distributive, compensatory, and social justice reasoning. At what age should this allocation be made? Why?
2. A group project:
   Discuss the pros and cons of the following proposed legislative bills from the point of view of distributive, compensatory, and social justice considerations. Vote for the one your group supports based on your reasoning.

Condition A is a progressive disease of the central nervous system. It first affects the spinal cord and in its later stages infiltrates the brain, resulting in progressive spasticity and later in multiple movement and thought disorders. It occurs primarily in white, middle-class men 40 to 55 years of age and leads to certain death within 15 to 20 years. The cause and course of the disease is well understood as an autoimmune condition. Recently, a medication has been discovered that can help to slow the progress of condition A dramatically. The cost of the medication needed for treatment is estimated to be about $5000 per month for each patient. About 7500 people in the United States have been diagnosed with the disease, and the incidence rate seems to be increasing. It is believed that many more cases will surface if the medication becomes available for any who need it.

Legislation has been introduced into the U.S. Congress to make possible the processing and administration of the drug to all patients "in the name of humanity." A conservative estimate is that the cost to U.S. taxpayers will be about $450 million per year.

When the bill is being debated, a counterproposal is introduced. Proponents propose that the funds be allocated to provide full annual physical examinations, free of charge, to any refugee child in the United States up to 12 years of age whose parents fall under the poverty line. This free service will be compartmentalized from other federal or state funding for medical care because some of those plans do not cover annual exams and some do not cover the children of undocumented (i.e., illegal) immigrants of whom some are refugees. The estimated total cost is close to that in the competing bill but "will serve 10 times as many, each of whom is equally deserving of services as the people in the competing bill." The core of the argument is that, in general, the latter individuals are discriminated against in the United States, that only the poorest among even that group has been targeted for public support, and that legislators and policymakers must take this factor into account in determining healthcare priorities.

3. James is a 29-year-old man who sustained a C3 spinal cord injury in a diving accident while on his company outing in Aruba. After several days in a coma from hitting his head on a rock, he woke up to the shock of having no movement from his neck down.

   James worked as an investment banker before his injury and saved a substantial amount given his 80-hour work week and single status. Most of these funds he placed in 401(k) retirement accounts. James has medical insurance; however, his medical bills are mounting, and the social worker recommends that he apply for state disability to receive additional coverage for long-term services that he will need but are not covered by his private insurer. James decides to do so and then realizes that to become eligible he must spend down his present dollar assets, including his 401(k) accounts. He is furious and yells at the social worker, "You've got to be kidding me. Do you think just because I'm crippled I don't want to retire comfortably? This is grossly unfair."

Given what you have studied in this chapter, what sources of support and at what cost to his personal savings do you think would meet the demands of a just allocation of resources for him and others like him?

References

1. Purtilo R: Social marginalization of persons with disability: justice considerations for Alzheimer disease. In Purtilo R, ten Have H, editors: *Ethical foundations of palliative care for Alzheimer disease*, Baltimore, 2004, Johns Hopkins University Press, pp 290–304.
2. Goffman E: Information control and personal identity. In Goffman E, editor: *Stigma: management of spoiled identity*, New York, 1963, Simon and Schuster, pp 41–105.
3. Notini L, Gillam L, Pang KC: Facial feminizzation surgery: private, personal identity, compensatory justice, and resource allocation, *Am J Bioethics* 18(12):12–21, 2018.
4. Dauda B, Denier Y, Dierickx K: What do the various principles of justice mean within the concept of benefit sharing? *Bioethic Inq* 13:281–293, 2016.
5. Fletcher B, Gapasin F: *Solidarity divided: the crisis in organized labor and a new path toward social justice*, Berkeley, CA, 2008, University of California Press.
6. Foraker RE, Bush C, Greiner MA, et al: Distribution of cardiovascular health by individual- and neighborhood-level socioeconomic status: findings from the Jackson Heart Study, *Global Heart* 14(3):241–250, 2019.
7. Bell D: Communitarianism. In Zalta EN, editor: *Stanford encyclopedia of philosophy*, 2016. Available at https://plato.stanford.edu/archives/sum2016/entries/communitarianism.
8. Rajczi A: Liberalism and public health ethics, *Bioethics* 30(2):96–108, 2016.
9. Green WS: Introduction. In Neusner J, Chilton B, editors: *Altruism in world religions*, Washington, DC, 2005, Georgetown University Press, pp x–xiv.
10. Powers M, Faden R: *Social justice: the moral foundations of public health and health policy*, New York, 2006, Oxford University Press.
11. United States Department of Health and Human Services: *National Partnership for Action to End Health Disparities: health equity and disparities*. Available at http://minorityhealth.hhs.gov/npa/templates/browse.aspx?lvl=1&lvlid=34.
12. Breunig M: Beings who are becoming: enhancing social justice literacy, *J Exper Educ* 42(1):7–21, 2019.
13. Gell NM, Mroz TM, Patel KV: Rehabilitation services use and patient-reported outcomes among older adults in the United States, *Arch Phys Med Rehabil* 98(11):2221–2227, 2017.
14. Williams MT, Rosen DC, Kanter JW, editors: *Eliminating race-based mental health disparities: promoting equity and culturally responsive care across settings*, Oakland, CA, 2019, Context Press.

15. Krahn GL, Walker DK, Correa-De-Araujo R: Persons with disabilities as an unrecognized health disparity population, *Am J Public Health* 105:S198–S206, 2015.
16. Disability as Inequality: Social disparities, health disparities, and participation in daily activities, *Social Forces* 97(1):157–192, 2018.
17. Namkung EH, Mitra M, Nicholson J: Do disability, parenthood, and gender matter for health disparities?: A US population-based study, *Disabil Health J* 12(4):594–601, 2019.
18. Sen A: *Inequality reexamined*, Cambridge, MA, 2004, Belknap Press of Harvard University.
19. Minow M: *Making all the difference: inclusion, exclusion and the American law*, New York, 1990, Cornell University Press, pp 20–21.
20. Centers for Disease Control and Prevention: *What is sickle cell disease*, Washington, DC, 2019, CDC National Center for Birth Defects and Developmental Disabilities. Available at http://www.cdc.gov/ncbddd/sicklecell/facts.html.
21. Anionwu E, Atkin K: *The politics of sickle cell and thalassaemia*, Philadelphia, 2001, Open University Press.
22. Luna F: Elucidating the concept of vulnerability: layers not labels, *Int J Fem Approaches Bioeth* 2(1):121–139, 2009.
23. Stanton JRR, Duran-Stanton AM: Vulnerable populations in disaster: residence, resilience, and resources, *Phys Asst Clin* 4(4):675–685, 2019.
24. Stiglitz J: *The price of inequality: how today's divided society endangers our future*, New York, 2011, W.W. Norton Company.
25. Anderson ES: What is the point of equality? *Ethics* 109:287–337, 1999.
26. Silvers A: The unprotected: constructing disability in the context of antidiscrimination law for individuals and institutions. In Francis LP, Silvers A, editors: *Americans with disabilities: exploring implications of the law for individuals and institutions*, New York, 2000, Routledge, pp 126–145.
27. Douwes R, Stuttaford M, London L: Social solidarity, human rights, and collective action: considerations in the implementation of the National Health Insurance in South Africa, *Health Hum Rights* 20(2):185–196, 2018.
28. Friesen P: Personal responsibility within health policy: unethical and ineffective, *J Med Ethics* 44(1):53–58, 2018.
29. Savulescu J: Golden opportunity, reasonable risk and personal responsibility for health, *J Med Ethics* 44(1):59–61, 2018.
30. Jha A, Dobe M: Personal vis-a-vis social responsibility for disparities in health status: an issue of justice, *Indian J Public Health* 60:216–220, 2016.

● 16

Health Professionals as Good Citizens: Responsibility and Opportunity

Objectives

The reader should be able to:

- Describe how the concepts of moral agency and professional responsibility apply to the health professional's role in addressing civic issues.
- Identify three spheres of moral agency that constitute a health professional's scope of professional responsibility.
- Discuss what a caring response entails when the "patient" is the public at large.
- Compare the focus of shared fate and self-realization careers in relation to your role as a professional involved in civic issues.
- Identify two ethical principles that apply to a health professional's participation in trying to resolve threats to health in the larger society.
- Examine the relevance of virtue theory in preparing professionals for participation in civic and larger global issues that threaten the health of individuals and populations.
- Describe four criteria of moral courage expressed by people who act courageously.
- Distinguish the idea of a civic self as an orienting notion when acting on behalf of the common good locally and globally.
- Reflect on how a basic respect for people may mean that the health professional becomes involved in pressing social issues outside healthcare.
- Define the term *rationing*.
- List and critique five criteria for a morally acceptable approach to rationing healthcare goods and services.
- Discuss situations in which random selection has been argued as a just approach to allocation and some arguments against this approach.
- Recognize the responsibilities of health professionals as global citizens within the context of worldwide health.

New terms and ideas you will encounter in this chapter

good citizenship	service ethic	dire scarcity
civic responsibility	public interest	proportionality
spheres of moral agency	common good	random selection
shared fate orientation	civic self	global citizens
self-realization	rationing	

Topics in this chapter introduced in earlier chapters

Topic	Introduced in chapter
Professional role	1
Professional responsibility	2
Agency	3
Moral agency	3
Moral distress	3
Utilitarian theory	4
Ethical reasoning	4
Duties and principles	4
Ethics of care	4
Virtue theory	4
Moral courage	6
Distributive justice	14
Solidarity	15
Resources allocation	14
Social justice	15
Inclusion	15

Introduction

As you come to the last chapter in this study of ethics, it is fitting that its focus is back on you, the health professional, and you, the citizen. *Good citizenship* is of course everyone's responsibility, and the activities that express good citizenship are captured in the idea of *civic responsibility*. Both "citizen" and "professional" are labels that carry assumptions about a person's role in society. Being a good citizen and being a good professional do have much in common. For example, each requires a measure of conscientiousness, engagement with societal needs, communication skills, and a willingness and ability to work with and on behalf of others.

There are certainly civic situations from which you are not exempt because you are a professional, such as paying taxes and jury duty. But there are also many interesting questions that surround this dual role. For example, does your professional training provide you with any special opportunities and imply any special duties and responsibilities as a citizen? What is your special role, if any, that makes you the most appropriate person to take leadership on a civic issue that affects your community? Do you owe anything to society because it has bestowed on you the privileges of being a "professional," a status that has always been held in high esteem in Western cultures? If asked, are you morally obligated to respond to a pressing civic need, or can you just say no? Are you a professional person 24/7, or can you blend into society as an ordinary citizen, leaving any special tugs on your moral conscience at your professional workplace? In this chapter, a framework is provided to address these types of questions.

To help focus the discussion, consider the following story.

 The Story of Two Health Professionals and the School Committee Chairperson

Michael Merrick is a pharmacist who works in Peetstown, a small town in the northeastern United States. He grew up in the beautiful hills 10 miles from where he now works, although for several years, he went to school and worked in New York City. He, his husband, and their two children moved back to Peetstown 2 years ago.

Recently, Michael and his family attended the fall school play at his 10-year-old son's, John's, elementary school. Michael went to use the rest room at intermission and on washing his hands noted that the water was slightly discolored with an odd odor. On exiting the restroom, he saw his husband holding up his 5-year-old to the water bubbler for a drink. He went to the fountain, noticing it too had a slightly odd odor. That evening Michael asked his son if he ever noticed anything weird about the water at school, to which he answered, "oh, I don't know, Dad, I can barely remember to wash my hands."

Michael suggested that the kids not use the water bubbler at school, instead only drinking from the canteens they brought in from home. The following evening when Michael picked up his son John from his afterschool program, he took a small jar and went back to collect a sample of the water from the bubbler. The next day, he drove 40 miles to visit a chemist friend who works in the chemistry department at the community college. The friend agreed to analyze the water and a couple days later called to say it tested positive for lead, an element known to be harmful to health in children, and high levels of trihalomethanes, a by-product of water disinfection. Alarmed, Michael told Sharleen Mays-Ramos, a physician colleague who makes biweekly visits to the local clinic in Peetstown, about his findings. The two decided to go to the chairperson of the school committee, who then promised to take care of the problem. "Let me know what happens," Sharleen said to the official as they left his office. "Sure will," said the man.

A month went by, and they heard nothing. Michael called the school committee's office with no success. Finally, he saw the man at the monthly Rotary Club meeting and asked him what was happening. The man took him aside and said, "Don't worry about it. I talked with the water and sewer commissioner and he said this happens from time to time in older pipes." Then he added, "You know this town has so many priorities for our schools. If we push the issue, the school may need to close and that means teacher layoffs and kids left out. Plus, the state tests the water, so you can just let the matter drop."

The next week, Michael returned to the school for a parent-teacher meeting. The bubbler looked and smelled the same. When he got back to the clinic, he called Sharleen and related his story. She said, "I guess we had better pursue this ourselves, Mike." That night after dinner, Michael discussed the matter with his husband. Both of them expressed concern about what lay ahead if they took on what now appeared to be a very unpopular issue with the town officials. Michael called Sharleen and told her he felt he had to pursue the matter as best he could because he was concerned about the effect of this toxin. She said, "It's the right thing to do. Count me in. I'll discuss it with my husband, but I couldn't live with myself if I knew you were out there tackling this problem alone. No level of lead exposure is safe for kids. We'll make a plan next week when I'm back in Peetstown."

Reflection

Does the action that this pharmacist and his physician colleague have taken so far demonstrate any special character traits that a good citizen would not also have (so that you would have to attribute it to their being health professionals)?

_____

_____

_____

_____

As you reflect on it further, is anything required of them as a duty because they are health professionals that would not also be required of any ordinary citizen?

_____

_____

_____

_____

Anyone reading about the situation probably feels that these two professional colleagues are responsible, caring citizens. Michael did not just ignore the worrisome thing he encountered, leaving a question about whether his children or other members in the community were at risk. But this does not in itself distinguish him from any other caring citizen. Nor does it answer the question as to whether there is anything in his and Sharleen's roles as health professionals that made them uniquely responsible to decide to pursue the matter over the responsibility of, say, a housewife, or chief executive officer of a small business in town, or a plumber who stumbled on to the same situation. Good thinking about this issue has been done, and key aspects of it are shared here to highlight when and why your civic responsibilities will emerge from, or combine with, the fact that you are a professional. You will also explore how in some situations your opportunity to contribute to society's well-being is enhanced because you are a health professional.

The Goal: A Caring Response

Two basic ethics notions presented early in this book help to provide a paradigm of understanding for what constitutes a professional's caring response to civic issues. The first is the idea of moral agency, accenting situations in which you can be expected to take charge. The second is the concept of professional responsibility.

Spheres of Moral Agency

As you recall from Chapter 3, agency means that you have an authoritative voice in a matter and society affirms that you are in a position to legitimately exercise that authority. Because of the moral dimensions of a professional's role, this agency is interpreted as moral agency. So that you do not think you are compelled to respond to every civic issue that comes your way, a helpful schema was developed by Gruen, Pearson, and Brenan to delineate *spheres of moral agency*, distinguishing different kinds of circumstances in which health professionals could become involved. Although their model was designed for physicians' and physician organizations' advocacy roles in public life, it is equally helpful for all health professionals (Fig. 16.1).[1]

Sphere One pertains to direct patient care decisions that fall within your area of professional expertise. Understandably, this remains the major focus of your moral agency in the clinic and beyond.

Sphere Two describes an area of moral authority that exists when you encounter a situation that is not direct patient care but you have important professional knowledge, insight, or skills that can help to effectively address the issue. In Sphere Two, the more your role as a professional prepares you better than any other group in society to address it, the more you will be looked to as an authority. For example, the more education a dietician has on the effects of

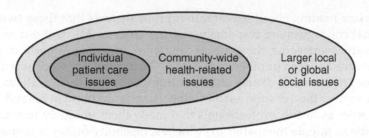

Spheres of Moral Agency

Fig. 16.1. Health professional responsibility and good citizenship. *(Modified from Gruen RL, Pearson SD, Brennan TA: Physician-citizens: public roles and professional obligations. JAMA 29[1]:94–98, 2004.)*

snack food on childhood obesity, the more other parents on the school Parent Teacher Association (PTA) board will look to her for advice regarding the proposed debate to institute a public mandate regulating the vending machine contents. And because of the moral role of the professional in society, the professional has the added power of being viewed as a moral agent who upholds deep societal values.

Sphere Three shifts the emphasis from your professional knowledge and skills base to the fact that professionals are held in high regard in society. Health professionals, lawyers, and religious leaders generally enjoy a high status, although they become the brunt of deep criticism when they do not stand up to society's realistic (or even unrealistic) expectations. Often the gravity or urgency of a situation is expressed more forcefully when professionals get behind the cause and provide leadership in endorsing it. This is seen in everything from television ads to appeals for financial contributions for societal issues. Your voice can influence the outcome by virtue of being a professional, although you may have little significant or unique professional knowledge regarding the issue under consideration. In this outermost sphere, you represent someone who is viewed as a moral leader simply because you are a professional.

These three spheres provide general guidelines for the relationship of your role as a professional to your role as a citizen. A commonsense conclusion is that the greatest pull on you is for issues in Sphere One. As you can probably quickly conclude, there are no hard and fast boundaries separating these three spheres. Your clinical expertise may be operative in any of them to some degree, and your position of high public trust supports your societal role as a moral agent with decision-making authority in all spheres. Still, as you move from issues that involve the first sphere to ones that involve the third sphere, the direct claim on you to exercise your authority lessens.

Professional Responsibility: Accountability and Responsiveness

Professional responsibility is a second relevant conceptual notion. It is essential in helping you to further fine-tune the boundaries of civic involvement.

Recall from Chapter 2 that responsibility as a professional must be cali-brated according to a combination of accountability and responsiveness to a situation. In society at large, the notion of responsibility is often viewed solely in terms of "accountability." In the health professions context, this re-duces responsibility to a duty that is inherent in the idea of professionalism. The standards of accountability by which you are measured range from the dictates of your professional codes, to patient care standards established by your profession and other licensing bodies, to institutional policies. You can see that in Sphere One of moral agency (concerned with direct patient care) they are appropriate standard bearers.

You also will recall that the companion idea of "responsiveness" is criti-cal to understanding professional responsibility. Being responsive means being sensitive to and understanding the other or others who will be im-pacted by your action. The urge to act must be balanced with detailed at-tention to the people involved, and with it a genuine humility reminding you that your accountability to professional standards designed for patient care alone does not always prepare you to be an effective advocate in every societal problem that crosses your path. As you continue outward toward Spheres Two and Three, your experience as a citizen and as a professional coincide more fully. In the second, you may quickly discern whether the type of health-related problem you encountered as a societal issue draws quite closely on what you know from your professional training. If so, you can more closely identify with the details of the situation and what should be done.

As you move into Sphere Three, you are increasingly acting as a citizen who is a health professional. Yet, others may view you primarily as a health professional because most people think of professionals as being a doctor, lawyer, pharmacist, or other professional 24/7. For example, if you have not already been prodded for your professional advice when someone recog-nizes you at a supermarket checkout counter, at a party, or elsewhere on the street, it is almost a guarantee that you will be. However, your professional identity is at work in Sphere Three is only as a member of a citizenry who is granted moral authority on the basis of your societal position. You are not drawing on the content of your professional training, and you will be acting more fully on what you can learn from the people involved and the issue concerning them in the same way that any other citizen does who becomes involved in that issue.

Summary

By combining three spheres of moral agency with your professional accountability and responsiveness to the relevant human implications of a situation, you have a general framework from which to analyze the morally correct course of action regarding involvement in civic issues.

The Six-Step Process in Public Life

Michael Merrick and Sharleen Mays-Ramos are not faced with a clinical situation. They may have no thoughts at this point about whether their decision to try to get at the root of a problem they believe is potentially causing harm to their community is related to their professional roles. If so, their lack of imagination or reflection on this point is understandable because the health professional's idea of "care" usually is thought of as being contained to situations between individuals. Yet they feel as if they should do something as citizens, and assumedly are driven in part by a motivation that they should be of service whenever they can. There is a lot of writing about this motivation among professionals, one aspect of which is presented briefly here through the lens of different kinds of careers.

We touched on the career choice issue in Chapter 15 when a part of Eino Maki's situation was analyzed from the point of view that he was in a job open to him as a worker with some societal strikes against him, and you met Jane Tyler, who was trying to increase her life options through the financial aid she had been granted to realize a career. All professionals fall within the category of having had an opportunity to choose a career, an option not open to most of the world's population. Having a career choice means that you are able to pursue your specific tastes, framing a life plan to suit your own character. Norman Care's classic article on the nature of careers suggests that people choose between two basic types of careers: those with a *shared fate orientation* and those oriented to *self-realization*. The former focuses on service to society, the latter solely on self-satisfaction.[2] Health (and other) professionals fall within both categories to some extent but primarily are in the shared fate category, with its straightforward *service ethic,* or inclination to be of service. This inclination again has been revisited and affirmed through a sociological analysis of the utility of the professions in the 21st-century workforce that you are entering or already a part of.[3]

In short, both from a personal leaning toward helping others and from a pragmatic consideration of our usefulness, the idea of service likely is deeply engrained in the two professionals who have decided to pursue the concerns they have about the water quality near their town. Such service also likely is informed by their awareness that their moral authority is a resource for them and that they have done sufficient thinking and homework to be prepared to exercise their professional responsibility.

Step 1: Gather Relevant Information

What information do you have as a result of their thinking and homework?

Michael and Sharleen know there is a hazardous toxin in the water in Michael's neighborhood school. Every action they have taken so far suggests that they know this is not a benign situation; rather, it is a problem that should arrest the attention of others. They surmise, although they do not have certainty, that something more is going on, perhaps an attempt by other leaders in the community to cover up any wrongdoing by government officials through improper monitoring or faulty testing. They are concerned just as any other good members of the community would be concerned.

However, these two individuals also are not like many other citizens in the community. It stands to reason that they have been exposed in their professional training to some understanding of how various environment pollutants affect health. As a pharmacist, Michael may have quite specific information about the toxic effects of lead. As part of their clinical training they may have explored the evidence on how environmental exposures in school buildings can affect student health, student thinking, and student performance.[4] At the very least, they have ready access to literature that will inform them in technical language they can more readily comprehend than many ordinary citizens. Whether or not they have direct knowledge of how contaminated water supplies are damaging the health of entire communities, is not known for sure. What is known is that lead in water is regulated by the Environmental Protection Association under both the Clean Water Act and Safe Drinking Water Act.[5] In addition, the World Health Organization has made water safety and quality a major focus worldwide, leading efforts to prevent transmission of waterborne disease and disseminating research findings regarding the link between public health and water quality to all health professions who provide direct patient care.[6] From just these facts alone, you can assume that Michael and Sharleen's moral agency falls more fully within Sphere Two of professional responsibility to become involved in this civic issue than if the issue involved failing infrastructure may be called into doubt by some members of the community.

You can also safely assume that this doctor and pharmacist are in a position to be heard if they speak up. The fact that the official took Michael aside and quietly implied that they not pursue the issue further suggests that he knew these two respected professionals would be heard if they called attention to the school committee's inaction and conduct. They work in a relatively small town, a type of closely knit community usually loyal to their professionals. Michael belongs to the Rotary Club, a social and service organization to which leaders in a community must be invited by other leaders. Their roles carry a certain amount of status and weight in relation to most citizens. So, all things being equal, they can be viewed as moral agents in this situation in Sphere Three by virtue of their status and role.

However, another human dimension informs Michael's situation. It depends on his having grown up in this community. In discerning his professional responsibility, accountability is one thing, but then there is responsiveness at a more detailed level. He can be sensitive to nuances of its people and residents that others would not be able to detect. For one thing, he knows how much the livelihood of this community does depend on public schools. Michael knows that, while he is "one of them," he also jumped ship and went to live in, of all places, New York City. Having come back, he is welcomed on the one hand as "a hometown boy who made good" but also may still be viewed with suspicion as an "outsider" who can be dismissed (and discriminated against) as a troublemaker. He and his family may become ostracized, even if his concern about the school committee and water commissioner is proven to be correct. So he is hesitant about what to do next not because he is ignorant of his or his colleague's power, but because they understand that pursuing this issue may be a messy business.

Finally, the two health professionals are faced with uncertainty about the outcome of their endeavor. They know they may be able to prove nothing because they independently tested the water and do not have full access to the routine testing data.

Reflection
Are there other types of information you consider relevant to their situation that have not been touched on? If so, what are they?

_____

_____

_____

Step 2: Identify the Type of Ethical Problem

This pharmacist and physician are facing an ethical problem in the form of moral distress. There is some uncertainty about the morally correct course of action, but for the most part, their distress is focused on the barriers, consistent with moral distress type A. They feel compelled to be sure this community has at least been warned that their water is contaminated and would like to be sure someone is taking care of the problem to prevent harm that may be befalling the townspeople.

Reflection
As far as you can imagine yourself in their situation, sketch out some details of the barriers causing their distress as they confront the realities of pursuing this civic action they want to take.

_____

_____

_____

Recall that an emotion of hesitance or fear can be a clue that you are encountering an ethical problem. These two health professionals are experiencing them as an interior barrier to action that combines with the external barrier of resistance from at least one powerful sector of the community. It is no wonder that they pause before moving ahead with doing what they believe is right. This situation highlights that moral distress is as helpful a tool for ethical analysis when a health professional's ethical problem calls for civic action as those which pertain to direct patient care or health policy challenges.

They may be faced with an ethical dilemma as well. Although they are not sure, Michael has raised concerns that his family or his and Sharleen's positions may be threatened because they have become "whistle-blowers." They know they have a duty to protect their families and the professional service they offer patients from harm, especially those who are vulnerable or disenfranchised. At the same time, they know that the harm of doing nothing will weigh heavily on them.

Step 3: Use Ethics Theories or Approaches to Analyze the Problem

Having identified their problem as one of moral distress with a background concern of an ethical dilemma, consider ethics theories or approaches that can help them in this delicate situation.

Utilitarian Reasoning

An approach based on utilitarian theory requires these moral agents to weigh all the consequences of their proposed action as far as they can determine them. What are they? Not to be underestimated is their feeling that their integrity depends on what they do or do not do. Other important factors have been discussed; among the most obvious are the potential harm of the lead to the children in the community if nothing is done and, if the issue is raised, the risk of the government official's retaliation either to these two moral agents or by closing the school and leaving hundreds of children at risk for educational loss. Benefits of their going ahead with their plan to pursue the truth of the matter include, of course, preventing harm (or further harm) from the toxic contaminants and being sure that those in positions of power in this community are held accountable for their conduct. There are other less obvious but important benefits, too, one being that the community can count on its knowledgeable professionals to try to help maintain a safe and flourishing environment.

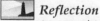 *Reflection*

Approaching this moral distress problem as a utilitarian, what other factors would you want to add if you were balancing the benefits and risks of the professionals pursuing a course of action designed to expose the presence of this toxin, its source, and a demand for governmental accountability?

_____

_____

_____

_____

Does your reasoning factor in the idea that their involvement is not around a Sphere One direct care issue but instead a Sphere Two issue (i.e., their professional role probably gives them insight into the clinical effects of the toxin) and a Sphere Three issue (i.e., they believe they can lend their authoritative voices as leaders in the community to help resolve the problem)?

_____

_____

_____

_____

Duties and Principles Approaches

Traditionally, oaths and codes of professional ethics depended heavily on deontological theory. They delineated the health professional's duties in direct patient care but said less about the professional's duties to society at large, except that patient care can be viewed as having a positive impact on the health of the larger society. Today, this focus on Sphere One duties only is changing in many professional codes of ethics.

Reflection
Check the code of ethics of your profession to look for ethical guidelines for your involvement in Sphere Two or Sphere Three activities. Jot them down here.

_____

_____

_____

_____

●   If Michael and Sharleen were using the code of your chosen
    profession as a tool for ethical reasoning, would they find guidance
    about how to proceed in their moral distress? If so, what are the items
    that address this type of situation?

    _____

    _____

    _____

    _____

As you should be aware of by now, the important guidance of your professional code of ethics does not give you the full answer to ethical problems.
Several ethics principles have been developed to help analyze the complex
situations health professionals now must face. Some of the principles come
to your aid when thinking about your moral agency and the extent of your
professional responsibility in civic matters.

The principles of nonmaleficence and beneficence apply to moral agency
you can exercise when the problem affects society in general, not just an
identified patient or client. Jennings, Callahan, and Wolf[7] distinguished two
types of societal involvement of professionals: the first is service that seeks
to promote the public interest, and the second is that which promotes the
common good. Both are instrumental in preventing harm in civic life and
in promoting beneficent outcomes that honor the ethical gold standard of
respect for all introduced in Chapter 1.

●   Legitimate use of your moral agency for Sphere One and Sphere Two
involvements are what Jennings, Callahan, and Wolf identified as *public
interest* activities. Public service that promotes the public interest includes
the profession's contribution of technical expertise to public policy analysis
and community problems. In other words, the value of your civic contribution is expanded by your technical and professional expertise.

Legitimate use of your moral agency for some Sphere Two and all Sphere
Three involvements focuses on issues that promote the *common good.* There
is interconnectedness between individuals and communities in pursuit of
the common good. As Scheffler stated:

> *even though we as individuals have diverse values and goals, and even though it is
> up to each of us to judge what we consider to be a good or worthy life, most of us
> pursue our goals and seek to realize our values within a framework of belief that as-
> sumes an ongoing humanity.*[8]

This includes the distinctive and critical perspective the various professions have to offer on basic human values and on facets of the human good
and the good life. It also includes the profession's contribution to what may

be called civic discourse—that ongoing conversation in a democratic society about our shared goals, our common purposes, and the nature of the good life in a just social order. Your influence is determined in large part by your social standing in the community as a professional.

Michael's and Sharleen's specific concern is with unclean water, but they are tapping into a deeper knowledge about health and its function in human flourishing. We are learning that among the most important values today is the safety of all living beings as a planet-wide, interdependent ecosystem: people, animals, and plants; and the air, water, and soil working together or being destroyed together. In Chapter 15, we discussed the ethical principle of solidarity and how it transforms our understanding of relationship. Here the notion of solidarity is expanded to include more than solely human life as a civic value. The development of a worldwide document titled The Earth Charter,[9] signed off on by leaders across the globe, highlights that we must become acutely aware of the fragility of ecosystems and of the deleterious effects of their imbalances on human and nature's healthfulness and survival. Viewed from this insight, the decision of the two health professionals in this chapter who enter the public arena to prevent or to remove harm to the entire community has more far-reaching health consequences than their direct patient care interventions. Their involvement provides an opportunity for us to reflect on what a caring response entails for today's health professionals, a theme heralded by Leonard Boff[10] in his piece *The Ethics of Care*: "Among so many other fine things, the Earth Charter proposes a new way of seeing that gives rise to a new ethic…" including its emphasis on care for the [whole] community of life, ecological integrity, and social and economic justice (Fig. 16.2).

What, does Boff conclude, is the result?

> *This sustainable way of life is equivalent to happiness in traditional versions of ethics deriving from the Greek, medieval and modern traditions. The supreme value now, that which must save the system of life… comes under the sign of care. It represents the new collective dream of humankind.*[10]

Virtue Theory and Civic Involvement: Moral Courage as a Model

A caring response directed to involvement in civic issues also provides an opportunity for us to assess the role of moral character and the virtues that support positive professional action. Many may apply in the case under discussion: compassion, a commitment to professional competence, integrity, honesty, and trustworthiness. All of these can come into play to help motivate action in any of the three spheres of moral agency.

However, recall that one of the barriers to action facing Michael and his physician colleague is their fear of what might happen if they go forward with what they believe is the morally appropriate thing to do. Their fear gives you an opportunity to explore the sometimes neglected resource of

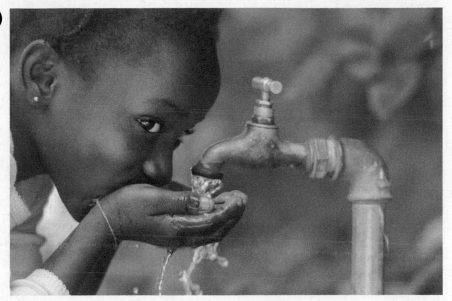

Fig. 16.2. A vision of care that includes each other and nature sustains human flourishing. *(Copyright iStock.com/borgogniels.)*

moral courage in health professionals' ethical decision making introduced in Chapter 6.

Moral courage is a readiness for voluntary, purposive action in situations that engender realistic fear and anxiety to uphold something of great moral value.[11] It is not surprising that this pharmacist and physician are having some fear about their proposed course. One way to view their reticence is that they are doing their homework by assessing the full picture of what they are up against. If they had no fear, they may bumble into the civic fray without thinking of the important by-products of their good intentions.

Courage can be built up by preparation for such moments. In her work with professionals and others who fought the injustices of the apartheid system in South Africa, Purtilo had the privilege of learning exemplars of courageous action. Several common themes emerged, among them the following ways in which courageous resisters identified the step-by-step process that allowed them to act courageously:

1. Name the seriousness of the situation. Do not pretend that what is happening, or not happening, is acceptable and that it will go away. It is not, and it will not. Michael and Sharleen increasingly seem convinced of that.
2. Believe that good will prevail over wrongdoing. (One might call this the optimism of courage, or "hoping courage.")

3. Take the opportunity to nurture and be nurtured by essential sources of support. Everyone emphasized this, no matter their individual circumstances in other regards. In this chapter, we see Michael, Sharleen, and their families as one "support coalition" that already is in place, and others will surely follow as the word gets out.
4. Become fully invested in the outcome. As one interviewee said, "The cause I started out to embrace eventually embraced me."[12]

There were other themes, but these four seem to fit Michael's and Sharleen's situation as they begin to stake out their strategies. Even if they find that their inquiries and probing reveal no wrongdoing, they will have prepared well and will benefit from the experience of having done so. In fact, in a report on their studies of moral development and moral agency in professionals, Bebeau, Rest, and Narvaez[13] attributed to Rest the idea of defining moral character as "having the strength of your convictions, *having courage*, persisting, overcoming distractions and obstacles, having implementing skills, [and] having ego strength." [Emphasis added.] He singles out moral courage as the attribute needed to turn disposition into moral action.[13]

 Summary

Moral courage is a virtue that, when cultivated, prods one to the right action, even in the face of fear or other difficulties.

Step 4: Explore the Practical Alternatives

With all of the information provided in this chapter about their situation, these two professional moral agents are still faced with the very personal decision about whether and how much to get involved. You have evidence from their story that they are motivated in part by a sense that their professional commitments should involve them in doing what they can in the larger society to make the world a better place.

They can, of course, reverse direction and do nothing, or Michael could decide to move his family out of town.

Some other alternatives that fall more fully into what appears to be consistent with their motivation to address the issue are available.

The health professionals can bypass (or first inform) the school committee chairperson and water commissioner and go directly to their mayor, governor, and state senator to be sure all levels of governmental leadership are aware of the water contaminants and report that the county official claims they know of the hazard. If there is a convincing positive response that this issue is being swiftly and adequately addressed, the professionals can link arms with governmental allies to plan a strategy to correct the situation. They also can help ensure that the plan includes an effective mechanism for compensating anyone with health threats that already may have resulted from the contaminated water supply and have a plan in place to address longer term negative effects of the poisoning.

The professionals can call local print and other media to avail them of the situation with the hope that they will provide leadership in exposing the health hazard.

Michael can share his concern during the next Rotary Club meeting, hoping that others of the town's leadership will take up the cause with him.

They can also build a coalition of professionals and other citizens who will work with them on a plan to address this issue before taking it to the broader public. But moral courage alone is not enough. One must be immersed in a supportive environment in which there are opportunities for action and reflection on the moral culture.[14] Western cultures often believe that, because we want to act responsibly, we must carry the moral weight of an issue on our individual shoulders. William May[15] pointed out in his book, *Beleaguered Rulers: The Public Obligations of the Professional*, that this is just one of the burdens we assume mistakenly. He reminds us that to cultivate strong, nurturing societies, we must cultivate a *civic self*:

> The civic self, as opposed to the imperial self, understands and accepts itself as limited and amplified by others. The civic self recognizes that it enjoys an expansion of its life in and through its participation in community.[15]

Finally, Michael and Sharleen can take some steps to further engage in self-understanding. This will fully prepare them for their task by affirming that their act is about who they, as professionals and citizens, want to be in spite of what they may or may not be able to do about resolving this serious societal situation. This preparation helps ensure they will go forward with integrity and the inner strength they need, whatever the outcome.

Reflection
What questions do you still want answered before deciding which of several practical alternatives that Michael and his physician colleague might follow will be the best one?

_____

_____

_____

_____

Steps 5 and 6: Complete the Action and Evaluate the Process and Outcome

Reflection

Which option would you take to best achieve a caring response? Why?

_____

_____

_____

_____

For purposes of our discussion, let's assume that Michael and the physician decide they will continue to pursue the issue.

Whichever of the alternatives they choose, they will have had the opportunity before taking action to consider their roles not only as traditional members of the health professions but also as citizens in one civic issue. After the fact, they will have an opportunity to use the three spheres of moral agency that they have as professionals combined with the idea of professional responsibility to help them reflect on the experience. What they learn will help them navigate through the many civic issues they will be asked to participate in. They will also have the opportunity to share what they have learned with their professional colleagues. Sharing their knowledge and reflections will widen the knowledge of others and may inspire moral courage.

When they are engaged in their reflection, they benefit by taking time to look outside their own immediate situation to be reminded of other examples that have allowed common, ordinary people to do remarkable things benefiting society.

Before you leave this exploration into the coherence between your professional role and the opportunity to participate effectively as a good citizen in society, the lens is turned to the questions of working in situations of crisis and the criteria for human-centered approaches to rationing, and some considerations regarding local versus global environments in which your moral agency can be effective.

Responding to Crises

Right now, health professionals all over the face of the globe are first responders or members of follow-up teams in situations of natural or human-made crises of mass proportion. Among the ongoing state of crisis globally are disasters caused by natural occurrences of flooding, fire, or earthquake;

armed conflict, terrorist attacks, and other more local outbreaks of violence; epidemics and pandemics. As this book goes to press, the headlines in newspapers and the "breaking news" in electronic media everywhere carry the story of yet another mass shooting and the call for more states (and the federal government) to adopt extreme risk protection orders, also known as "Red Flag" gun laws.[16] These laws allow police and certain others, but not health professionals, in specific states to petition a district criminal court to remove gun license and guns from dangerous people. As the debate around dangerousness, immunity, and failure to report continues the news of one mass shooting will fade and be replaced by another disaster situation, but the human suffering caused by injury and other health-related needs will continue.

Whether by choice or chance, many health professionals today find themselves in such crisis situations locally or in a locale outside their home area. Some readers have no inclination to seek such situations, knowing they may be putting themselves in harm's way or feeling compelled to honor responsibilities and loyalties that prevent such ventures. Even when chance places one in a situation, such as hundreds of New York City health professionals experienced when the terrorist attack on the Twin Towers struck that city, some may shirk from involvement; however, most find it part of "who they are" to respond immediately. The call to service discussed previously in this chapter often takes over, and opportunities in all three spheres of professional involvement present themselves immediately or during reconstruction efforts.

Rather than fully analyze the ethical issues that confront professionals in such a situation, let us focus your attention on yet another expression of justice that brings some different lines of reasoning into the themes presented in Chapters 14 and 15 when faced with emergent situations of mass proportions.

Rationing: Allocation and Dire Scarcity

Having given careful attention in Chapter 14 to the way the general principle of distributive justice works, consider the companion notion of *rationing*. Some use the term rationing to denote any intentional method of distributing a desired good when there are far too many qualified claimants for a good, or the good is much too costly for all to have it. As you will recall, this is a general principle guiding allocation. Traditionally, rationing decisions were made when there was a *dire scarcity*, a severe shortage, of the good. Currently, an active discussion about this type of rationing focuses on the sobering prospect of a desperately inadequate supply of lifesaving equipment or basic quality-of-life interventions, often set within a context in which time is in essence. Ethical decision-making frameworks for medical scarcity have increased in need within the United States and globally. Drug and medical product shortages, because of disruptions in supply chains and

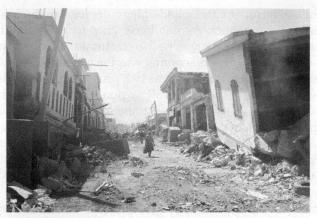

Fig. 16.3. Natural or human-made disasters create chaos that may require triage and rationing of resources. *(Copyright istockphoto.com/Claudiad.)*

other factors, have become common place in the United States and globally. These shortages have led to medical scarcity requiring organizations to work collaboratively as interprofessional care teams to develop proactive policies that encourage a fair and unbiased approach when a drug or medical product is in short supply.[17] In light of the recent increases, the American Society of Health-System Pharmacists recently took a proactive approach establishing guidelines for managing drug product shortages. These guidelines provide health professionals and policymakers with guidance for the complex and challenging nature of the drug shortage problem. They are supported by ethical frameworks taking into consideration transparency, relevance, appeals and revisions, enforcement, and fairness.[18]

Climate change and extreme weather events also have been occurring with increased frequency in the United States and globally. These events negatively impact health and well-being, in particular in vulnerable populations and communities. In large urban areas, such as the location of the recent earthquake in Katmandu or hurricanes that ravaged Dominica, Puerto Rico, disaster thrusts an entire population into a sudden position of dire scarcity of personnel, appropriate equipment, and other basic health-related resources (Fig. 16.3). Every major medical center knows that there is no way to stockpile sufficient supplies to effectively combat such a situation. Who should be admitted into emergent care or into the hospital and other medical facilities? Who should be admitted after the first wave of emergent care?[19]

Criteria for a Morally Acceptable Approach to Rationing
Several criteria have been developed to assist in the difficult, usually tragic, situation occasioned by the severe shortage of an essential life-sustaining or pain-relieving good or service.

● *A demonstrated need.* There must be proof that rationing is necessary. At times, politicians and others have declared that rationing of a particular good or service is necessary because of "dire scarcity." Any use of this powerful argument not based on data-driven decision making is just plain wrong. Rationing means that some groups who would benefit will not receive any of a desperately needed service or good. In contrast, the one who would benefit is the essential focus of clinical decisions. The widespread idea that healthcare responds to a basic human need requires that the burden of proof be placed on anyone declaring that it is necessary to ration some aspect of healthcare.

A last-resort move. It follows from the preceding criterion that every other approach must be exhausted before the decision is made to exclude from care individuals who would benefit. But when rationing is required after such alternatives have been exhausted, the argument is that the entire society is at such a risk of total breakdown that priority must be given to those who are the most likely to be able to help the group or society get back on its feet, not necessarily those with the most clinical need. The aftermath of the terrible natural disasters illustrates the deep quandary of healthcare providers in this kind of situation. For this reason, some have said that rationing in the face of dire scarcity turns usual understandings of justice upside down because it may be that the least medically needy are the ones to receive priority.

An established standard of care. For some order to be brought into these desperate kinds of situations, an agreed-on standard of care must be established. Many groups have attempted to establish a baseline level to help ensure equity for everyone, even in these extreme circumstances. If the situation becomes so desperate, at least a standard was set. Many nations have used a set of basic benefits everyone must receive as a bottom-line standard, no matter how minimal. Although applaudable in spirit, the practical downside of this criterion is that, in some instances, there is so little to go around that no one benefits.

An inclusive and transparent process. Representatives and advocates for all groups that will be affected should participate in the allocation process if possible. This is not always possible in crises situations such as we have been describing, but even the smallest group of persons waiting to be treated may recommend that an older person or child take priority over themselves, which can help the group exercise their moral agency or show compassion for those they judge are in most need. The process should also be documented and shared with health professionals and patients so that all stakeholders understand the decisions made, alternatives, and actions impacting care delivery.

Proportionality and reversibility. Beneficial services that are withheld must be proportional to the actual scarcity. *Proportionality* means that just enough, but no more, constraint is adopted to meet the difficult demands

Box 16.1   Criteria for a Morally Acceptable Approach to Rationing of Healthcare Resources

1. Rationing is necessary.
2. Rationing is a last-resort move.
3. A high standard is the goal.
4. The process is inclusive and transparent.
5. The cuts are proportionate and reversible.

of severe scarcity in the situation. Moreover, cuts or cutbacks are justifiable only as long as true and serious scarcity exists so that the constraints on care can be reversed as soon as the dire scarcity situation no longer exists. Box 16.1 summarizes all five criteria for rationing.

The Issue of Random Selection

In the unthinkable possibility of eliminating some people from receiving resources altogether, a process of *random selection* has been suggested by some as a procedure that can help to make a decision more just when the claim is for an essential lifesaving treatment unavailable to everyone who needs it.

In random selection, a prior medical judgment of medical need and suitability has been made, and the patient's freedom to refuse possible treatment has been ascertained. In an attempt to be as unbiased as possible in selecting who is to receive treatment among those still found eligible, "rolling the dice" has been suggested as a model. In extreme circumstances, such as an earthquake, terrorist attack, or other horrendously tragic situations, the method has been upheld in the courts of the United States as a procedure that expresses an equal consideration of the equal right of each person to life *(United States v. Holmes)*.[19] The actual situation that led to this decision was around the tragic moment in which survivors of a shipwreck, while lost at sea, realized that all would die if one or more were not "sacrificed." They decided among themselves to draw lots, and those who lost were thrown overboard. Eventually, the remainder were rescued and had to stand trial regarding the death of their life raft mates. The court's conclusion was that under extreme life-threatening circumstances, drawing lots was a just solution.

Nonetheless, not everyone agrees that random selection is the most humane way of proceeding instead of the criteria of rationing. They argue that once patients have been selected as being similarly situated in terms of medical need, it makes sense to give weight to such merit-related social factors as the likelihood of future service to society, the extent of past services, severity of illness, or family responsibilities. These positions take seriously into account that people are seldom viewed in isolation but rather in context as members of their larger communities. The conclusion also is that even in the most extreme situations persons are capable of moral agency and should be included in the decision if possible.

> ### Summary
>
> Random selection attempts to remove the opportunity for bias and discrimination in situations of dire scarcity, but some criticize its deeply impersonal nature.

Analyses that address basic healthcare needs and a dire scarcity of resources do not all do so in the context of a big blowout like a dirty bomb or major flood or deprivation from a worldwide growth of extreme poverty. Even with the wealth and resources in the United States, there are some who project a more gradual but persistent move into an unsustainable healthcare system as we know it today. Among the most prevalent themes are arguments that concern how to address healthcare needs across populations or constituencies. A recent example is the demands of a growing number of children in some segments of the United States against the demands of an aging society. In 2018, the United States spent $3.6 trillion on healthcare.[20] Previous estimates suggested that roughly a third of healthcare expenditures were spent on those over 65 years old, although they constituted only about 10% of the population. Combining this with the advent of post–World War II baby boomers now coming into retirement age, the 2010 figure of 38 million "senior citizens" over 65 years old will proliferate to more than 75 million just 15 years later (2025).[21] These types of data raise serious questions about how justice can be sustained across both populations and diagnoses. If rationing becomes necessary under these progressive conditions, the criterion of rationing discussed previously can serve to contain the harm that a move to such an approach would entail.

Good Citizenship: Local or Global?

Finally, this chapter concludes with some good citizenship considerations that are hinted at in the examples offered. There is a popular adage designed to liberate caring citizens from trying to be all things to all people: "Think global, act local." The wisdom of this phrase seems self-evident insofar as it suggests correctly that having a "global" awareness of how a local need connects to the larger human condition is a valuable resource. It also reflects that because many health professionals are by nature adventurers, wanting to save the world (while seeing the world), they can ignore their professional responsibility to be effective moral agents in their local environment in which they may actually be of much more service. Their responsibility is limited to accountability to the larger world that beckons them. The idea that professional responsibility requires responsiveness to the deeper human needs of a community finds support in the idea of acting locally when the need is there under your nose. Generally speaking, professionals usually can more fully comprehend the needs of a familiar community and assess what they can do to help in any of the three spheres of moral agency than if working in a geographic and social environment that is foreign. For instance, we assumed that Michael, the hometown boy who returned, had an advantage insofar as he knew these townspeople and how they might respond.

That being said, your generation of health professionals will be *global citizens*, requiring new paradigms in education and practice that replace current ones based primarily on the idea of local versus global preparation and service. Some of you have come from areas that were homogeneous ethnically, religiously, and in other ways, only to see the population mix dramatically shift in your lifetime. The globe is at your doorstep and, to some degree, at everyone's doorstep, everywhere. Some trends that point to an increasingly globalized world that will require our deep interdependence with others worldwide and make all health professionals global citizens include:

- An increase in the number of community-based disease prevention and health promotion programs in all parts of the world that can more efficiently be administered as international initiatives and that require knowledge of deeply diverse health-related issues and cultural competence of all health professionals.
- Convincing evidence of the relationship of the spread of poverty worldwide and the power of even simple on-the-ground solutions involving basic healthcare and clean drinking water to help minimize or reverse this fundamental source of human suffering. Such solutions already are inspiring many health professionals to seek service in poverty-immersed areas locally and globally.[22]
- The health professions' response to the need for global preparedness to combat new viral strains such as Ebola disease, drug-resistant infections to common diseases such as malaria, and the health effects of bioterrorism, none of which are confined to national boundaries.
- The global call to health professionals to protect the health of current and future populations given the exponential increase of injuries, illnesses, and deaths as a result of climate change (e.g., extreme weather events such as floods, storms, droughts, and heat and cold waves) impacting morbidity and mortality; most significantly, nutrition and mental health.[23]
- Increased reliance worldwide on information technology for sharing effective diagnostic, research, and clinical interventions, and, as a result, an increased need for systems to prevent cyberattacks and healthcare data breaches.
- More movement across nations and continents by unprecedented numbers of immigrants and refugees along with millions of global tourists and businesspeople annually.

- Advancement in biomedical technologies, including the limitations and promises of the use of artificial intelligence in healthcare delivery, and the impact of technology on health equity.[24]

Given these realities, the idea of "citizen" is comprehensible only in the context of being a global citizen. Understanding our mutual interdependence as "global civic selves" allows us not only to call on our colleagues and others worldwide to resolve problems they are more suited to handle, but also to count on their support for addressing our challenges. The paradigm that combines the three spheres of moral agency along with awareness of the dual aspects of responsibility is useful for determining in a general way where and around what issues you should seek involvement. Your moral agency potentially can be exercised in your hometown, at the national level, or literally anywhere else in the world, depending on where you feel at home professionally.

Reflection
Of the many places you may find yourself using your professional expertise, do you imagine it being exercised locally or also nationally or internationally?

_____

_____

_____

_____

Summary

In this final chapter, you have had an opportunity to see yourself as a moral agent in regard to important societal issues that face the larger human community locally and beyond. You will find a niche where your expertise, skills, standing in the community, interests, and the urgency of the needs will help you set priorities. Attentiveness to how and when to become involved depends in part on understanding the characteristics of moral agency in the three spheres of opportunity in which you can express your professional responsibility. The tools of ethical reasoning along with key character traits, such as moral courage and resilience, will expand your bandwidth of effectiveness. Your readiness to be a positive force in civic society, whatever the circumstances, is a resource well worth cultivating as a part of the larger role you have as an informed citizen, health professional, and advocate.

Questions for Thought and Discussion

1. Because you cannot become involved in every societal issue that comes along, it is a good idea to choose the issues that hold some interest for you. If you were to become involved in trying to solve three societal problems today, what would they be? Do they fall within Sphere One, Two, or Three of your moral agency?

2. You work at Metro Central Hospital, which was recently designated as a regional center for treatment of any person admitted with symptoms of Ebola virus because of its 16-unit intensive care unit (ICU) that was outfitted for biocontamination measures and its highly trained ICU staff and support personnel. The recent outbreak in East Africa with Ebola virus had taken the lives of more than 10,000 people, but the few cases brought to the United States were easily absorbed by three or four existing biocontamination centers. Evaluating its preparedness, the U.S. government is taking this opportunity to think preventively should this virus mutate and spread into new populations including the United States and also to augment measures to respond to a possible bioterrorist attack.

   So it came as a shock that almost simultaneously Ebola symptoms began to show up in patients in five U.S. cities, including yours, about 2 weeks ago. Twenty-four people have been admitted to hospitals designed for Ebola treatment across the United States, stressing the resources of every other existing unit designed to treat them.

   Professionals in Metro Central Hospital are placed on high alert. All professional employees are asked to indicate their willingness to be a member of the core group of volunteers to become part of the interprofessional care team to treat patients with Ebola. Each is asked also to discuss the matter with loved ones before arriving at this decision. Not knowing exactly what the medical center is facing, you are asked to consider the possibility that, under the worst-case scenario, a triage network will be set up to include—and exclude—some victims for desperately needed attention. Will you volunteer? On what factors do you base your decision? How will you advise and support your interprofessional coworkers in their decisions?

3. You have been invited to become a member of a commission in your town/city that will examine how to best use public space (parks, gardens, beaches, parking areas, playgrounds, and so on) for the welfare of the citizens. They have asked you because they think "your expertise as a health professional is needed." What, if anything, do you think you can bring to such a commission from the point of view of your health professional training and expertise?

4. You are thrilled to be selected for a 6-month fellowship to serve as a member of a primary care interprofessional care team that will establish a public health campaign for immunization compliance in school age children.

Recent data suggest that many in the community have been swayed by the antivaccine movement and there have been two documented cases of measles in the town where you live. What questions do you have regarding the vaccination rate? As of today, what do you think you will bring with you to the analyses of this complex problem? What approach will you suggest?

References

1. Gruen RL, Pearson SD, Brennan TA: Physician-citizens: public roles and professional obligations, *JAMA* 29(1):94–98, 2004.
2. Care N: Career choice, *Ethics* 94(2):283–302, 1984.
3. Sullivan WM: *Work and integrity: the crisis and promise of professionalism in America*, New York, 2004, Jossey-Bass Publishing Company.
4. Eitland E, Allen J: school buildings: the foundation for student success, *State Educ Stand* 19(1):35–38, 2019.
5. Environmental Protection Association: Lead regulations. Available at https://www.epa.gov/lead/lead-regulations#water.
6. World Health Organization: *Guidelines for drinking-water quality: fourth edition incorporating the first addendum*. Geneva: World Health Organization, 2017. License: CC BY-NC-SA 3.0 IGO. Available at https://apps.who.int/iris/bitstream/handle/10665/254637/9789241549950-eng.pdf;jsessionid=063319A09E548FABDF15215797478A22?sequence=1.
7. Jennings B, Callahan D, Wolf S: The professions: public interest and the common good, *Hastings Cent Rep* (Suppl):3–11, 1987.
8. Scheffler, S: *The importance of the afterlife. Seriously.* Available at https://opinionator.blogs.nytimes.com/2013/09/21/the-importance-of-the-afterlife-seriously/?mtrref=www.google.com&gwh=8FDB6DB3A3A9BB132258A3E5A4E86883&gwt=pay&assetType=REGIWALL Accessed October 1, 2019.
9. United Nations Commission on Environment and Development: *The earth charter*, Paris, 1994, UNESCO Headquarters. Approved 2000. Available at www.earthcharter.org. Accessed May 5, 2015.
10. Boff L: The ethics of care. (Berryman P, translator). In Corcoran PB, Wohlpart AJ, editors: *A voice for Earth: American writers respond to the Earth Charter*, Athens, GA, 2008, University of Georgia Press, pp 29–145.
11. Purtilo R: Moral courage in times of change: visions for the future, *J Phys Ther Educ* 14(3):4–7, 2000.
12. Purtilo R: Step up, speak out, stand firm! Moral courage: lessons from South Africa, *Creighton Mag Fall*:20–25, 1999.
13. Bebeau M, Rest T, Narvaez D: Beyond the promise: a perspective on moral education, *Educ Res* 28(4):22, 1999.
14. Rodeheaver MD, Gradwell JM: "We are Dumbledore's army": forging the foundation for future upstanders, *J Int Soc Studies* 4(2):57–72, 2014.

15. May WF: *Beleaguered rulers: the public obligation of the professional*, Louisville, KY, 2001, Westminster John Knox Press, pp 188–189.
16. Rosmain D: *Massachusetts' 'Red Flag' gun law needs an update*. Available at https://www.wbur.org/cognoscenti/2019/08/21/massachusetts-extreme-risk-protection-order-red-flag-gun-law-david-rosmarin, August 21, 2019.
17. Beck JC, Smith LD, Gordon BG, et al: An ethical framework for responding to drug shortages in pediatric oncology, *Pediatr Blood Cancer* 62(6):931–934, 2015.
18. Fox ER, McLaughlin MM: ASHP guidelines on managing drug product shortages, *Am J Health Syst Pharm* 75(21):1742–1750, 2018.
19. *United States v. Holmes:* 1842.26 F Case 36 (No 15, 383) C.C.E.D. Pa.
20. Centers for Medicare and Medicaid Services. *National Health Expenditure Data: NHE fact sheet*. Available at https://www.cms.gov/research-statistics-data-and-systems/statistics-trends-and-reports/nationalhealthexpenddata/nhe-fact-sheet.html.
21. Gawande A: The cost conundrum: what a Texas town can teach us about health care, *The New Yorker*, June 1, 2009. Available at http://www.newyorker.com/reporting/2009/06/01/090601fa_fact_gawande.
22. Sachs JD: *The end of poverty: economic possibilities for our time*, New York, 2006, Penguin Books, pp 233–234.
23. Rosa WE, Schenk E, Travers JL, et al: Climate change and health consequences: engaging public health nursing within the framework of the United Nations sustainable development goals, *Pub Health Nurs* 36(2):107–108, 2019.
24. National Academies of Sciences, Engineering, and Medicine: *Framework for addressing ethical dimensions of emerging and innovative biomedical technologies: a synthesis of relevant National Academies reports*, Washington, DC, 2019, The National Academies Press.

Index

Note: Page numbers followed by *b* refer to boxes; page numbers followed by *f* refer to figures; and page numbers followed by *t* refer to tables.

Standards
  national, 244
  physiological, 339
  probability, 339
  quality-of-life, 339
State interests, 23
Statutes, 21
Statutory law, 21
Stigma, 385
"Stop-look-listen!" reactions, 16
Story, getting straight, 106, 107b
Story or case approaches, 78
  ethics of care and, 82
Stresses
  coping with, 310
  sources of, 310f
  types of, 310
Student life, special challenges of, 121, 124b
Substituted judgment standard, 272
Suicide, clinically assisted, 346, 347b, 348b
Supererogation, 335
Surrogate or proxy consent, 272

T
Team(s), 156
  effects of, 302f, 302
  interprofessional, 11, 151, 298
Team and family, trust between, 302f
Team communication, 246
Team loyalty, as relevant information, 159, 160b
Technical competence, 36, 37b
Technologies
  communicating with, 246, 247b
  digital, 220
Teleological theories, deontological and, 94
Teleology, 97, 98t
Theory
  teleological, 94, 95b, 96f
  virtue, 82
Therapeutic research, 277
Time-limited trial, 114
Tottle, Beth, 231b, 231
Traditional arrangements, 60
Traits, character, 83
Trust, 205
  between team and family, 302f
Type A moral distress, 305, 306f
Type B moral distress, 306f, 306

U
Unintended effect, of principle of double
    effect, 342
Unjust practices, limited resources and, 43, 45b
Usual and customary treatments, 337
Utilitarianism, 97
Utilitarian reasoning, 307b, 307, 417b, 417
  in organization ethics, 189, 192b
Utilitarians, rule, 97
Uwilla, Mrs., 231b, 231

V
Value-based transfer, 243
Values, 7
Veracity, 93, 129
Very important person (VIP), 370
Virtue, 7
  compassion as, 334b, 334
Virtues associated with caring, 266
Virtue theory, 82, 420
Virtuous organization, right to, 198
Voluntariness, 261, 263
Voluntary medical euthanasia, 348
Vulnerability, 393, 396, 397b
Vulnerable populations, 277, 396

W
Weighting duties, 96f
Well-being, clinician, 140, 141f
Whistle-blowers, 169, 170
Whistle-blowing, 169, 170
Williams, Helen, 283b
Worker's compensation, 386
Wrongdoing
  address others, 131
  cooperation with, 144
  reporting, 169
  right any, 131b, 131

Y
Yourself
  duties to, 138
  improving personally, 142
  responsibilities to, 140
  self care, 134, 138